OTHER BOOKS BY DR. MARGARET R. O'LEARY AND DR. DENNIS S. O'LEARY

Tragedy at Graignes: The Bud Sophian Story (2011)

Adventures at Wohelo Camp: Summer of 1928 (2011)

R. D. O'Leary: Notes from Oxford, 1910–1911 (2014)

R. D. O'Leary: Notes from Mount Oread, 1914–1915 (2015)

Raphael Dorman O'Leary: The English Professor (2016)

The Kansas City Meningitis Epidemic, 1911–1913: Violent and Not Imagined (2018)

THE TEXAS MENINGITIS EPIDEMIC

(1911-1913)

Origin of the Meningococcal Vaccine

Margaret R. O'Leary, MD

Dennis S. O'Leary, MD

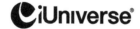

THE TEXAS MENINGITIS EPIDEMIC (1911–1913)
ORIGIN OF THE MENINGOCOCCAL VACCINE

iUniverse books may be ordered through booksellers or by contacting:

iUniverse
1663 Liberty Drive
Bloomington, IN 47403
www.iuniverse.com
1-800-Authors (1-800-288-4677)

ISBN: 978-1-5320-5433-4 (sc)
ISBN: 978-1-5320-5434-1 (hc)
ISBN: 978-1-5320-5432-7 (e)

Library of Congress Control Number: 2018908575

Print information available on the last page.

iUniverse rev. date: 11/2/2018

The authors dedicate this book to the following people who played roles in addressing the Texas meningitis epidemic of 1911 to 1913 (in alphabetical order):

Robert Percy Babcock (1881–1966)
Mrs. Jesse Barnes
Miss Frankie Bettis (1892–1912)
Dr. James Harvey Black (1884–1958)
Dr. William McDuffie
Brumby (1866–1959)
Dr. Manton Marble Carrick (1879–1932)
Thomas Mitchell Campbell (1856–1923)
Oscar Branch Colquitt (1861–1940)
Dr. Willus Gurden Cook (1866–1963)
Dr. John Spencer Davis (1881–1947)
Mr. George Bannerman
Dealey (1859–1946)
Dr. John Caleb Erwin (1857–1951)
Henry Arthur Finch (1853–1934)
Dr. Simon Flexner (1863–1946)
Dr. Henry Charles Hartman (1881–1963)
George Herder Sr. (1863–1934)
Mr. William "Willie" Meredith
Holland (1875–1966)
Joseph Clark Hunt (1857–1913)
David C. Kelley (1856–1913)
Dr. Samuel Newton Key (1886–1956)
Albert Leroy "Lee"
Killingsworth (1859–1913)

Archer W. Koons (1892–1913)
Dr. Henry Kern Leake (1847–1916)
The McCallum Family
Thomas McNeal (1849–1913)
Dr. Albert Ware Nash (1883–1934)
Dr. John M. Neel (1863–1921)
Miss Rose Emma Nielsen (1891–1934)
Dr. William Hallock Park (1863–1939)
Fisher Younger Rawlins (1892–1913)
John Elijah Rosser (1882–1960)
Dr. William Worthington
Samuell (1878–1937)
Clyde Duff Smith (1874–1912)
Miss Jessie Smith (1888–1971)
Dr. Abraham Sophian (1885–1957)
Dr. Ralph Steiner (1859–1926)
Dr. Arthur Marston Stimson (1876–1953)
Chester Hunter Terrell (1882–1920)
Dr. Alfred Edward Thayer (1863–1953)
Dr. John Shade Turner (1866–1936)
Dr. Rudolph Hermann von
Ezdorf (1873–1916)

CONTENTS

PREFACE

The Texas Meningitis Epidemic, 1911–1913: Origin of the Meningococcal Vaccine is the historical account of the monstrous yet strangely forgotten cerebrospinal meningitis epidemic that swept through the state of Texas during the unusually cold and rainy months of 1911–1912 and 1912–1913. Before the decade of the 1940s, when antibiotics first became available to treat the disease, cerebrospinal meningitis was one of the most malignant, rapacious, non-discriminating, unpredictable, and difficult to control of all the contagious-disease epidemics afflicting humans. The Texas version of the epidemic personified the disease's savage reputation for harming individuals and communities.

The Texas cerebrospinal meningitis epidemic garnered our attention after a spectacular, fourteen-inch-tall, three-handled sterling-silver Texas loving cup came into our possession in 2001. Engraved on one of its rounded sides are the following words: "To Doctor Abraham Sophian in recognition of his unselfish devotion to the cause of science and in appreciation of his masterly leadership in preventing the spread of disease and in saving lives among us. This token is given by grateful citizens, Dallas, Texas, February First, Nineteen Hundred Twelve." Dr. Abraham Sophian (1885–1957) was then a celebrated American public health clinician and researcher. He later became a pioneering, commanding, erudite, fastidious, and tireless internist in Kansas City in a career that spanned the first half of the twentieth century and was also the maternal grandfather of Dr. Dennis Sophian O'Leary, a co-author of this book.

We knew little about the early period of Dr. Sophian's long professional career and spent two years unearthing information about it. One of our discoveries was Dr. Sophian's important role in stemming the Texas cerebrospinal meningitis epidemic of 1911 to 1913 and his contribution to the origin of the meningococcal vaccine.

We have dedicated many years of our lives to the care of patients suffering from severe diseases such as cerebrospinal meningitis, one of us doing so in emergency medicine (Dr. Margaret Rose O'Leary) and the other in internal medicine (Dr. Dennis S. O'Leary). We have written copiously—both separately and together—for all of our professional lives as physicians (see "About the Authors" at the end of this book). During our almost forty years of marriage, writing has been a shared rewarding experience for us.

Telling the story of the Texas cerebrospinal meningitis epidemic of 1911 to 1913 involves technical concepts and terminology that may be new to some readers. We have introduced the book with a brief history of cerebrospinal meningitis and its treatment to facilitate readers' understanding of the subsequent events in the course of this epidemic. Carefully reading the introduction will probably be a good investment for most readers.

The Texas Meningitis Epidemic, 1911–1913: Origin of the Meningococcal Vaccine identifies all the major Texas cities with a high prevalence of the disease during those years. However, the book focuses on Dallas and Austin, because the former was the state's cerebrospinal meningitis epicenter (1911–1912) and the latter was the site of the deaths from the disease of a number of Texas legislators who were working in the Texas State Capitol building when they became ill (1913).

For the purpose of this book, the adjectives "communicable," "infectious," "contagious," and "transmissible," as used to modify the word disease, mean the same thing—that is, a specific disease, such as cerebrospinal meningitis, is capable of traveling from one person to another. Different jurisdictions in the United States during the past century have used one or another of these adjectives to describe their experiences.

Margaret R. O'Leary, MD
Dennis S. O'Leary, MD
Fairway, Kansas
September 3, 2018

ACKNOWLEDGMENTS

We appreciate the assistance of the following professionals in preparing this book: Michelle Lambing, graphics coordinator, Texas State Preservation Board, Austin, Texas; Claire Duncan, director, Texas Medical Association Knowledge Center, Texas Medical Association, Austin, Texas; Rebecca Schulte, university archivist, Kenneth Spencer Research Library, University of Kansas Libraries, Lawrence, Kansas; Kathy A. Lafferty, coordinator/copy services manager, public services department, Kenneth Spencer Research Library, University of Kansas Libraries, Lawrence, Kansas; Elizabeth Shepard, interim head of archives, Weill Cornell Medicine, Medical Center Archives of New York-Presbyterian/ Weill Cornell, Samuel J. Wood Library, New York, New York; Greg Bailey, university archivist and Clements curator, Cushing Memorial Library and Archives, University Libraries, Texas A&M University; Teri Watkins, senior publishing service associate, iUniverse, Bloomington, Indiana; and Alison Holen, artist and cover design supervisor, WestBow Press.

A BRIEF HISTORY OF CEREBROSPINAL MENINGITIS AND ITS TREATMENT, 1805-1908

The written history of cerebrospinal meningitis dates to a description by Dr. Gaspard Vieusseux[1] of a meningitis epidemic in Geneva, Switzerland, during February, March, and April of 1805.[2-3] The distinctive and lethal nature of the disease startled the region's physicians. Dr. Vieusseux wrote,

> Though the illness that reigned during the recent spring in and around Geneva was not considerable by the number of those afflicted and those who died [there were thirty-three deaths] and that endured for three months before disappearing in the summer, it nevertheless was remarkable by the symptoms that distinguished it from all the other fevers that presented to physicians who had exercised their art in their cities for more than 30 years.[2]

Dr. Vieusseux continued,

> The outbreak began in a suspicious and scary manner a very small distance from the city in a

dirty quarter habituated by poor people and others vulnerable to the development of all contagious diseases ... At the end of January [1805], in a family composed of a woman and three children, two of the children were attacked and died in less than 48 hours.

Dr. Vieusseux described the disease's clinical presentation:

There appears suddenly a severe prostration, accompanied by a feeble pulse—small and fast, sometimes almost gone, and in a few cases, hard and elevated. It manifests itself with a violent headache, especially over the forehead, followed by heart pain or the vomiting of greenish material, [and] of stiffness of the spine. In the fatal cases, the course was extremely rapid, lasting only 12 hours in some cases, in others from one to five days. In children there were convulsions. In those who died within 24 hours of the onset, the larger proportion had an eruption of violet spots[4] upon the body.[2]

The disease crossed the Atlantic Ocean to reach the eastern shore of the United States in 1806. In that year, Dr. Elisha North[5] reported an epidemic in Goshen, Litchfield County, Connecticut, describing it as "a flood of mighty waters, bringing along the horrors of a most dreadful plague."[6-7] The disease ricocheted unremittingly among cities and towns in Europe and the eastern half of the United States for the next four decades.[7]

In 1847, Dr. François Louis Isidore Valleix[8] in Paris named the disease described by Dr. Vieusseux and Dr. North as "simple acute meningitis" to distinguish it from "tuberculosis of the meninges"[9] (tubercular meningitis). Simple acute meningitis, said Dr. Valleix, typically gave no warning before its rapid onset. Its symptoms included a severe headache, suffusion of the face, photophobia, and vomiting. The progress of the disease was continuous and its duration short, usually from one to six days, rarely longer. Tubercular meningitis, by contrast, featured antecedent symptoms of tuberculous disease, such as the cough, fever, weight loss, and night sweats associated with pulmonary tuberculosis. The symptoms of tubercular meningitis were more subdued, slower and more insidious in onset, longer in duration, and more prone to remissions than were those of simple acute meningitis.[9] In 1847, no one knew the cause of either simple acute meningitis or tubercular meningitis.

Two decades passed, as cerebrospinal meningitis continued its deadly forays into cities and towns in the United States, frustrating physicians who stood by helpless to alleviate their afflicted patients' intense suffering. In 1868, Dr. Meredith Clymer,[10] an estimable American clinician, renamed simple acute meningitis as "cerebro-spinal meningitis," describing it as

> an acute specific disorder, commonly happening as an epidemic, general or limited, and, rarely, sporadically; caused by some unknown external influence; of sudden onset, rapid course, and very fatal; its chief symptoms, referable to the cerebrospinal axis, are great prostration of the vital powers, severe pain in the head and along the spinal column, delirium, tetanic, and occasionally clonic, spasms, and cutaneous hyperaesthesia, with, in some cases, stupor, coma, and motor paralysis; attended frequently with cutaneous haemic spots; its morbid anatomical characters being congestion and inflammation of the membranes of the brain and spinal cord, particularly the pia mater, although there is reason to believe that the evidence of these changes may be wanting, even in cases of long duration.[11]

Also, in 1868, Dr. William Aitken,[12] a Scottish pathologist and a younger colleague of Dr. Clymer's, described cerebro-spinal meningitis as a malignant epidemic fever of an acute specific character, of sudden invasion, attended by painful contraction of the muscles of the neck and retraction of the head. In certain epidemics it has been frequently accompanied by a profuse purpuric eruption, and occasionally be secondary effusions into certain joints. Lesions of the brain, the spinal cord, and their membranes, are found on dissection. The course of epidemic cerebro-spinal meningitis is rapid and very fatal, attended with great prostration of the powers of life, severe headache, and pain along the spine.[13]

In 1872, a fierce cerebrospinal meningitis epidemic struck the old city of New York City (Manhattan and the Bronx boroughs), killing 782 residents. (Henceforth, New York City refers to the Manhattan and Bronx boroughs combined unless otherwise noted). Epidemiologically-speaking, the number 782 is called a *death count*. Health officials obtained the death count number in every way possible, including by death certificates, by report of physicians and institutions, and by complaints of citizens and others.

Cerebrospinal meningitis was not a reportable disease in 1872, so New York City health department officials lacked information about the total number of persons with the disease (the total number of persons with the disease includes both those people who had died from the disease and those who had survived it). However, health department officials did know that the population size of New York City in 1872 was 968,710 residents.[14] With this information, they divided the death count (782) by the size of the population (968,710) to produce a *mortality rate* of *8.07 deaths per 10,000 New York City residents*.[14] The mortality rate allowed health department officials to compare the disease's death impact across populations, places, times, and other diseases.

Meanwhile, the cause of cerebrospinal meningitis during the epidemic of 1872 in New York City remained elusive. Dr. Clymer, expressing the consensus of his peers, noted that disease's cause was "beyond physical and bodily conditions [and was] outside of the degree of heat, moisture, etc., and the constitutional state of the individual." He concluded, "We are forced to take refuge in the assumption of an unknown special morbific agent as the aetic factor."[15]

Another decade passed. In 1882, bacteriologist Dr. Robert Koch[16] in Berlin first identified the tubercle bacillus (*Mycobacterium tuberculosis*), an acid-fast[17] microorganism, as the cause of tuberculosis. His discovery finally settled the question of the cause of tubercular meningitis. Three years later (1885), bacteriologist Dr. Anton Weichselbaum[18] at the University of Vienna, identified a Gram-negative[19] microorganism as the cause of cerebrospinal meningitis. He named the microorganism *Diplococcus intracellularis meningitidis* after its tendency to reside in flattened pairs inside the inflammatory cells of infected cerebrospinal fluid. Dr. Weichselbaum isolated the meningococcus from six of eight specimens of cerebrospinal fluid collected and submitted to him by Central European physicians who had collected the specimen from their patients with meningitis.[20-22] Dr. Weichselbaum published his discovery in *Fortschritte der Medizin* in 1887.[23] In 1901, Dr. Heinrich Albrecht and Dr. Anton Ghon renamed Weichselbaum's microorganism *Neisseria meningitides*, the moniker that holds today.[24]

Nearly two more decades passed after the discovery of the *Neisseria meningitidis* bacteria, also known as the meningococcus. In 1904, New York City suffered its worst cerebrospinal meningitis epidemic in terms of loss of life since the cerebrospinal meningitis epidemic of 1872.[25] Of the 2,318,831 New York City residents in 1904, 1,083 succumbed to the disease, resulting in a mortality rate of *4.6 cerebrospinal meningitis deaths per 10,000 New York City residents*.[26] The mortality rates for cerebrospinal meningitis in New York City for the years 1866 through 1907 are listed in the following table.[26] The bolded numbers are mentioned in the text.

Table 1: Number of Cases and Deaths from Cerebrospinal Meningitis in the Old City of New York (Present Boroughs Manhattan and Bronx), 1866–1907, Inclusive[26]

Year	Population (Manhattan and the Bronx combined)	No. of Deaths from Cerebrospinal Meningitis	Mortality Rate per 10,000
1866	767,979	18	.23
1867	808,489	33	.40
1868	851,137	34	.39
1869	896,034	42	.47
1870	943,300	32	.34
1871	955,921	48	.50
1872	**968,710**	**782**	**8.07**
1873	981,671	290	2.95
1874	1,030,607	158	1.53
1875	1,044,396	146	1.40
1876	1,075,532	127	1.18
1877	1,107,597	116	1.05
1878	1,140,617	97	.85
1879	1,174,621	108	.92
1880	1,209,196	170	1.41
1881	1,244,511	461	3.70
1882	1,288,857	238	1.86
1883	1,390,388	223	1.69
1884	1,356,764	210	1.55
1885	1,396,388	202	1.45
1886	1,437,170	223	1.55
1887	1,479,143	203	1.37
1888	1,522,341	173	1.14
1889	1,566,801	145	.93

Year	Population (Manhattan and the Bronx combined)	No. of Deaths from Cerebrospinal Meningitis	Mortality Rate per 10,000
1890	1,612,559	136	.84
1891	1,659,654	189	1.14
1892	1,708,124	230	1.35
1893	1,758,010	469	2.67
1894	1,809,353	213	1.18
1895	1,873,201	204	1.09
1896	1,906,139	178	.93
1897	1,940,553	232	1.20
1898	1,976,572	258	1.31
1899	2,014,330	287	1.42
1900	2,055,714	201	.97
1901	2,118,209	201	.94
1902	2,182,836	190	.87
1903	2,249,680	195	.86
1904	2,318,831	1,083	4.60
1905	2,390,382	1,511	6.30
1906	2,464,432	600	2.50
1907	2,541,471	471	1.80

In 1904, physicians still did not know how cerebrospinal meningitis was transmitted. However, in general, they believed that it was not highly contagious. For example, Bellevue Hospital physicians in 1904 year admitted persons afflicted with cerebrospinal meningitis to the hospital's general wards, reasoning that the disease was only mildly contagious and that no afflicted patient had ever communicated his or her disease to a Bellevue physician or nurse, with one exception. That exception was Dr. Joseph F. McCarthy,[30] an attending physician and Bellevue Hospital who contracted the disease and became a patient at Bellevue Hospital but did not know how he had acquired the disease.[27] Dr. Thomas Darlington[28], the New York City health commissioner in 1904, concurred with the Bellevue physicians' assessment, proclaiming that cerebrospinal meningitis was not "directly contagious," and "if meningitis [was] contagious it [was] in slight degree."[25]

The next year (1905), cerebrospinal meningitis returned with a vengeance to New York City, killing 1,511 persons of the 2,390,382 persons making up the population that year. The mortality rate calculated to *6.30 deaths per 10,000 New York City residents*, as compared with the mortality rate of *4.60 per 10,000 New York City residents* the previous year (1904) (see Table 1).[26] The disease also erupted in other cities in 1905, including Philadelphia, where it killed Dr. Albert Burns Craig.[30] The death of this relatively young Philadelphia physician and the rising death count and mortality rate associated with cerebrospinal meningitis in New York City between 1904 and 1905 so alarmed Dr. Darlington that he convened a New York City commission[31] of medical experts[32] to study the disease. The medical experts included Dr. Simon Flexner,[33] director of the fledgling Rockefeller Institute for Medical Research,[34] and Dr. Hermann Michael Biggs,[35] the chief medical officer of the New York City Board of Health[36] and its Research Laboratory.[37] Dr. Darlington tasked the commission with evaluating the disease's degree of communicability, its modes of transmission, and the possibilities for its control.

Dr. Flexner determined, through experimentation with his laboratory monkeys, that cerebrospinal meningitis was indeed contagious.[38] Dr. Charles Bolduan,[39] a bacteriologist with the Research Laboratory, confirmed earlier studies that identified a healthy meningococcal carrier state. This state was identified through the culturing of meningococci from the noses and throats of healthy individuals during cerebrospinal meningitis epidemics.[40] A theory of infection was that the meningococci entered the body by way of the nose and throat, where they lived without producing an illness, and that, in a small proportion of cases, the meningococci gained access to the bloodstream, which delivered them to the meninges, where they caused meningitis.[4]

Based on the commission's findings, the New York City Board of Health declared cerebrospinal meningitis a communicable disease (an infectious disease transmissible from one person to another by various means) and henceforth "required reporting of all cases by physicians, enforcement of quarantine, isolation of patients, exclusion of other children in the family from school, and disinfection of premises and bedding on termination of the disease."[41] One case of cerebrospinal meningitis was defined as one person with cerebrospinal meningitis. Reports of cases of cerebrospinal meningitis began to flow to the New York City Board of Health, thereby making possible for the first time a *case count*. A case count consisted of a running tally of the number of cases counted. The case count provided health department officials with a better grasp of the activity of the disease. As noted above, this total number was made up of the people who had died from the disease and the people who were surviving, or had survived, the disease. The case count permitted the identification of disease patterns and control planning.

Health department officials subsequently figured out that a case count divided by the size of the population from which the case count arose could provide a frequency rate useful for comparing the extent of the disease's presence (prevalence) in different populations, places, and times. *Prevalence*[42] (prevalence rate) is the case count of all persons with a health condition in a given population during a specified period of time. For example, the cerebrospinal meningitis case count in Greater New York City in 1906 was 1,032, according to the *Journal of Experimental Medicine*.[43] Using this case count, the prevalence rate for cerebrospinal meningitis in 1906 in Greater New York City calculated to *4.2 cerebrospinal meningitis cases per 10,000 Greater New York City residents*.

As early as 1905, researchers in the United States and Europe (where the disease also was prevalent) sought a cure for cerebrospinal meningitis. The major research laboratories[44] were the Research Laboratory of the New York City Board of Health and the Rockefeller Institute for Medical Research,[45] both in New York City; the laboratory of Drs. Wilhelm Kolle and August von Wasserman at the Institute for Infectious Diseases in Berlin, Germany[46]; and the laboratory of Dr. Georg Jochmann at the Medizinische Klinik of Breslau, Germany.[47]

The cure developed by the four researchers was an antimeningitis serum produced by immunizing horses with the meningococcus. Dr. Flexner, after experimenting as to the safest and most humane way to immunize his horses, settled on the subcutaneous route. He injected his horses with live meningococci and autolysate (i.e., the disintegration products of meningococcal cultures) at seven-day intervals. He used many different strains of the meningococci to prepare the living cultures and autolysate. He gradually increased the dose of living meningococci injected into his horses over six to twelve months. He then harvested, purified, and bottled the horse serum for use in humans.[48]

In 1905, Dr. William Hallock Park,[49] the director of the Research Laboratory of the New York City Board of Health, sent vials of his laboratory's antimeningitis serum for subcutaneous injection in twenty desperately-ill cerebrospinal meningitis patients in Hartford, Hartford County, Connecticut. Dr. Park and the Hartford physicians requesting the antimeningitis serum for their patients hoped that it might have the same beneficial effect on persons with cerebrospinal meningitis as did the subcutaneous administration of diphtheria antitoxin in patients with diphtheria. Unfortunately, the use of the antimeningitis serum in Hartford produced uncertain results. As a result, Dr. Park withheld further antimeningitis serum from distribution.[50] Despite the disappointing results of the subcutaneous injection of antimeningitis serum in persons with cerebrospinal meningitis, Dr. Park never gave up the idea that the approach could work, referring to the "somewhat favorable" results achieved by Dr. Kolle and Dr. Wassermann in Berlin in their cerebrospinal meningitis patients administered subcutaneous antimeningitis serum.[51]

In April and May 1906, Dr. Georg Jochmann first experimented with the *intraspinal* injection of antimeningitis serum in thirty-eight infected persons at the Medizinische Klinik of Breslau. He injected ten to twenty cubic centimeters of antimeningitis serum directly into the inflamed meninges of his patients, noting a prompt beneficial response. During the course of the year (1906), he used the intraspinal antimeningitis serum in thirty more afflicted patients. He then compared the health outcomes of cerebrospinal meningitis patients treated with intraspinal antimeningitis serum to the cerebrospinal meningitis patients not so treated. Twenty-seven percent of his patients who received the intraspinal antimeningitis serum died, while 52 percent of his patients who did not receive the intraspinal antimeningitis serum died.[52] The administration of intraspinal antimeningitis serum apparently had rendered the disease less lethal.

The 27 percent and 52 percent figures noted above are called *lethality rates*, better known as *case fatality rates*.[42] The case fatality rate is the proportion of persons with a disease who die from it. It is calculated by dividing the death count by the case count during a specified period of time. It is always expressed as a percentage. The case fatality rate is not the same as the mortality rate, even though both rates contain the death count in their numerators. In a mortality rate, the denominator is the size of the population at risk; in a case fatality rate, the denominator is the case count of persons infected with the disease. With the advent of antimeningitis serum, the case fatality rate became an important measure of the efficacy of intraspinal antimeningitis serum in persons with cerebrospinal meningitis.

Dr. Flexner carefully followed news of Dr. Jochmann's experiments. In August 1906, he proclaimed the latter's intraspinal injection innovation premature, writing in the *Journal of the American Medical Association*, "I do not think that the injection into the spinal canal of man of alien sera should be undertaken until their physiologic action has been worked out in more detail in monkeys."[53] Dr. Flexner then tested and established to his satisfaction the efficacy and safety of the intraspinal antimeningitis serum route of administration in his laboratory monkeys. In 1907, he offered his antimeningitis serum to physicians for use in humans in New York City; Philadelphia; Cleveland, Castalia, and Akron, Ohio; Edinburgh, Scotland; and Belfast, Ireland.[54]

Dr. Flexner collected outcome data on forty-seven patients with cerebrospinal meningitis who received his antimeningitis serum via the intraspinal route. Of the forty-seven persons, thirty-four recovered (72.3 percent), and thirteen (27.6 percent) died.[55]

Dr. Flexner was pleased with the data but quickly foresaw the need for a larger human clinical test group. To accomplish this goal, he supplied antimeningitis serum free of charge directly to physicians throughout the United States and world. In return for the free antimeningitis serum, he required physicians to meet certain conditions and to return specified cerebrospinal meningitis outcome data to him.[56] Three physicians in Fort Worth, Tarrant County, Texas, applied for and received some vials of antimeningitis serum from Dr. Flexner in October 1908.[57] They guarded their treasure while awaiting the first case of cerebrospinal meningitis to appear in their county.

INTRODUCTION NOTES

1 Gaspard Vieusseux, "*Mémoire sur La Maladie Qui a Règne à Genève, au Printemps de 1805*," *Journal de Médecine, Chirurgie, Pharmacie, etc.* xii (1806): 163–82; and "Gaspard Vieusseux: The Disease Which Raged in Geneva during the Spring of 1805," in Ralph Hermon Major, ed., *Classic Descriptions of Disease* (Springfield, IL: Charles C. Thomas, 1959): 188–90.

2 Dr. Gaspar Vieusseux (1746–1814), a native of Geneva, Switzerland, obtained his medical doctorate from the University of Leiden (the Netherlands) in 1766. After studying medicine in Edinburgh and London, he returned to Geneva to practice medicine in 1770. He quickly embraced vaccination as a preventive or mitigatory of smallpox and published *Traité de la Nouvelle Méthode d'Inoculer La Petite Vérole* in 1773. He was providing smallpox vaccinations twenty-three years before Dr. Edward Jenner (1749–1823) "discovered" the practice in England in 1796. In 1805, Dr. Vieusseux gave the first modern description of what is now known as cerebrospinal meningitis in "*Mémoire sur La Maladie Qui a Règne à Genève, au Printemps de 1805*," which he published in the *Journal de Médecine, Chirurgie, Pharmacie, etc.*, xii (1806): 163–82. In January 1808, Dr. Vieusseux developed a neurological syndrome consisting of vertigo, unilateral facial numbness, loss of pain and temperature appreciation in the opposite limbs, dysphasia and hoarseness, minor tongue involvement, hiccups, and eyelid drop. He visited London (1810–1811) to communicate his clinical situation to his friend Dr. Alexander Marcet (1770–1822), a native of Geneva who lived in London. Dr. Marcet published Dr. Vieusseux's communication in "History of a Singular Nervous or Paralytic Affection Attended with Anomalous Morbid Sensations, Communicated by Dr. Marcet, Read Dec. 28, 1810," *Medico-Chirurgical Transactions* 2 (1811): 215–33. Dr. Vieusseux had another stroke in 1813 and died in the fall of 1814 at the age of forty-eight years.

3 Eduard-Rudolf Müllener, "Six Geneva Physicians on Meningitis," *Journal of the History of Medicine and Allied Sciences* 20, no. 1 (January 1965): 1–26; and R. Bruce Low, "Epidemic Cerebrospinal Meningitis," *Transactions of the Epidemiological Society of London, New Series* 18 (January 20, 1899): 53–85.

4 Physicians as early as Dr. Vieusseux in 1806 noted that some of their patients, in whom they otherwise suspected cerebrospinal meningitis

because of a fever and a headache, also developed a violet-colored pinprick-sized (petechial) rash that spread over their bodies. These individuals usually died within twenty-four to forty-eight hours of the appearance of the rash. In the early 1940s, physicians called this disease presentation and entity meningococcemia, meaning a blood infection with *Neisseria meningitidis*. Researchers today attribute the rash of meningococcemia to a heavy bacterial load of meningococci that enters the bloodstream, spreads, and colonizes peripheral blood vessels, resulting in vascular leakage. The leakage produces the petechiae that may also coalesce to form purpura, or pools of blood, beneath the skin. On account of this rash, cerebrospinal meningitis earned the names spotted fever, petechial fever, purpuric fever, neuro-purpuric fever, purpura maligna, infectious purpura, purpura contagiosis, purple fever, and malignant purple fever. See Marcel van Deuren, Petter Brandzaeg and Jos W. M. van der Meer, "Update on Meningococcal Disease with Emphasis on Pathogenesis and Clinical Management," *Clinical Microbiology Reviews* 13, no 1 (January 2000): 144–166; and Mathieu Coureuil, Olivier Join-Lambert, Hervé Lécuyer, et al., "Pathogenesis of Meningococcemia," *Cold Spring Harbor Perspectives in Medicine* 3, no. 6 (June 2013).

5   Dr. Elisha North (1771–1843) was born in Goshen, Litchfield County, Connecticut, about fifty miles west of Hartford, as one of the nine children of Dr. Joseph North Jr. (1737–1806) and Lucy Cole (1747–1829). He studied medicine with his father and with Dr. Lemuel Hopkins (1750–1801) of Hartford. He then practiced medicine in Goshen to earn money to attend the University of Pennsylvania Medical School in Philadelphia where he studied under Dr. Benjamin Rush (1746–1813) in 1793. He returned to Goshen before earning his medical diploma and resumed his medical practice. Cerebrospinal meningitis was a new and obscure disease at the time. It struck Goshen during the winters of 1806–1807 and 1808–1809. Dr. North wrote about the epidemic in *A Treatise on a Malignant Epidemic Commonly Called Spotted Fever* (New York: T and J. Swords, 1811), an early American medical classic. He described the clinical findings of the disease: "A great, surprising, and sudden loss of strength, is a constant and prominent symptom ... Violent pain of the head, and many times of the limbs, is among the first symptoms ... There is loss of appetite, and sickness at stomach, and vomiting." He added, "The worst form this disease ever assumes, particularly in children, is that of coma, or cholera morbus. It frequently assumes the form

of a violent mania at the time, or within a few hours of the attack, particularly in sanguine young men. Sometimes delirium is among the first symptoms; sometimes coma; and many times, petechia [*sic*]." Dr. North described petechiae as variable in size and in color, from a bright red to a bright purple. He did not believe that the presence of petechiae occurred often enough to warrant naming the disease after them. He said, "Unless the patient recovers, he commonly dies within the first 12, 24, or 48 hours. Death is ushered in by the gradual giving up of the powers of life, by syncope, by the febrile apoplexy, or by convulsions." He noted that the appearance of petechiae marked the worst form of the disease and that petechiae occurred in almost every case during the 1806–1807 Goshen epidemic but only rarely in the 1808–1809 Goshen epidemic. Dr. North married Hannah Beach (1775–1862); they had eight children. He died at the age of seventy-two years. See "Elisha North," in Ralph Hermon Major, ed., *Classic Descriptions of Disease* (Springfield, IL: Charles C. Thomas, 1959), 188–90; and "North, Elisha," in *Appletons' Cyclopedia of American Biography, 1600–1889* (New York: D. Appleton and Company, 1888), 4:533–34.

6   Elisha North, *A Treatise on a Malignant Epidemic Commonly Called Spotted Fever* (New York: T and J. Swords, 1811).

7   A bibliography of works (1768–1902) about cerebrospinal meningitis is available at Cecil Wall, "On Acute Cerebro-Spinal Meningitis Caused by the Diplococcus Intracellularis of Weichselbaum: A Clinical Study," *Medico-Chirurgical Transactions* 86 (1903), 77–79. See also "Epidemic Cerebro-Spinal Meningitis," in William Aitken and Meredith Clymer, *The Science and Practice of Medicine* (Philadelphia, PA: Lindsay and Blakiston, 1868), 445–60; Eduard-Rudolf Müllener, "Six Geneva Physicians on Meningitis," *Journal of the History of Medicine and Allied Sciences* 20, no. 1 (January 1965): 10n30; Lothario Danielson and Elias Mann, "The First American Account of Cerebrospinal Meningitis," *Review of Infectious Diseases* 5, no. 5 (September–October 1983), 969–72; and Alexander Crever Abbott, *The Hygiene of Transmissible Diseases* (Philadelphia, PA: W. B. Saunders, 1899), 119–20.

8   Dr. François-Louis-Isidore Valleix (1807–1855) was born in Toulouse, Haute-Garonne, France. He moved to Paris to study medicine and was an extern (1829) and an intern in Parisian hospitals (1831–1833). He received his medical diploma in 1835. He was an ardent disciple of Pierre-Charles-Alexandre Louis (1787–1872), who first

developed the numerical method, the forerunner to epidemiology, the modern clinical trial, and evidence-based medicine. While an intern in Parisian hospitals, Dr. Valleix became attracted to the diseases of infancy. In 1838, he turned his attention to the investigation of nervous diseases. In 1836, he became a physician at the Bureau central des Hôpitaux de Paris. Between 1844 and 1848, he produced *Guide du Médecin Praticien or Résumé Général de Pathologie Interne et de Thérapeutique Appliqués*, a work in ten volumes, including one (tome IX) on the nervous diseases. He died in 1855 after contracting diphtheria from a child; he was forty-nine years old. See "M. Valleix," *Boston Medical and Surgical Journal* 53, no. 17 (November 22, 1855): 352–53; "Valleix, François Louis Isidore," *Comité des travaux historiques et scientifiques*, accessed April 2, 2018, http://cths.fr/an/savant.php?id=106004.

9   François-Louis-Isidore Valleix, *Guide Médecin Praticien or Résumé Général de Pathologie Interne et de Thérapeutique Appliqués* (Paris: J. B. Billière, 1847), 6:219.

10 Dr. Meredith Clymer (1816–1902) was born in London, England (while his parents were traveling), as the eldest of the two sons of Mary (Marie, Maria) Gratiot (O'Brien) (1790–1853) and George W. Clymer (1785–1848). He was the grandson of George Clymer Sr. (1739–1813), a signer of the United States Declaration of Independence on Saturday, July 20, 1776. Meredith Clymer earned his bachelor's degree from the University of Pennsylvania in 1835 and his medical degree from the University of Pennsylvania Medical School in 1837. In 1839, he studied abroad before returning to Philadelphia to practice medicine for ten years, during which time he consulted at the Philadelphia Hospital (1843–1846) and served as physician in chief at the Cholera Hospital and as a professor of medicine at the Hampden-Sidney College in Richmond, Virginia. He moved to New York City in 1851 to become a professor of the practice of medicine at the University of the City of New York. He specialized in diseases of the nervous system and the mind. During the American Civil War, he served as a surgeon in the United States Volunteers and as medical director of the Department of the South (1864–1865) at Hilton Head, Beaufort County, South Carolina. In 1871, he became a professor of mental and nervous diseases at Albany Medical College (1871–1874) in Albany, Albany County, New York. During his time in Albany, he studied the severe cerebrospinal meningitis epidemic 150 miles to the south in New

York City in 1872. He was the author of many works on medicine, including *The Pathology, Diagnosis, and Treatment of Fevers* (1846); *Notes on the Physiology and Pathology of the Nervous System, with Reference to Clinical Medicine* (1868); *Lectures on Palsies and Kindred Disorders* (1870); *Ecstasy and Other Dramatic Disorders of the Nervous System* (1870); *Hereditary Genius* (1870); *Epidemic Cerebro-Spinal Meningitis* (1872); and others. He married Virginia Margaret Garesche (Gareschi) (1827–1849) of Wilmington, New Castle County, Delaware, in 1843 and Eliza "Lily" ("Lillie") Strong Snelling (1838–1922) in 1856. He had no children. He died at home in New York City at the age of eighty-six years. See "Necrology: Meredith Clymer," *Alumni Roster of the University of Pennsylvania* 6, no. 9 (June 1902): 481; "Death List: Meredith Clymer," *New York Times*, April 21, 1902, 9; and "Obituary, Dr. Meredith Clymer," *British Medical Journal* 1, no. 2159 (May 17, 1902): 1,243.

11 "Epidemic Cerebro-Spinal Meningitis," in William Aitken and Meredith Clymer, *The Science and Practice of Medicine* (Philadelphia, PA: Lindsay and Blakiston, 1868), 2:445–60.

12 Dr. William Aitken (1825–1892) was born in Dundee, Angus, Scotland, as the eldest of the three children of Dr. William Aitken Sr. (1800–1854) and Ann Paterson (1801–1869). He received his early formal education at the Dundee High School, followed by an apprenticeship with his father while taking courses at the Dundee Royal Infirmary. In 1842, he entered the University of Edinburgh, earning his medical diploma in 1848. He served as a demonstrator of anatomy at the University of Glasgow and subsequently as a pathologist to the Glasgow Royal Infirmary until 1855. He then travelled to the Crimea as an assistant pathologist in a commission led by Dr. Robert Spencer Dyer Lyons (1826–1886). The purpose of the commission was to determine the diseases afflicting British Isles soldiers fighting there. In 1860, Dr. Aitken became professor of pathology at the Army Medical School at Fort Pitt, Chatham, Kent, England. He held this appointment for the next thirty-two years, resigning in 1892 because of failing health. He married Emily Clara Allan in 1884, six years before his death at the age of sixty-seven years. He wrote the first edition of *Handbook of the Science and Practice of Medicine* in 1857, describing meningitis as "inflammation of the arachnoid and pia mater." He did not use the term *cerebro-spinal meningitis* in the early editions of his textbook. His book saw seven editions, the last in 1880. He was knighted

on the occasion of Queen Victoria's Golden Jubilee in 1887. He pioneered the use of the thermometer as a means of determining the temperature of the body in cases of a fever. An image of Dr. Aitken is available at https://brianaltonenmph.com/gis/more-historical-disease-maps/1872-william-aitken-book/, accessed April 1, 2018. See "Obituary, Sir William Aitken, MD," *British Medical Journal* 2 (July 2, 1892): 54–55.

13 "Epidemic Cerebro-Spinal Meningitis," in William Aitken and Meredith Clymer, *The Science and Practice of Medicine* (Philadelphia, PA: Lindsay and Blakiston, 1868), 2:442.

14 Charles Bolduan, "Cerebrospinal Meningitis from the Standpoint of Public Health," *Medical Times* 36, no. 7 (July 1908): 193; and Centers for Disease Control and Prevention, "Introduction to Epidemiology: The Epidemiologic Approach," *Principles of Epidemiology in Public Health Practice, Third Edition*, accessed August 12, 2018, https://www.cdc.gov/ophss/csels/dsepd/ss1978/lesson1/section5.html.

15 Meredith Clymer, *Epidemic Cerebro-Spinal Meningitis* (Philadelphia, PA: Lindsay and Blakiston, 1872), 33.

16 Dr. Robert Koch (1843–1910) was born in Clausthal, a small mining town in Hanover, Germany, as one of the eighteen children of Hermann Koch (1814–1877), a mining engineer, and Mathilde Julie Henriette Biewend (1819–1871). He earned his medical degree from the University of Göttingen (Göttingen, Lower Saxony, Germany) in 1866; worked at a mental hospital in Langenhagen, Lower Saxony, Germany; moved to Niemegk (Potsdam-Mittelmark, Brandenburg, Germany) to practice medicine in 1868; moved again in 1869 to Rakwitz, near Posen, Prussia; served in the German Army during the Franco-German War in 1870; served as the district physician in Wollstein (Rhineland-Palatinate, Germany) in 1872; became a staff member of the Imperial Health Office in Berlin in 1880; gave his famous address on the discovery of the tubercle bacillus in Berlin on Friday, March 24, 1882; articulated Koch's postulates in 1883; became professor of hygiene at the University of Berlin in 1885; opened the Robert Koch Institute for Infectious Diseases in 1900; and received the Nobel Prize for Physiology or Medicine for his investigations and discoveries in relation to tuberculosis in 1905. Dr. Koch married Emilie Adolfine Sophie Fraatz (1847–1913) in 1867; they had one child and divorced in 1893. He married Edwig Emma Franziska Freiberg (1872–1945) in 1893. He died of heart disease after failing health for a year; he was sixty-seven years old.

See Robert Koch, *Die Ätiologie der Tuberkulose* (Berlin: Verlag von August Hirschwald, 1884): 1–88; Thomas D. Brock, *Robert Koch: A Life in Medicine and Bacteriology* (Berlin: Springer-Verlag, 1988); and "Koch Dies Martyr; Famous Bacteriologist Victim of Exposure in Africa; Discovered Tuberculin; One of World's Leaders in Fight Against Consumption; Recipient of Many Honors; Member of Medical Bodies the World Over and Given a Title by the Kaiser," *Evening Star* (Washington, DC), May 28, 1910, 8.

17 *Mycobacterium tuberculosis* resists staining by the Gram-stain method of bacterial differentiation devised by the Danish bacteriologist Hans Christian Gram (1853–1938). However, *Mycobacterium tuberculosis* is stainable by a special bacteriological dye (the Ziehl-Neelsen stain) originally developed by Dr. Robert Koch (1843–1910) in 1882 and modified by the bacteriologist Franz Ziehl (1859–1926) in 1882 and 1883 and by the pathologist Friedrich Neelsen (1854–1898) in 1883. See "R. C. Ellis and L. A. Zabrowarny, "Safer Staining Method for Acid Fast Bacilli," *Journal of Clinical Pathology* 46 (1993): 559–560.

18 Dr. Anton Weichselbaum (1845–1920) was born in Schiltern, Krems-Land, Lower Austria, as the son of a barrel maker. He attended the Krems gymnasium (1855–1863) and studied medicine at the Imperial Medical Surgical Military Hospital (Vienna) and at the University of Vienna, where he earned his medical doctorate in 1869. He subsequently assisted the Bohemian pathologist Dr. Carl Freiherr von Rokitansky (1804–1878) and the Austrian anatomist Dr. Josef Engel (1816–1899) at the University of Vienna. After serving as a military physician, he ascended the ranks at the University of Vienna to become a full professor in 1893 and the rector of the university in 1912. He was among the first physicians to recognize the importance of bacteriology for pathological anatomy and to embrace the science of serology. He trained Dr. Karl Landsteiner (1868–1943), who discovered interagglutination between serum and blood cells, and Dr. Anton Ghon (1866–1936). See K. Cartwright, "Microbiology and Laboratory Diagnosis," *Methods of Molecular Medicine* 67 (2001): 1–8; Anton Weichselbaum, *The Elements of Pathological Histology* (London: Longmans, Green, and Company, 1895); "Anton Weichselbaum," accessed March 3, 2018, http://www.whonamedit.com/doctor.cfm/2874.html; and "Anton Weichselbaum," *Wikipedia*, accessed March 3, 2018, https://en.wikipedia.org/wiki/Anton_Weichselbaum.

19 A Gram-negative bacterium will not retain the crystal violet stain used in the Gram-staining method of bacterial differentiation. The Danish bacteriologist Hans Christian Gram (1853–1938) devised the Gram-staining method in 1884 while he was studying in the laboratory with Carl Friedländer (1847–1887) in Berlin. A few years later, Dr. Carl Weigert (1845–1904) added a final step of staining with safranin, which turned the colorless Gram-negative bacteria red. See Kaivon Madani, "Dr. Hans Christian Jaochim Gram: Inventor of the Gram Stain," *Primary Care Update for OB/GYNS* 10, no. 5 (September–October 2003): 235–37.

20 Cecil Wall, *On Acute Cerebro-Spinal Meningitis Caused by the Diplococcus Intracellularis of Weichselbaum; A Clinical Study* (London: Royal Medical and Chirurgical Society, 1993), 36–37, 39.

21 Of note, Dr. Weichselbaum isolated the Gram-positive pneumococcus microorganism (now known as *Streptococcus pneumoniae*) from two of the eight submitted cases. A Gram-positive bacterium retains the crystal violet stain used in the Gram-staining method of bacterial differentiation. Thus, this group of bacteria stain blue.

22 The pneumococcus was independently first described in 1881 by Dr. George Miller Sternberg (1838–1915) in the United States and Dr. Louis Pasteur (1822–1895) in France. The microorganism exists as lancet-shaped pairs of coccoid bacteria, also known as diplococci. Pneumococci stain blue, whereas meningococci stain red, using the Gram method of bacterial differentiation. In 1886, the organism was called the pneumococcus because of its propensity to cause pulmonary disease. It was renamed *Diplococcus pneumoniae* in 1920 and *Streptococcus pneumoniae* in 1974. The pneumococcus is a bacterial cause of meningitis. See David Watson, Daniel M. Muser, James W. Jacobson, et al., "A Brief History of the Pneumococcus in Biomedical Research: A Panoply of Scientific Discovery," *Clinical Infectious Diseases* 17, no. 5 (November 1993): 913–24.

23 Anton Weichselbaum, "Über die Ätiologie der Akuten Meningitis Cerebrospinalis," *Fortschritte der Medizin* 5 (1887): 573–83.

24 Heinrich Albrecht and Anton Ghon, "About the Etiology and Pathological Anatomy of Meningitis Cerebrospinalis Epidemica," *Vienna Klinische Wochenschrift* 14 (1901): 984–96; and "Neisseria Meningitidis," in NCBI Taxonomy, *EOL Encyclopedia of Life*, accessed March 3, 2018, http://eol.org/pages/996566/names/synonyms.

25 "Spotted Fever Record; Largest Number of Cases Since Epidemic of 1872," *New York Tribune*, May 12, 1904, 1; John S. Billings, "Cerebrospinal Meningitis in New York City during 1904 and 1905," *Journal of the American Medical Association* 46, no. 22 (June 2, 1906): 1,670–76; and "Cerebro-spinal Meningitis in the United States, etc." *Public Health Reports* 20, no. 15 (April 14, 1905): 655.

26 How to calculate the 8.07 mortality rate:
$782/968{,}710 = x/10{,}000$; $x = 8.07$. See Charles Bolduan, "Cerebrospinal Meningitis from the Standpoint of Public Health," *Medical Times* 36, no. 7 (July 1908): 193.

27 Dr. Thomas Darlington (1858–1945) was born in the Williamsburg neighborhood of Brooklyn, New York, as the fourth of the eight children of Thomas Darlington (1826–1903), a sawyer [*sic*], and Hanna Anne Goodliffe (1830–1900). He received his early formal education in the Brooklyn public schools and at Newark High School in New Jersey. He studied science and engineering at the College of the City of New York before earning his medical diploma from the College of Physicians and Surgeons of New York City in 1880. He practiced medicine in Newark, New Jersey (1880–1882); in the Kingsbridge neighborhood of the Bronx (1882–1888); in Bisbee, Cochise County, Arizona Territory (1888–1891); and in Kingsbridge (1891–1904), until Mayor George B. McClellan Jr. (served 1904–1909) appointed him New York City health commissioner on Friday, January 1, 1904. He was the first man with medical training to occupy the position. The next New York City mayor, William Jay Gaynor (1849–1913), did not reappoint Dr. Darlington as health commissioner. Dr. Darlington subsequently practiced medicine and served as a member of the mayor's committee on sanitation and harbor pollution. He married Josephine Alice Sergeant (1864–1890) in 1886; they had two children. He died at the age of eighty-three years. "Sketches of Appointees: Dr. Thomas Darlington," *New York Tribune*, January 1, 1904, 5; Frances M. Rackemann, "Dr. Thomas Darlington," *Transactions of the American Clinical and Climatological Association* 58 (1946): lvii–lix; and "Thomas Darlington," in Frances E. Quebbeman, *Medicine in Territorial Arizona* (Phoenix, AZ: Arizona Historical Foundation, 1966), 337.

28 See "Health Commissioner Darlington Recommends Hot Baths and Sedative Medicine for Scourge of Cerebro-Spinal Meningitis— Disease Not Directly Contagious," *Evening World*, March 18, 1905,

5; "Disease Not Caught from Patient," *New York Tribune*, March 16, 1905, 14; and "Fresh Air for Meningitis: Dr. Darlington Says It Has Proved Better than Serums," *New York Times*, May 6, 1905, 16.

29 Dr. Joseph F. McCarthy (1874–1965) was born in Yonkers, Westchester County, New York, as the son of Jeremiah McCarthy and Honorah Moynihan. He attended a local parochial school; worked in a drugstore beginning at the age of fifteen years; earned his pharmacy degree from the New York College of Pharmacy (1896); earned his medical degree from the College of Physicians and Surgeons of New York City (1901); and served as a house staff surgeon Bellevue Hospital (1901–1903) and as an attending physician for a year. He developed cerebrospinal meningitis while serving as an attending physician at Bellevue Hospital. He survived the disease; traveled to the urologic clinics of Berlin, Vienna, and Paris in 1904; and returned to the United States to work at the New York Postgraduate Medical School and Hospital as a professor of urology (1917). He also taught at other medical schools. He developed urologic instruments and surgical procedures and became a renowned urologist. He married Katherine F. Ewald. They had no children. He lived to ninety years of age. See "Joseph Francis McCarthy MD, 1874–1965," William P. Didusch Center for Urologic History, accessed August 15, 2017, http://www. urologichistory.museum/content/collections/uropeople/mccarthy/ p1.cfm; and "Joseph Francis McCarthy," accessed August 15, 2017, http://prabook.com/web/person-view.html?profileId=1111777.

30 Dr. Albert Burns Craig (1867–1905) was born in Auxvasse, Callaway County, Missouri, as the middle child of the nine children born to Joseph L. Craig (1832–1926), a farmer, and Mary Elizabeth Jones (1832–1920). He moved to eastern Washington, taught school in Spokane, and served as the principal of the Medical Lake schools in Medical Lake, Spokane County, Washington. Thereafter, he served for two years as the steward of the Eastern Washington Hospital for the Insane at Medical Lake under Dr. John McFarland Semple (1857–1932), the hospital's superintendent and a graduate of Bellevue Hospital Medical College in 1886. Albert Craig entered the Jefferson Medical College of Philadelphia in 1897 and graduated as valedictorian of the class of 1901; he was thirty-four years old. He married Frances Boyd Foster (1880–1925) on October 12, 1904, at her parents' home in Newton, Middlesex County, Massachusetts. After the wedding, they moved to Philadelphia. At the time of his death, Dr. Craig was assistant editor of *American Medicine* and

assistant demonstrator in surgery and anatomy at his alma mater. He was also building a medical practice. See "Dr. Crig [*sic*] Dies a Hero; Former Medical Lake Asylum Steward Victim to Cerebro Spinal Meningitis; Contracted the Disease from Friend—Was Known by Teachers of Eastern Washington," *Evening Statesman* (Walla Walla, Washington), March 25, 1905, 2; "City Will Put Ban on 'Spotted Fever'; Dr. Craig's Death Induces Authorities to Enter upon Strenuous Campaign against Pestilential Cerebrospinal Meningitis," *Philadelphia Inquirer*, March 17, 1905, 1; "Contagion in Horrible Form; Deaths from Cerebrospinal Meningitis; Two Recent Deaths in Philadelphia Have Developed the Medical Theory that the Disease Is Highly Contagious," *Baltimore American* (Baltimore, MD), March 16, 1905, 14; "Doctors Mourn at Craig's Bier; Impressive Funeral Services on Body of Dr. Albert B. Craig, Who Gave Life for a Friend," *Boston Journal* (Boston, MA), March 17, 1905, 3; "Craig's Doctors out of Danger; Those Who Attended Cerebro-Spinal Victim Not Infected; Body of Late Physician Taken to Newton, Mass., after Services in This City," *Philadelphia Inquirer*, March 16, 1905, 16; "Dr. Albert B. Craig, Who Gave His Life in Aiding Friend," *Boston Journal*, March 17, 1905, 3; and "Spotted Fever in Contagion Test; Philadelphia Physicians Watch with Great Interest Persons Exposed through Dr. Craig," *St. Louis Post-Dispatch*, March 22, 1905, 7.

31 See "Plans War on Meningitis. Dr. Darlington Alarmed at Spread—Board Asks Fund for Inquiry," *New York Times*, March 2, 1905, 16; "To Probe Spinal Fever. Health Board Wants Commission to Investigate—Spread Alarming," *New York Tribune*, March 2, 1905, 5; "To Study Meningitis; Dr. Darlington Names Commission Provided for by Board of Estimate," *New York Times*, March 19, 1905, 6; and "79 Spotted Fever Deaths in 2 Months and 18 Days; Dr. Darlington Names Experts—Nature of Cerebro-Spinal Meningitis So Far as Known," *Brooklyn Daily Eagle*, March 18, 1905, 2.

32 The commission members were Dr. Thomas Darlington, Dr. Hermann M. Biggs, Dr. W. K. Draper, Dr. E. K. Dunham, Dr. Simon Flexner, Dr. Walter B. James, Dr. William L. Polk, Dr. William P. Northrup, Dr. Joshua Van Cott, and Dr. W. J. Elser. At its first meeting on March 24, 1905, the commission separated into a bacteriological section and a clinical section. See Wade W. Oliver, *The Man Who Lived for Tomorrow: A Biography of William Hallock Park, MD* (New York: E. P. Dutton, 1941), 231.

33 Dr. Simon Flexner (1863–1946) was born in Louisville, Jefferson County, Kentucky, as the fourth of the nine children of German immigrants Moritz "Morris" Flexner (1820–1882), a peddler, and Esther Abraham (1835–1905). Simon graduated from the two-year lecture program at the University of Louisville College of Pharmacy, worked as a druggist, earned a medical diploma following graduation from the two-year program of lectures at the University of Louisville Medical Department in 1889, and won a place in the pathology program, headed by Dr. William Henry Welch (1850–1934), at the Johns Hopkins School of Medicine in Baltimore in 1890. In 1892, 1893, and 1899, he studied the cerebrospinal meningitis epidemic in Maryland, medicine in Europe, and tropical diseases in the Philippines, respectively. He subsequently won a research professorship at the University of Pennsylvania. In 1904, John Davison Rockefeller (1839–1937), the oil magnate and philanthropist, recruited him to direct the fledgling Rockefeller Institute for Medical Research in New York City. See James Thomas Flexner, *An American Saga: The Story of Helen Thomas and Simon Flexner* (New York: Fordham University Press, 1993); George Washington Corner, *A History of the Rockefeller Institute, 1901–1953: Origins and Growth* (New York: Rockefeller Institute Press, 1964); and "Rockefeller Money and Medical Science: A Social Investment," in E. Richard Brown, *Rockefeller Medicine Men: Medicine and Capitalism in America* (Berkeley, CA: University of California Press, 1979), 105–11. For images of the Rockefeller Institute Laboratory in 1912, visit "Founder's Hall and the Hospital" webpage, Rockefeller University, accessed March 3, 2018, http://digitalcommons.rockefeller.edu/ hospital-of-institute/15/ngs. For images of Dr. Simon Flexner, visit the National Library of Medicine webpage, accessed March 3, 2018, https://collections.nlm.nih.gov/?utf8=%E2%9C%93&PID=nlm%3 Anlmuid-56431240R-bk&q=flexner.

34 John Davison Rockefeller Sr. (1839–1937) was born in Richford, New York, as the second child and eldest son of William Avery Rockefeller (1810–1906), a peddler, and Eliza Davison (1813–1889). The family moved frequently before settling in Cleveland, Cuyahoga County, Ohio, where John D. Rockefeller became a bookkeeper at the age of sixteen years (1855), an oil refiner at the age of twenty years (1859), and a founder of Standard Oil Company at the age of thirty-one years (1870). He founded the University of Chicago in 1890 and the Rockefeller Institute for Medical Research in Manhattan in June

1901. See Ron Chernow, *Titan: The Life of John D. Rockefeller Sr.* (New York: Vintage, 1984); and George Washington Corner, *A History of the Rockefeller Institute, 1901–1953: Origins and Growth* (New York: Rockefeller Institute Press, 1964).

35 Dr. Hermann Michael Biggs (1859–1923) was born in Trumansburg, Tompkins County, New York as one of the two sons Joseph Hunt Biggs (1827–1877), a merchant, and Melissa A. Biggs (1826–1910). He attended Cornell University in Ithaca, Tompkins County, New York (1879–1882) and earned his medical diploma from the Bellevue Hospital Medical College (1883). He served as an interne at Bellevue Hospital (1884) before studying medicine in Europe. He helped establish and director the first municipal bacteriological laboratory in the United States. From 1901 to 1914, he served as the general medical officer of the New York City Board of Health. In 1914, he accepted an appointment as the state health commission, a position that he held until his death. He married Frances Richardson Gibbs (1869–1931) in 1898; they had two children. Dr. Biggs died at the age of sixty-four years. Charles-Edward Amory Winslow, *The Life of Hermann M. Biggs, Physician and Statesman of the Public Health* (Philadelphia, PA: Lea and Febiger, 1929).

36 The Research Laboratory of the New York City Board of Health originated as the Diagnostic Bacteriological Laboratory of the New York City Board of Health on May 4, 1893. The Diagnostic Bacteriological Laboratory was the first public health diagnostic bacteriological laboratory in the United States. Dr. Hermann Biggs (1859–1923), chief of the newly created Division of Pathology, Bacteriology, and Disinfection of the New York City Board of Health, founded the laboratory to assist the city in controlling the diphtheria epidemic. Dr. William Hallock Park (1863–1939), the bacteriological diagnostician of diphtheria recruited by Dr. Hermann Biggs, directed the laboratory in the Laboratory and Division Office of the New York City Board of Health at 42 Bleecker Street. The laboratory soon moved to larger laboratory space in the Criminal Court Building at 100 Centre Street in Lower Manhattan. The number of bacteriologists and technicians employed for the laboratory examinations of diphtheria and tuberculosis specimens increased to twelve to handle the volume of incoming specimens designated for culture. On December 23, 1894, the New York City Board of Health received funds to manufacture diphtheria antitoxin; the first antitoxin produced by Dr. Park and Dr. Anna

Williams (1863–1954). The diphtheria antitoxin became available for distribution on January 1, 1895. The New York City Board of Health distributed the diphtheria antitoxin free of charge to private physicians in New York City at diphtheria culture stations organized by Dr. Park to collect swabs for culture from the throats of patients. In February 1895, the staff of the Division of Pathology, Bacteriology, and Disinfection expanded to include an assistant pathologist, an assistant chemist, four assistant bacteriologists, several additional laboratory assistants, and a collector of culture tubes. In October 1895, Dr. Park and his staff moved from the Criminal Court Building to the second floor of the Willard Parker Hospital Disinfecting Station on the west side of Willard Parker Hospital, itself located on East Sixteenth Street, Manhattan, near the East River. The Diagnostic Bacteriological Laboratory became known as the Hospital Laboratory. In 1905, the Hospital Laboratory moved out of the Willard Parker Hospital Disinfecting Station into a new six-story building called the Laboratory Building, which sat on the east side of Willard Parker Hospital. The Hospital Laboratory in the Laboratory Building subsequently became known as the Research Laboratory (also Research Laboratories). Dr. Park directed the Research Laboratory and the municipal production of all vaccines, antitoxins, and sera for use by the physicians and patients of New York City. He sold surplus antitoxin to other cities to raise funds to support the work of the Research Laboratory. In 1908, the New York City municipal government purchased acreage in Otisville, Orange County, New York, to erect a municipal tuberculosis sanatorium. In 1909, the municipal government gave some of the acreage to the Research Laboratory to build facilities for stabling the horses and other animals used in the production of sera, antitoxins, and vaccines. See Charles-Edward Amory Winslow, *The Life of Hermann M. Biggs, Physician and Statesman of the Public Health* (Philadelphia, PA: Lea and Febiger, 1929); Wade W. Oliver, *The Man Who Lived for Tomorrow: A Biography of William Hallock Park, MD* (New York: E. P. Dutton, 1941); Hermann M. Biggs, *Brief History of the Campaign against Tuberculosis in New York City: Catalogue of the Tuberculosis Exhibit of the Department of Health, City of New York, 1908* (New York: Department of Health, 1908), 12–13; and Ben Freedman, "The First State Board of Health Laboratories in the United States," *Public Health Reports* 69, no. 9 (September 1954): 868.

37 See Charles F. Bolduan, "Over a Century of Health Administration in New York City," *Department of Health of the City of New York Monograph Series* 13 (March 1916): 23–24; and Arthur Bushel, *Chronology of New York City Department of Health (and Its Predecessor Agencies) 1655–1966* (New York: New York City Health Department, March 1966), accessed April 3, 2018, https://www1.nyc.gov/assets/doh/downloads/pdf/history/chronology-1966centennial.pdf.

38 See Simon Flexner, "Experimental Cerebrospinal Meningitis and Its Serum Treatment," *Journal of the American Medical Association* 47, no. 8 (August 25, 1906): 560–66; and Simon Flexner, "Experimental Cerebro-Spinal Meningitis in Monkeys," *Journal of Experimental Medicine* 9, no. 2 (March 14, 1907): 142–67.

39 Dr. Charles Frederick Bolduan (1873–1950) was born as the son of William Bolduan and Juliane Caroline Dreibholz in Bielefeld, Ostwestfalen-Lippe, North Rhine-Westphalia, Germany. In 1879, he immigrated to the United States, where he attended Brooklyn public schools before moving to Berlin to earn a pharmacy doctorate. He next returned to the United States, became a naturalized citizen (1894), earned a medical degree from the College of Physicians and Surgeons of New York City (1901), and joined the New York City Board of Health (1904). He organized the board's bureau of education (1914) and directed it for decades. From 1918 to 1928, he was associated with the US Public Health Service. In 1906, he married Adele Jonsson; they had one child. His second wife was Herma Engelsdorff, whom he married in 1928. He died at Bellevue Hospital at the age of seventy-seven years. See John Shrady, *The College of Physicians and Surgeons, New York, A History* (New York: Lewis Publishing Company, 1903), 2:529; and "Dr. C. F. Bolduan, Health Official," *Brooklyn Daily Eagle*, July 5, 1950, 15.

40 William Hallock Park and Charles Bolduan, "The Communicability of Cerebro-Spinal Meningitis," *Public Health Reports* 31, Pt 1 (1905): 359–63.

41 "Quarantine for Meningitis; New York Health Official Thinks the Disease is Communicable," *Democrat and Chronicle* (Rochester, NY), April 22, 1905, 2; and Wade W. Oliver, *The Man Who Lived for Tomorrow: A Biography of William Hallock Park, MD* (New York: E. P. Dutton, 1941), 232.

42 Centers for Disease Control and Prevention, "Measures of Risk," *Principles of Epidemiology in Public Health Practice, Third Edition,*

accessed August 12, 2018, https://www.cdc.gov/ophss/csels/dsepd/ss1978/lesson3/section2.html.

43 Simon Flexner and James Wesley Jobling, "An Analysis of Four Hundred Cases of Epidemic Meningitis Treated with the Anti-Meningitis Serum," *Journal of Experimental Medicine* 10, no. 5 (September 5, 1908): 691–692.

44 Wade W. Oliver, *The Man Who Lived for Tomorrow: A Biography of William Hallock Park, MD* (New York: E. P. Dutton, 1941), 300.

45 Simon Flexner, "Experimental Cerebrospinal Meningitis and Its Serum Treatment," *Journal of the American Medical Association* 47, no. 8 (August 25, 1906): 560–66.

46 Wilhelm Kolle and August Wasserman, "Versuch zur Gewinnung und Wertbestimmung eines Meningococcenserums," *Deutsch Medizinische Wochenschrift* 32 (1906): 609–12.

47 Gustaf Jochmann, "Versuche zur Serodiagnostic und Serotherapie der epidemischen Genickstarre," *Deutsch Medizinische Wochenschrift* 32 (1906): 788–93.

48 Simon Flexner and James Wesley Jobling, "Serum Treatment of Epidemic Cerebro-Spinal Meningitis," *Journal of Experimental Medicine* 10, no. 1 (January 1, 1908): 194–95.

49 Dr. William Hallock Park (1863–1939) was born at 164 West Eleventh Street, Manhattan, as one of the three sons of Rufus Park (1813–1896), a merchant, and Hannah Joanna Hallock (1835–1881). Rufus Park had been widowed twice before marrying Hanna Hallock and had three children by his previous wives, including one daughter, Julia, with whom William was close throughout his life. William H. Park attended the Boys' Public School on West Thirteenth Street and completed in 1883, at the age of twenty years, the five-year combined secondary-collegiate program at the College of the City of New York. He earned his medical degree from the College of Physicians and Surgeons of New York City in 1886; performed postgraduate work at Roosevelt Hospital in New York City, 1886–1889, advancing from surgical dresser to senior assistant to house surgeon and then to house surgeon; studied medicine in Europe for a year; returned to New York City to run a private medical practice for a year; and joined the staff of Dr. T. Mitchell Prudden's laboratory (1890–1892) at the College of Physicians and Surgeons of New York City to study diphtheria. At the same time, he was associated with Bellevue Hospital, the Vanderbilt Clinic of the College of Physicians and Surgeons, Roosevelt Hospital, and Manhattan Eye and Ear

Hospital as a laryngologist. In 1892, Dr. Park published his first scientific paper describing his method of diagnosing diphtheria by demonstrating diphtheria bacilli in cultures. In 1893, Dr. Hermann Biggs recruited him as the bacteriological diagnostician of diphtheria of the Diagnostic Bacteriological Laboratory of the New York City Board of Health. Dr. Park steadily advanced to become director of the Research Laboratory of the New York City Board of Health. He never married and had no children. He died suddenly of heart disease in 1939; he had worked for the New York City Board of Health for forty-three years. See William H. Park and Alfred Beebe, "Diphtheria and Allied Pseudo-Membranous Inflammations, A Clinical and Bacteriological Study," *Medical Record* 42 (July 30 and August 6, 1892): 113–25, 141–47; Wade W. Oliver, *The Man Who Lived for Tomorrow: A Biography of William Hallock Park, MD* (New York: E. P. Dutton, 1941); Page Cooper, *The Bellevue Story* (New York: Thomas Y. Crowell Company, 1948), 135–43; Harry Filmore Dowling, "Field, Ward, and Laboratory: Where the Infectious Disease Physician Worked," *Journal of Infectious Diseases* 153, no. 3 (March 1986): 390–96; "Dr. William Park, Health Official," *Brooklyn Daily Eagle*, April 6, 1949, 15; and Hans Zinsser, "William Hallock Park 1863–1939," *Journal of Bacteriology* 38, no. 1 (July 1939): v-3–3.

50   Wade W. Oliver, *The Man Who Lived for Tomorrow: A Biography of William Hallock Park, MD* (New York: E. P. Dutton, 1941), 300. See also Simon Flexner, "Experimental Cerebrospinal Meningitis and Its Serum Treatment," *Journal of the American Medical Association* 47, no. 8 (August 25, 1906): 560–66; Clemens F. von Pirquet and Béla Schick, *Serum Sickness* (Philadelphia, PA: Williams and Wilkins, 1951); and "A Communication: Serum Sickness," *Texas State Journal of Medicine* 7, no. 12 (April 1912): 335–36.

51   August Wassermann, "Über die Bisherigen Erfahrungen mit dem Meningococcen-Heilserum bei Genickstarre-kranken," *Deutsch Medizinische Wochenschrift* 33 (1907): 1,585–87.

52   See Georg Jochmann, "Versuche zur Serodiagnostik und Serotherapie der Epidemischen Genickstarre," *Deutsche Medizinische Wochenschrift* 1, no. 1 (1906): 788–93; Abraham Sophian, *Epidemic Cerebrospinal Meningitis* (St. Louis, MO: C. V. Mosby Company, 1913), 175; and Wade W. Oliver, *The Man Who Lived for Tomorrow: A Biography of William Hallock Park, MD* (New York: E. P. Dutton, 1941), 303.

53 Simon Flexner, "Experimental Cerebrospinal Meningitis and Its Serum Treatment," *Journal of the American Medical Association* 47, no. 8 (August 25, 1906): 566.

54 Simon Flexner and James Wesley Jobling, "Serum Treatment of Epidemic Cerebro-Spinal Meningitis," *Journal of Experimental Medicine* 10, no. 1 (January 1, 1908): 141–203.

55 Ibid., 196.

56 Ibid., 202.

57 See "Physicians Are Arming against Meningitis (Fort Worth)," *Abilene Semi Weekly Farm Reporter* (Abilene, TX), October 8, 1908, 7; and "Treatment of Meningitis; Valuable Serum Is Received from New York Institute," *Dallas Morning News*, October 31, 1908, 9.

CHAPTER 1

HARBINGER: A TEXAS FAMILY
FALLS ILL, JANUARY 1909

During the wee hours of Tuesday, January 5, 1909, nine-year-old Mattie Darcus McCallum,[1] a tenant farmer's daughter, awoke with a chill and a headache in her family's farmhouse near McKinney,[2] Collin County in North Central Texas. Mattie McCallum had felt well the previous evening when she had gone to sleep with her fourteen-year-old sister Ossie Barron McCallum, her three-year-old sister Mary Lou McCallum, her two-year-old brother Edward "Eddie" Owenby McCallum, and her forty-one-year-old widowed mother, Mrs. Lizzie McCallum.[3-4]

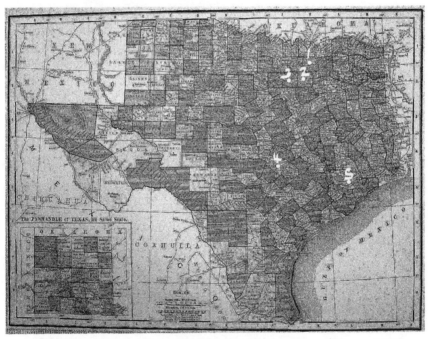

Rand, McNally, and Company's business atlas map of Texas, 1909; Rand, McNally and Company, Chicago, Illinois, #E 14435, Feb. 16, 1909. The location of the following cities is highlighted with numbers: #1: McKinney, #2: Dallas, #3: Fort Worth, 4: #Austin, 5: Houston.

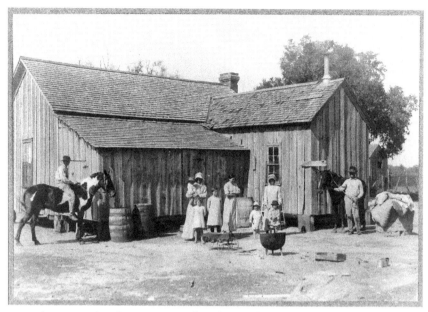

An example of an itinerant family at a farmstead rented from J. W. Vaughn, Corsicana, Navarro County, Texas, October 1913. Photographer: Lewis Wickes Hine (1874–1940). The image is held at the Library of Congress Prints and Photographs Division, Washington, DC.

When Mattie's condition worsened at noon that same Tuesday, her mother contacted Henry Arthur Finch, the farm's owner.[5] Mr. Finch telephoned Dr. John Caleb Erwin,[6] who motored over dirt roads from his medical office in downtown McKinney to the McCallum family's farmhouse. He found Mattie McCallum lying deathly still in bed in a darkened room. Her temperature was 102 degrees Fahrenheit and her pulse rate was ninety beats per minute. Her neck was stiff to flexion and her pupils were sluggish to light stimulation. Tiny, deep purple spots covered her body. At six o'clock that evening, Mattie's temperature spiked to 104 degrees and her body rattled. At a half hour past midnight on Wednesday, January 6, 1909, she sank.[7] She had been ill for less than twenty-four hours.

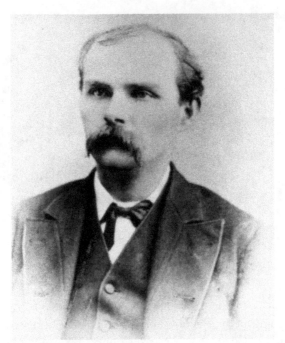

Honorable Henry Arthur Finch (1853–1934), Texas State Legislature House of Representatives, circa 1883. The image is a detail from the 18th House Composite (CHA #1989.5411). The image is courtesy of the Texas State Preservation Board, Austin, Texas.

Dr. Erwin tentatively diagnosed Mattie's cause of death as cerebrospinal meningitis, basing his clinical diagnosis on her fever, rigid neck, rash, mental-status changes, and rapid demise. Dr. Erwin knew that the only way to reliably establish the cause of Mattie's meningitis was to perform a lumbar puncture procedure, obtain a sample of her cerebrospinal fluid, examine the fluid under the microscope lens, and look for *Neisseria meningitidis* bacteria.[8] In 1909, few Texas physicians, including Dr. Erwin, performed the lumbar puncture procedure well or performed it at all.[9–10]

Several hours after Mattie died, Henry "H. R." Robinson,[7,11] a fourteen-year-old orphan living with the McCallum family, developed a chill and a fever.[12] On Thursday, January 7, 1909, he complained of a headache and a backache so painful that Mrs. McCallum again called Mr. Finch, who again called Dr. Erwin. After finding Henry in bed with a temperature of 101 degrees but no rash or specific neurological findings, Dr. Erwin diagnosed an ordinary malarial chill,[7] treated Henry with a full dose of the purgative calomel,[13] and noted good results by three o'clock that same afternoon (Thursday, January 7, 1909).[7] An hour later, however, Henry's temperature rose to 102 degrees and he vomited and shook. Dr. Erwin injected morphine and atropine to treat Henry's convulsion and head and back pain[7] and to help him sleep.[14] Henry did sleep through the night. On Friday morning, January 8, 1909, Henry's temperature was normal, and Dr. Erwin expressed optimism for Henry's recovery. Several hours later, however, Henry became delirious, plunged into a coma, and died. The duration of his illness was about seventy-two hours from the time of his first chill.[7] Dr. Erwin wrung his hands.

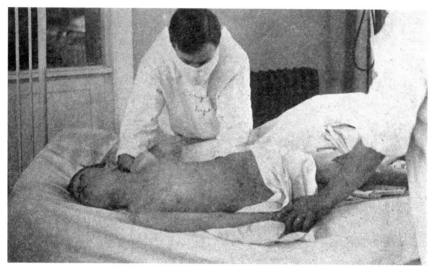

A young male with cerebrospinal meningitis, 1912–1913. The original caption of this image is: "Boy of eleven, ill forty-eight hours with epidemic meningitis. He was actively delirious so that he had to be held for the photograph. Note the posture. The head markedly retraced, back bowed." The photographer is unknown. Date: circa 1912–1913. The image was scanned from Abraham Sophian, *Epidemic Cerebrospinal Meningitis* (St. Louis, MO: C. V. Mosby, 1913), 73.

On the morning of Monday, January 11, 1909, Dr. Erwin returned to the McCallum farmhouse to evaluate fourteen-year-old

Ossie Barron McCallum, who was complaining of a chill and intense pain in her right knee joint, head, and back. Her temperature was 101 degrees, her pulse rate was 110 beats per minute, and her right knee was swollen and tender. She lacked any rash or specific neurological findings. About three o'clock in the afternoon of that same day, her left knee joint also became painful and her head and back pain worsened. She vomited, seized, slipped into a coma, and died. The duration of her illness was about seventy-two hours from the time of her first chill.[7]

Dr. Erwin feared he was witnessing an incipient epidemic of cerebrospinal meningitis. He had read about Flexner antimeningitis serum, a promising treatment developed by Dr. Simon Flexner at the Rockefeller Institute for Medical Research in New York City.[15-16] The treatment consisted of infusing Dr. Flexner's antimeningitis serum directly into the cerebrospinal fluid space—also known as the subarachnoid, intrathecal, or intraspinal space—located within the bony spinal column.[17] Dr. Erwin wondered where he might obtain antimeningitis serum and instructions on its use. In January 1909, a Texas State Board of Health did not yet exist[18] to provide the antimeningitis serum or training in its use.

Soon Dr. Erwin recalled that three Fort Worth physicians— Dr. Willus Gurden Cook,[19] Dr. Ira Carleton Chase,[20] and Dr. Khleher Heberden Beall[21]—had procured a small supply of Flexner antimeningitis serum from the Rockefeller Institute for Medical Research in October 1908.[22-23] Dr. Erwin hoped to obtain some serum from these Fort Worth physicians if another person in or around McKinney developed the illness that he feared was cerebrospinal meningitis.

Dr. Erwin brightened when no further patients developed the dread affliction between Monday, January 11, 1909, and Sunday, January 17, 1909. However, on Monday, January 18, 1909, he was back at the McCallum farmhouse tending to little Eddie Owenby McCallum, who had developed a chill and a fever at eleven o'clock the previous night.[7] Dr. Erwin, certain that Eddie had the same disease that had killed his two older sisters and the orphan Henry

Robinson, called Dr. Willus G. Cook in Fort Worth to request some Flexner antimeningitis serum.

Dr. Cook asked Dr. Erwin whether he had confirmed the diagnosis of cerebrospinal meningitis by obtaining and examining cerebrospinal fluid from Eddie and the three previous patients with the same clinical presentation and course. Dr. Erwin said no. Dr. Cook explained that Dr. Flexner had released the antimeningitis serum to him and his two colleagues on three conditions. First, physicians using the antimeningitis serum must fill out and promptly return to the Rockefeller Institute for Medical Research a medical report containing evidence that the patient receiving the serum had cerebrospinal meningitis and not some other disease. To reliably prove this fact required performance of a lumbar puncture procedure and a microscopic and culture analysis of the patient's cerebrospinal fluid to confirm that the culprit was *Neisseria meningitidis*. Second, physicians could levy no monetary charges to the patient for the antimeningitis serum. Third, physicians could not discriminate among individuals selected to receive the antimeningitis serum based on their economic status, race, or other characteristics.[23] Dr. Cook then invited Dr. Erwin to transport Eddie McCallum to St. Joseph's Infirmary[24] in Fort Worth for further evaluation and possible treatment with antimeningitis serum. Dr. Erwin bundled up Eddie McCallum, boarded a train with Mrs. McCallum and her sick son, and arrived at St. Joseph's Infirmary about two o'clock on Tuesday morning, January 19, 1909.[7]

The jostling train ride between McKinney and Fort Worth (about fifty miles) and the brisk winter air apparently invigorated Eddie, as he appeared so much better by Tuesday morning at breakfast that Dr. Cook and Dr. Erwin agreed to postpone the lumbar puncture procedure. Dr. Erwin, who was needed in McKinney, urged Dr. Cook to perform a lumbar puncture procedure and administer the Flexner antimeningitis serum at the first clinical signs of meningitis shown by Eddie.[7] Dr. Cook agreed and Dr. Erwin returned to McKinney.

About twelve hours later, Mrs. McCallum frantically called Dr.

Erwin in McKinney to plead for his immediate return to Fort Worth, as Eddie was refusing fluids, arching his back, and intermittently shaking. Dr. Erwin instructed Mrs. McCallum to call Dr. Cook at once. She did and Dr. Cook quickly arrived at St. Joseph Infirmary, diagnosed Eddie with probable clinical cerebrospinal meningitis, performed a lumbar puncture procedure, removed turbid cerebrospinal fluid, identified *Neisseria meningitidis* through the microscope lens, and infused antimeningitis serum directly into Eddie's inflamed meninges. In this way, little Eddie McCallum became the first person in Texas to receive antimeningitis serum.[23] Eddie received a second spinal infusion of antimeningitis serum about forty-eight hours later and steadily improved.[7]

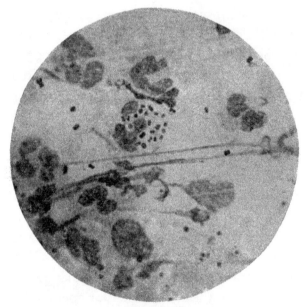

Fig. XX.

Meningococci and inflammatory cells in cerebrospinal fluid seen through a microscopic lens, 1912–1913. The original caption of this image is: "Stained sediment of cerebrospinal fluid removed from a case of epidemic meningitis at the beginning of the disease, before serum treatment was instituted. Note the presence of intra- and extracellular diplococci and pus-cells." The photographer is unknown. The image was scanned from Abraham Sophian, *Epidemic Cerebrospinal Meningitis* (St. Louis, MO: C. V. Mosby, 1913), 245.

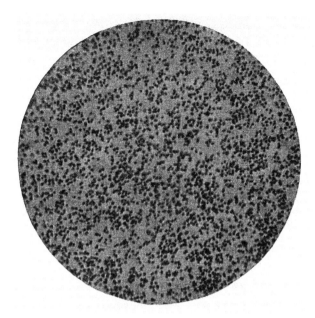

A pure meningococcal culture as seen through a microscope lens. The original caption of this image is: "Pure culture of meningococcus, 36 hours old. Note the irregular staining, the arrangement in pairs of the biscuit-shaped organisms and the approximation of the flat surfaces of the individual bacteria. Note that the division between the individual cocci cannot be determined in many instances." The photographer is unknown. The image was scanned from Abraham Sophian, *Epidemic Cerebrospinal Meningitis* (St. Louis, MO: C. V. Mosby, 1913), 21.

Soon after Dr. Erwin in McKinney spoke with Mrs. McCallum in Fort Worth, he learned that Mary Lou McCallum had developed pain in her head and back. Dr. Erwin hurried to the McCallum family farmhouse. By six thirty in the evening on Wednesday, January 20, 1909, Dr. Erwin was holding blanket-wrapped Mary Lou on his lap on a train barreling along the railroad tracks to Fort Worth. Dr. Cook was waiting for them at the Fort Worth Union Depot at about three o'clock on the morning of Thursday, January 21, 1909. On reaching St. Joseph's Infirmary, Dr. Cook and Dr. Erwin together performed a lumbar puncture procedure, withdrew thirty cubic centimeters of cerebrospinal fluid, and administered about the same amount of antimeningitis serum directly into Mary

Lou's inflamed meninges. Her cerebrospinal fluid was positive for meningococci. Dr. Cook slipped two fifteen-cubic-centimeter bottles of serum into Dr. Erwin's pocket to use in McKinney. Dr. Erwin thanked him and returned to McKinney.[7]

The McKinney community rallied around Mrs. Lizzie McCallum's remaining healthy sons—John Chester, Willie Jessee, Watus Bucephalous, and Obediah Franklin.[24] For example, Mr. and Mrs. Finch did everything possible for the boys. John Thomas Couch,[25] a piano store owner; Adolphus Barbee Mayes,[26] a wealthy retired farmer; and Dr. Eustace Eugene King,[27] a Baptist minister, visited and consoled the boys.

On Saturday morning, January 23, 1909, cerebrospinal meningitis struck a different family in McKinney. Dr. Erwin treated an eleven-year-old girl complaining of chills and head and back pain. Her temperature was 104.5 degrees, her pulse rate was 120 beats per minute and weak, her respirations were around thirty-two breaths per minute, her pupils were unreactive to light, and her neck was stiff to flexion. Dr. Erwin sedated her with morphine and atropine and applied cold compresses to reduce her temperature. She slipped into a coma as a purple rash spread across her body. Dr. Erwin performed a lumbar puncture procedure, withdrew twenty cubic centimeters of slightly turbid cerebrospinal fluid, and injected fifteen cubic centimeters of the antimeningitis serum given to him by Dr. Cook. The same night, his patient's temperature fell to about 100.5 degrees. Dr. Erwin identified meningococci in his patient's cerebrospinal fluid and sent a sample of the fluid to Dr. Cook, who verified the finding, cultured the specimen, and filled out a medical report to send to Dr. Flexner. Dr. Erwin's eleven-year-old patient rapidly improved.[7]

Mary Lou McCallum at St. Joseph's Infirmary in Fort Worth required only one lumbar puncture procedure and one antimeningitis serum treatment to recover. In early February 1909, Mrs. McCallum returned home with Eddie and Mary Lou McCallum, who made full recoveries. Local newspapers, the Tarrant County Medical Society, and the Texas State Medical Association trumpeted the successful health outcomes of the two children treated with Flexner antimeningitis serum at St. Joseph's Infirmary in Fort Worth.[28] Dr. Erwin continued to care for additional patients with cerebrospinal meningitis in and around McKinney.[7]

When the cerebrospinal meningitis outbreak in McKinney finally ended with the onset of hot weather in 1909, Dr. Erwin organized and published his experience in diagnosing and treating thirteen patients with the disease.[7] Of the thirteen patients, seven received intraspinal antimeningitis serum. Of the seven patients who received the treatment, four made complete recoveries, and three died. Of the three who died, two received the antimeningitis serum late in the course of their illnesses—one because his mother objected to the serum and the other because the patient was moribund when Dr. Erwin identified him as a candidate for the antimeningitis serum. Dr. Erwin subtracted these two cases from the seven who received intraspinal antimeningitis serum. One of the remaining five patients died, yielding a case fatality rate of 20 percent. Of the six patients who did not receive intraspinal antimeningitis serum, the case fatality rate was 100 percent. Dr. Erwin became an ardent supporter of intraspinal antimeningitis serum in victims of cerebrospinal meningitis.[7] He noted in his report that the only other epidemic of meningitis in the McKinney area occurred in 1870, when the town had forty-two cases and forty deaths.[7]

In October 1909, Dr. Flexner published the antimeningitis serum outcome data sent to him by physicians from throughout the United States and world between April 1907 and April 1909. Dr. Flexner received approximately 1,000 reports, of which 712 contained a bacteriologic diagnosis of cerebrospinal meningitis. Of the 712 individuals represented by these 712 reports, 488 recovered, and 224 died, resulting in a case fatality rate of 31.5 percent.[29]

CHAPTER 1 NOTES

1 McCollum and McCollom are variant spellings of McCallum in the historical literature.

2 McKinney, Collin County, Texas, is located near the East Fork Trinity River in the Texas Blackland Prairies, a broad, temperate grassland ecoregion named for its rich, dark soil. The tract runs about three hundred miles from the Red River at the Texas-Oklahoma border, through the Dallas-Fort Worth area, and into Southwestern Texas. The human population of McKinney in 1910 was about 4,700, as compared to the populations of San Antonio (97,000), Dallas (92,000), Fort Worth (73,000), Austin (30,000), and Waco (26,000). McKinney is about thirty miles north of Dallas, about 225 miles north of Austin, and about sixty miles northeast of Fort Worth. See *Texas Almanac: City Population History of Selected Cities, 1850–2000*, accessed December 8, 2017, https://texasalmanac.com/sites/default/files/images/CityPopHist%20web.pdf; Julia L. Vargo, *McKinney, Texas—The First 150 Years* (Virginia Beach, VA: Donning Company Publishers, 1997); Ryan Barnhart and Ryan Estes, *McKinney* (Charleston, SC: Arcadia Publishing, 2010); United States Department of Agriculture, *The Agriculture, Soils, Geology, and Topography of the Blacklands Experimental Watershed, Waco, Texas* (Washington, DC: Government Printing Office, 1942); Harrell J. Budd Jr., "Geology of the McKinney Area, Collin County, Texas" (master's thesis, Southern Methodist University, Dallas, TX, 1950); "Collin McKinney, Signer of the Texas Declaration of Independence," in Samuel Houston Dixon, *The Men Who Made Texas Free* (Houston, TX: Texas Historical Publishing Company, c. 1924), 259–64; Zachary Taylor Fulmore, "Collin," in *The History and Geography of Texas as Told in County Names* (Austin, TX: Texas Historical Association, 1915), 73; J. Lee Stambaugh and Lillian J. Stambaugh, *A History of Collin County, Texas* (Austin, TX: Texas State Historical Association, 1958); Harold Beam, "A History of Collin County, Texas" (master's thesis, University of Texas, Austin, 1951); and *1910 United States Census: Volume 7; Agriculture, 1909 and 1910, Reports by States, with Statistics for Counties* (Washington, DC: Government Printing Office, 1913), 626–27, 682.

3 Mary Elizabeth "Lizzie" Pendergrass McCallum (1868–1945) was born in Baton Rouge, Chester County, South Carolina, as the eldest

of the four children of Watus Pendergrass (1841–1912), a farmer, and Mary Belle Worthy (1850–1873). Lizzie was five years old when her mother died. In 1887, nineteen-year-old Lizzie wed thirty-two-year-old William "Bill" Jefferson McCallum (1855–1908). Bill McCallum was also a native of Baton Rouge, Chester County, South Carolina, and was one of the seven children of William McNeil McCallum (1826–1884), a farmer, and Darcus Adeline Darby (1832–1873). After marrying, Bill and Lizzie moved a thousand miles to the west to settle in Dallas County, Texas. They farmed there from 1889 to 1905 and moved to nearby Collin County to farm acreage owned by the Henry Arthur Finch (1853–1934). Between 1889 and 1909, Lizzie and Bill had eight children. In addition, an orphan, Henry Robinson, lived with them. Fifty-three-year-old Bill died in June 1908 after becoming paralyzed from an undiagnosed ailment a month earlier. Lizzie McCallum died in University Park, Texas, at the age of seventy-seven years. She was buried next to Bill in McLarry Cemetery in McKinney. See "Multiplied Misfortunes, Home North of Town Enshrouded in Deepest Gloom," *Courier Gazette* (McKinney, TX), January 13, 1909, 1; and "No title" (a brief article about Bill McCallum's illness), *Courier Gazette*, May 19, 1908, 2.

4   Mrs. Lizzie McCallum's children in 1909 were John Chester (1889–1925), Willie Jessee (1890–1952), Watus Bucephalous (1892–1962), Ossie Barron (1894–1909), Mattie Darcus (1899–1909), Obediah "Obe" Franklin (1901–1965), Mary Lou (1905–1949), and Edward "Eddie" Owenby (1907–1980) McCallum. Henry Robinson (1895–1909) was the orphan who lived with the McCallum family until his death from cerebrospinal meningitis in 1909.

5   Henry Arthur Finch (1853–1934) was born in Brandon, Rankin County, Mississippi, as the only child of Dr. William Jasper Finch (1831–1916) and Ellen Elizabeth Gibson (1836–1901). Henry was named after his father's slave, Henry Arthur, who saved Dr. Finch's life by carrying him off the battlefield at Shiloh, Hardin County, Tennessee, in 1862. Henry Finch completed his collegiate education in the law department of Cumberland University in Lebanon, Wilson County, Tennessee, after attending the University of Mississippi in Jackson, Mississippi, for three years. In January 1876, he moved to McKinney, opened a law practice, and represented Collin and Denton Counties in the Eighteenth Legislature (1883–1885) of the Texas State House of Representatives and the Twenty-Second

Legislature (1891–1893) of the Texas State Senate. Both legislatures met in the Texas State Capitol in Austin, Travis County, Texas, about 225 miles south of McKinney. Henry Finch also served as McKinney's mayor (1917–1921), whence he oversaw the erection of McKinney's first hospital—a three-story, forty-bed facility that cost $100,000. In 1923, the hospital met the high "Minimum Standard" developed and required by the American College of Surgeons for hospital accreditation. This was an unusual achievement at the time. During his professional life, Mr. Finch acquired wealth, purchased agricultural land near McKinney, and rented acreage to farming families, including the McCallum family in 1905. Henry R. Finch married Laura Frances "Fannie" Shipe (1866–1942), a teacher, in 1890; they had seven children, of whom two died in childhood. See "Henry A. Finch," *Legislative Reference Library of Texas*, accessed October 14, 2017, http://www.lrl.state.tx.us/legeleaders/members/memberdisplay.cfm?memberID=3698; "Henry Arthur Finch," in Lewis E. Daniell, *Personnel of the Texas State Government with Sketches of Representative Men of Texas* (San Antonio, TX: Maverick Printing House, 1892), 195–96; "McKinney City Hospital," *Collin County, Texas History*, accessed October 14, 2017, http://www.collincountyhistory.com/mckinney-hospital.html; "State-Wide Tribute Paid to Late Collin Senator," *Dallas Morning News*, January 12, 1934, 5; and "The 1919 'Minimum Standard' Document," American College of Surgeons, accessed March 4, 2018, https://www.facs.org/about-acs/archives/pasthighlights/minimumhighlight.

6   Dr. John Caleb Erwin (1857–1951) was born near Charlotte, Mecklenburg County, North Carolina, as the eldest of the seven children of Reverend Thomas Washington Erwin (1827–1911) and Elizabeth Phillips Douglas (1830–1912). He graduated from the Bingham Military Academy at Mebane Station, Orange County, North Carolina; earned his medical diploma from the University of Louisville Medical Department (also called the University of Louisville Medical Institute and the University of Louisville Medical College) in 1884; moved to McKinney, Collin County, Texas, in 1886; and formed a practice with Dr. Calvin McCauley and later with Dr. John E. Gibson (1847–1928). He led the founding of the Collin County Medical Association in 1891 and held its meetings in his medical office in downtown McKinney for years. He served as a delegate to the Texas State Medical Association in 1893 after the

Collin County Medical Association received recognition as a chapter of the Texas State Medical Association; established the McKinney Collegiate Institute, a boarding and day school for girls and boys, in 1893; sold his medical office building in 1911 to the Union Telephone Company (he moved across the street) so that the town had proper telephone service; headed, in 1913, the Collin County Good Roads Association, which oversaw the building of new roads in McKinney; and helped to establish McKinney's first hospital with Mayor Henry Arthur Finch in 1921. He owned farms near McKinney. He delivered three thousand babies before retiring around 1940. He married Evelyn Wilson (1865–1948) in 1886; they had four children. He was an elder of the First Presbyterian Church of McKinney for sixty-three years. When he developed colon cancer and could no longer attend church, he listened to worship services through a speaker system connected from the church to his bedroom across the street from the church. He died in 1951 at the age of ninety-three years. See "Obsequies Held Here Monday for Dr. J. C. Erwin Sr.," *Courier Gazette* (McKinney, TX), May 7, 1951, 8; "Dr. J. E. [*sic*] Irwin [*sic*] Sr. Dies at His McKinney Home," *Dallas Morning News*, May 6, 1951, 15; "Honor to Whom Honor Is Due," *McKinney Weekly Democrat-Gazette* (McKinney, TX), December 18, 1913, 3; and "Home Folks Now," *Courier Gazette*, October 28, 1911, 5.

7   John Caleb Erwin, "Report of Ten Cases of Epidemic Meningitis, Treated with Flexner Antimeningitis Serum," *Texas State Journal of Medicine* 5, no. 3 (July 1909): 124–25.

8   Dr. Heinrich Ireneaus Quincke (1842–1922), a German internist and pathologist, invented the spinal needle, or Quincke needle, in 1891 to perform a lumbar, or spinal, puncture procedure to relieve the pressure resulting from hydrocephalus and to obtain cerebrospinal fluid for bacterial diagnosis and culture. See Heinrich Quincke, "Die Lumbalpunktion des Hydrocephalus," *Verhandl Kong Innere Medizinisch Wiesbaden* 10 (1891): 321–31; and Heinrich Quincke, "Über Lumbalpunktion," *Berliner Klinische Wochesnschrift* 32 (1895): 861–62, 929–33. The earliest American print articles on the lumbar puncture procedure include George W. Jacoby, "Lumbar Puncture of the Subarachnoid Space," *New York Medical Journal* 62 (December 28, 1895): 813–18; Lewis A. Conner, "The Technique of Lumbar Puncture," *New York Medical Journal* 71 (May 12, 1900): 723–25; Alfred Hand Jr., "A Critical Summary of the Literature on the Diagnostic and Therapeutic Value of Lumbar Puncture,"

American Journal of the Medical Sciences 120 (October 1900): 463–69; Henry Heiman, "The Technics of Lumbar Puncture in Children: With Particular Reference to the Pressure of the Cerebrospinal Fluid," *Mount Sinai Hospital Reports* 5 (1905–1906): 114–23; and Samuel Joseph Kopetzky, "Lumbar Puncture: A General Review of Its Value and Applicability," *American Journal of the Medical Sciences* 131 (April 1906): 648–74.

9   See John T. Moore, "The Laboratory of Clinical Pathology and Its Relation to the Practice of Medicine and Surgery," *Texas State Journal of Medicine* 2, no. 2 (June 1906): 61–62; and Marvin L. Graves, "Some Remarks on Cerebrospinal Meningitis," *Texas State Journal of Medicine* 3, no. 10 (February 1908): 261–63.

10 Dr. Ira Carleton Chase, "Flexner's Antimeningitis Serum," *Texas State Journal of Medicine* 5, no. 3 (July 1909): 105; I. J. Jones, "The Epidemic of Cerebrospinal Meningitis in Texas during the Years 1898–1899," *Transactions of the Texas State Medical Association, Thirty-Third Annual Session Held at Galveston, Texas* (Austin, TX: Von Boeckmann, Schutze, and Company, 1899), 183–85; and William R. Blailock, "Meningitis in Texas and Indian Territory during First Three Months of 1899," *Transactions of the Texas State Medical Association, Thirty-First Annual Session Held at San Antonio, Texas* (Austin, TX: Von Boeckmann, Schutze, and Company, 1899), 121–38.

11 "Henry Robinson," in "Vital Statistics," *McKinney Courier* (McKinney, TX), February 18, 1909, 6.

12 The term *chills and fevers* was a nineteenth-century description of an illness (or ague) that afflicted many settlers in the interior lowlands of the United States. Dr. Daniel Drake (1785–1852), the author of *Systematic Treatise on the Principal Diseases of the Interior Valley of North America (1850–1854)*, ascribed the chills and fevers to a organisms living in decaying vegetation. In combatting the chills and fevers, Texas physicians often prescribed Peruvian bark (quinine) and the purgative calomel (mercurous chloride or mercury[l] chloride associated with cinnabar mined in the Terlingua District of Brewster County, Texas). See Harvey Scribner, *Memoirs of Lucas County and the City of Toledo* (Madison, WI: Western Historical Society, 1910), 1:498–99; H. C. Fisher, "Malaria—Its Treatment," *Southern Illinois Journal of Medicine and Surgery* 1, no. 7 (February 1901): 247–50; and W. F. Hillebrand and W. T. Schaller, "The Mercury Minerals from Terlingua, Texas: Kleinite, Terlinguaite, Eglestonite,

Montroydite, Calomel, Mercury," *Journal of the American Chemical Society* 29, no. 8 (1907): 1,180–94.

13 See William Fuller, "Treatment of Meningitis," *Canada Medical Record* 5 (June 1877): 237–39; and Luther B. Creathe, "Gelsemium," *Texas State Journal of Medicine Transactions* 17 (1885): 140–41.

14 Phebe L. DuBois, "Differential Diagnosis and Treatment of Epidemic Cerebrospinal Meningitis," *Journal of the American Medical Association* 60, no. 11 (March 15, 1913): 822.

15 Flexner antimeningitis serum was named for Dr. Simon Flexner (1863–1946), the director of the Rockefeller Institute for Medical Research in New York City, 1904–1935. He developed a version of antimeningitis serum for the treatment of cerebrospinal meningitis. From his efforts, the serum soon bore his name. Synonyms for Flexner antimeningitis serum include Flexner's antimeningitis serum, Flexner's serum, antimeningitis serum, meningitis serum, meningococcal serum, meningococcic serum, antimeningococcal serum, and antimeningococcic serum. See James Thomas Flexner, *An American Saga: The Story of Helen Thomas and Simon Flexner* (New York: Fordham University Press, 1993); George Washington Corner, *A History of the Rockefeller Institute, 1901–1953: Origins and Growth* (New York: Rockefeller Institute Press, 1964); and "Rockefeller Money and Medical Science: A Social Investment," in E. Richard Brown, *Rockefeller Medicine Men: Medicine and Capitalism in America* (Berkeley, CA: University of California Press, 1979), 105–11.

16 Dr. Simon Flexner worked on manufacturing and testing an antimeningitis serum at the Rockefeller Institute for Medical Research during the New York City cerebrospinal meningitis epidemic (1904–1907), as described in the introduction of this book. Beginning in April 1907, he recruited physicians from across the United States, Canada, Europe, and elsewhere to voluntarily administer his serum to their patients with cerebrospinal meningitis to test the serum's efficacy and safety in humans. Reports in the medical and lay media about Dr. Flexner's quest to establish the safety and efficacy of the antimeningitis serum abounded, and physicians flocked to participate in Dr. Flexner's clinical trials using the serum. See Simon Flexner, "Concerning a Serum Therapy for Experimental Infection with *Diplococcus intracellularis*," *Journal of Experimental Medicine* 9, no. 2 (March 14, 1907): 168–85; Simon Flexner and James Wesley Jobling, "Serum Treatment of Epidemic Cerebrospinal Meningitis,"

Journal of Experimental Medicine 10, no. 1 (January 1, 1908): 141–203; and Simon Flexner and James Wesley Jobling, "An Analysis of Four Hundred Cases of Epidemic Meningitis Treated with the Antimeningitis Serum," *Journal of Experimental Medicine* 10, no. 5 (September 5, 1908): 690–733. Texas print articles about Flexner antimeningitis serum, April 1907–July 1909, included "Cure for Meningitis; Wealth of Rockefeller Said to Have Discovered Serum," *Dallas Morning News*, April 7, 1907, 2; "Spinal Meningitis Cure; Dr. Simon Flexner Declines to Discuss His Serum," *Dallas Morning News*, April 10, 1907, 4; "Dr. Flexner's Monkey Life Savers; How the Missing Link Has Saved the Scourge of Spotted Fever," *San Antonio Express*, January 5, 1908, 21; "Physicians Are Arming against Meningitis," *Abilene Semi Weekly Farm Reporter*, October 8, 1908, 7; and "New Serum a Success," *Dallas Morning News*, July 11, 1909, 20. Print articles about Flexner antimeningitis serum from elsewhere in the United States included "Spotted Fever Serum Wanted," *San Francisco Call*, April 5, 1905, 3; "May Test Meningitis Serum," *New York Tribune*, April 8, 1907, 1; "Serum for Meningitis, Head of Rockefeller Institute Has Not Tried It Yet on Man," *Evening Star* (Washington, DC), April 9, 1907, 18; and "Rockefeller Serum Saves Dying Children," *Salt Lake Telegram*, April 24, 1907.

17 The cerebrospinal fluid space is the area surrounding, bathing, and nourishing the spinal cord—the long, thin bundle of nervous tissue and support cells that extends from the medulla oblongata of the brainstem to the lumbar region of the back. The cerebrospinal fluid space is also known as the subarachnoid space, which lies between the arachnoid mater and the pia mater—two of the coverings of the spinal cord (the pia lies closest to the spinal cord itself). The cerebrospinal fluid space is also known as the thecal sac, the membranous tube of dura mater—the third and outermost covering of the spinal cord. The two terms used to describe the administration of medication directly into the cerebrospinal fluid space are *intraspinal* (within the spinal column) and *intrathecal* (within the theca).

18 See chapter 2.

19 Dr. Willus Gurden Cook (1866–1963) was born in Grand Blanc, Genesee County, Michigan, as one of the seven children of Joseph Pierson Cook (1828–1902), a farmer, and Julia H. Slaght (1828–1918). He earned his bachelor of science degree from the University of Michigan; served as a teacher and principal at a high school in Flint, Michigan; and earned his medical degree from the University

of Michigan Medical School in Ann Arbor, Washtenaw County, Michigan, in 1899. Thereafter, he moved to Fort Worth, Tarrant County, Texas, with his lifelong friend Dr. John Delamater Covert (1876–1951), a graduate of the University of Michigan Medical School in 1900. They opened a medical practice called Cook and Covert. In addition to running a medical practice, Dr. Cook taught chemistry at Fort Worth University and served as the health supervisor of the Fort Worth public schools. He married twice: Carrie E. Hasse (1871–1910) in 1902 and Mrs. Harriet "Hallie" Peacock Graham (1876–1965) in 1929. He had no children. He practiced medicine for six decades in Fort Worth and died at the age of ninety-seven years. See *University of Michigan General Catalogue of Officers and Students, 1837–1901* (Ann Arbor, MI: University of Michigan, 1902), 106; and "Deaths," *Fort Worth Star-Telegram*, March 20, 1910, 13.

20 Dr. Ira Carleton Chase (1868–1933) was born in Oberlin, Lorain County, Ohio, as one of the two children of Malvena Dayton (1848–1914) and Reverend Edward Richard Chase (1840–1874), a Presbyterian minister who studied theology at the Union Theological Seminary in Chicago, Illinois, only to die three years after ordination as a pastor. After earning his bachelor's degree from Oberlin College in 1891, Ira Chase traveled to Texas on business, where he developed typhoid fever. He remained in Texas after his recovery, finding work as a professor at Fort Worth University and serving as the dean of its medical school beginning in 1892. In 1899, he earned his medical diploma from the University and Bellevue Hospital Medical College in New York City. He began serving as the editor of the *Texas State Journal of Medicine* around 1906. He was elected the president of the Texas State Medical Association in 1920. He introduced radiological equipment to Fort Worth and x-rayed exuberantly without shield protection, eventually developing general carcinomatosis of his hand and arm, which originated from x-ray burns. His hand and arm required amputation in 1932. The following year, he died at the age of sixty-four years. His marriage in 1910 to Helene Delaney Keating (1871–1933) in Manhattan, New York, ended in divorce; they had two children. See W. J. Maxwell, *General Alumni Catalogue of New York University* (New York: New York University, 1916), 505; "Fort Worth Doctor Dies; Martyr to Profession," *Bonham Daily Favorite* (Bonham, TX), June 22, 1933, 3; "Physician Victim of Disease; He Spent Years in Seeking Cure," *Messenger* (Marshall, TX), June 20,

1933, 1; and "Chase, Edward R.," John McClintock and James Strong, *McClintock and Strong Biblical Cyclopedia* (New York: Harper and Brothers, 1880).

21 Dr. Khleher Heberden Beall (1878–1946) was born in Fort Worth, Tarrant County, Texas, as one of the six children of Dr. Elias James Beall (1834–1914) and Frances Cooke van Zandt (1842–1935). Khleher Beall earned his bachelor of science and master of science degrees from the University of Texas at Austin in 1899. He earned his first medical degree from Fort Worth University in 1900 and his second medical degree with honors from Johns Hopkins University in Baltimore, Maryland, in 1905. He served an internship at the Johns Hopkins University Hospital before returning to Fort Worth to open a medical practice. He was the medical director and physician in chief of Cook Memorial Hospital in Fort Worth and the treasurer of the State Medical Association of Texas continuously from 1923 to 1946. He married Camilla Weir Labatt (1888–1992) in 1911; they had two children. He died of myocardial infarction at the age of sixty-eight years. See *Johns Hopkins University Circular* 24, no. 174–182: 81, 644, 676; and "Dr. K. H. Beall, 68, Dies at Fort Worth," *Dallas Morning News*, November 22, 1946, 7.

22 See "Physicians Are Arming Against Meningitis (Fort Worth)," *Abilene Semi Weekly Farm Reporter* (Abilene, TX), October 8, 1908, 7; and "Treatment of Meningitis; Valuable Serum Is Received from New York Institute," *Dallas Morning News*," October 31, 1908, 9.

23 "New Serum Treatment Given Little Son of Mrs. McCollum [sic]— First in Texas," *Courier Gazette*, January 19, 1909, 1.

24 "Serum Treatment Success, Two McKinney Children Treated in Fort Worth for Meningitis," *Courier Gazette*, January 26, 1909, 1.

25 James Thomas Couch (1871–1947) was born in Basin Springs, Grayson County, Texas, as one of the seven children of Sidney Pinkney Couch (1833–1920), a farmer, and Nancy Jane Norwood (1844–1880). He moved to McKinney in 1896 from Union Springs, Wise County, Texas, to open a piano and organ business. He married Sallie Mills Bingham (1873–1956) in 1897; they had six children. He was active in the Baptist church and Boy Scouts. See "Last Rites Held Here Tuesday for James T. Couch," *Courier Gazette*, June 24, 1947, 6.

26 Adolphus Barbee Mayes (1844–1919) was born in Adair (Green) County, Kentucky, as the youngest of the four children of Dr. Robert

B. Mayes (1798–1865) and Nancy Barbee (1811–1893). Dr. Robert B. Mayes moved his family to Collin County, Texas, in 1852 and settled his family on land ten miles west of McKinney. After serving as a Confederate soldier during the American Civil War, Adolphus married Calpurnia "Pernie" Ann Allen (1844–1921). They lived on a farm near Frisco, Collin County, Texas, until 1886, when they moved to a house in McKinney. They had eight children. After moving into the city, Adolphus Mayes chaired the United Charity work in McKinney and devoted much of his time to looking after the needy of the city. See "The Mayes and Foster Families," *Courier Gazette*, October 1, 1915, 1; "Recalling the Days of Sixty-One; A. B. Mayes of McKinney Renews Associations of Long Ago," *Courier Gazette*, February 9, 1915, 1; and A. B. Mayes, 75, Ex-Confederate Veteran, Is Dead," *Democrat-Gazette* (McKinney, TX), July 3, 1919, 1.

27 Dr. Eustace Eugene King (1850–1919), a Baptist minister, was born in Raymond, Hinds County, Mississippi, as one of the five sons of Joseph Monroe King (1808–1857), a planter at King's Point, near Natchez, and Margaret Williams (1856–1919). His parents died when he was seven years old. He was converted to Christianity at the age of thirteen years and joined the Baptist church two years later. He earned his bachelor's degree from the Academy of Mississippi College in 1873 and received his doctor of divinity degree from Baylor University in 1890. He spent two years in the Southern Baptist Theological Seminary at Greenville, Greenville County, South Carolina. He preached for nearly fifty years in five pastorates. The first three pastorates were in Senatobia, Starksville, and Greenville, Mississippi. The second two were the First Church, San Antonio, Texas, and the First Church of McKinney, Collin County, Texas. During his professional life, Dr. King was one of the most widely known Baptist ministers in the South. He married Eleanor Augusta Frink (1854–1920) in 1877; they had four children. He died of cancer at the age of sixty-eight years. See "Dr. E. E. King to Rich Reward; Veteran Baptist Pastor Died Here Today," *Daily Courier-Gazette*, March 11, 1919, 1.

28 See "Serum Proves Successful on Test; Two Meningitis Cases Treated at St. Joseph's Cured—Report Sent to Rockefeller Institute," *Fort Worth Star-Telegram*, 6; "Meningitis Cured; Medical Society Hears Report on Serum Treatment Here," *Fort Worth Star-Telegram*,

March 9, 1909, 12; and "The Tarrant County Medical Society," *Texas State Journal of Medicine* 4, no. 12 (April 1909): 336.

29 Simon Flexner, "The Present Status of the Serum Therapy of Epidemic Cerebrospinal Meningitis," *Journal of the American Medical Association* 53, no. 18 (October 30, 1909): 1,443–45.

CHAPTER 2

A NEW TEXAS HEALTH BOARD, 1909-1911

News about the cerebrospinal meningitis outbreak in McKinney, Texas, during the first five months of 1909 attracted the attention of Texas Governor Thomas Mitchell Campbell[1] and Dr. William McDuffie Brumby,[2] the head of the Texas State Department of Health and Vital Statistics.[3] Together, they were concerned about the return of cerebrospinal meningitis in Texas, possibly with greater virulence, and reach during the cold months of 1909–1910. The compliance of Texas county clerks, county and city health officers, physicians, midwives, and undertakers in reporting vital statistics to Dr. Brumby was variable and generally poor, thereby constraining the state's ability to detect, monitor, and respond to communicable-disease flares.[4]

To correct the situation, Governor Campbell signed into a law in April 1909 the Texas State Board of Health Act, which replaced the feeble Texas Department of Public Health and Vital Statistics with the more robust Texas State Board of Health.[5-6] Dr. Brumby and his associates wrote most of the act.[7] The new act authorized the Texas State Board of Health to develop a Texas Sanitary Code,[8] which contained the state's rules and regulations governing a wide array of public health functions, including the reporting of vital statistics (births, deaths, and specified communicable [contagious] diseases).

On Tuesday, September 14, 1909, Dr. Brumby and his fellow members of the Texas State Board of Health used the authority of the Texas State Board of Health Act to adopt the Texas Sanitary Code they had written. The code still required Governor Campbell's signature to become effective.[9] The Texas Sanitary Code's preamble stated that its rules and regulations had "the absolute force of law" and that "any persons violating any of its rules and regulations [were] guilty of a misdemeanor and upon conviction liable to a penalty of not less than $10 nor more than $1,000." Rule 1 of the sanitary code, reproduced immediately below, required physicians to report all cases of contagious disease to their local health officials who were to report the case to the president of the State Board of Health.

> Every physician in the state of Texas shall report in writing or by an acknowledged telephone communication to the local health authority immediately after his or her first professional visit, each patient he or she shall have or suspect of suffering with any contagious disease, and if such disease is of a pestilential nature, he shall notify the president of the State Board of Health at Austin by telegraph or telephone at State expense, and he or she shall report to said health authority every death from such disease immediately after it shall have occurred.[8]

The reportable contagious diseases listed in Rule 1 of the Texas Sanitary Code were Asiatic cholera, bubonic plague, typhus fever, yellow fever, smallpox, scarlet fever (scarlatina), diphtheria (membranous croup), *epidemic cerebrospinal meningitis* [emphasis added], dengue, typhoid fever, epidemic dysentery, trachoma, tuberculosis, and anthrax.[8] All reportable disease cases would be entered into a case count database in Austin.

Soon after the adoption of the Texas Sanitary Code by the Texas State Board of Health in September 1909, some observers questioned the legality of the code on the grounds that the Texas State Constitution assigned all legislative authority to the Texas State Legislature and not to any state board. Thus, the enactment of the Texas Sanitary Code by a state board of health could not be made the basis of an indictment since the state board of health was not a legislative body.[10]

As the legality of the Texas Sanitary Code underwent further discussion and analysis, Dr. Brumby and his new state registrar of vital statistics, Mr. Clyde Duff Smith,[11] worked diligently to collect[12] birth, death, and communicable-diseases data from authorized individuals during the fiscal year August 31, 1909, to August 31, 1910. They continued to encounter problems obtaining the data, especially case reports of contagious diseases. However, they were able to gather enough birth and death reports to publish in late November 1910 "the first annual report of health conditions in Texas which this State has ever had furnished."[13] They counted eighty-eight deaths from meningitis (the type of meningitis was not necessarily specified) from among the 3,896,542 persons[14] making up the Texas population in 1910, resulting in a cerebrospinal meningitis mortality rate of *.23 deaths per 10,000 Texas residents* for the fiscal year 1909 to 1910. This rate was tiny compared to the mortality rate of *6.7 deaths per 10,000 Texas residents* for pulmonary tuberculosis (2,600 deaths, 1909–1910), the state's leading cause of death that year. The low case count for meningitis relieved Governor Campbell and Dr. Brumby, who concluded, correctly, that the return and spread of cerebrospinal meningitis during the cold months of 1909–1910 had not materialized.

In January 1911, Oscar Branch Colquitt,[15] also known as Little Oscar, Little Napoleon, and Little Warrior,[16] succeeded Thomas M. Campbell as the new Texas governor. He appointed Dr. Ralph Steiner,[17-18] an otolaryngologist in private practice in Austin, Travis County, Texas, to succeed Dr. Brumby as the Texas state health officer and president of the Texas State Board of Health. Governor Colquitt also appointed six prominent physicians to the Texas State Board of Health.[19] On Saturday, January 28, 1911, Dr. Steiner hired John Elijah Rosser,[20] a newspaper reporter, as the state registrar of vital statistics.[21] At the first meeting of the Texas State Board of Health on Tuesday, February 7, 1911, Dr. Ralph Steiner and the board voted to adopt some of the recommendations proposed by Dr. Brumby and his board.[22] For example, Dr. Steiner moved the commissioner of the Texas Department of the Food and Dairy from Denton to Austin.[23]

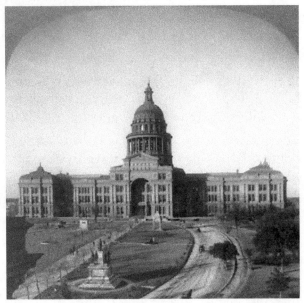

The Texas State Capitol at Austin, Texas. The original caption of this image is: "The proud state capitol of Austin, Texas." Creator: Keystone View Company, Meadville, Pa, circa 1909. The image is held at the Library of Congress Prints and Photographs Division, Washington, DC.

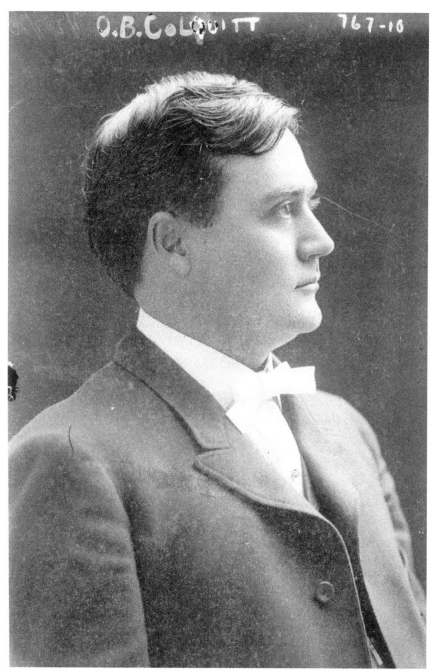

Texas Governor Oscar Branch Colquitt (1861–1940), 1910, Bains News Service. The image is held at the Library of Congress Prints and Photographs Division, Washington, DC.

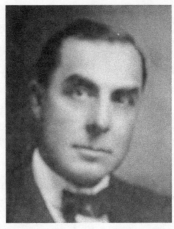

Dr. Ralph Steiner (1859–1926), 1914, from "The Buzzing Nuisance,
by Dr. Ralph Steiner, Austin, State Health Officer," *Courier-Gazette*
(McKinney, Texas), August 26, 1914, p. 3. The photographer is unknown.

Dr. Steiner next undertook lobbying the Thirty-Second
Texas Legislature to enact into law the Texas Sanitary Code as
amended, which supposedly addressed the charges that the code
was unconstitutional.[24] On Saturday, March 11, 1911, the Thirty-
Second Texas Legislature enacted into statute the Texas Sanitary
Code, which the Texas State Board of Health already had adopted
at its meeting in September 1909, as noted above. Objections,
however, persisted about the code's lack of definitions of certain
general terms, its failure to provide means for the county or city
registrars to manage vital statistics records, and its heavy-handed
levying of a misdemeanor charge against violators. Opponents of
the code complained that the misdemeanor charge was heavier than
the character of the violation justified, since a great majority of the
violations of the vital statistics section of the Texas Sanitary Code
were due to carelessness without any criminal intent.[9,25] The section
of the code on vital statistics is available elsewhere.[25] Governor
Colquitt signed the bill into law on Friday, March 24, 1911.[26]

Emboldened by the new law, Mr. Rosser issued a warning to
county clerks and local registrars to "observe the notices of births
and deaths printed in the papers, with a view to securing the
names of those physicians and undertakers who persist in violating

the law." For example, his February 1911 vital statistics report contained no reports of cases of meningitis,[27] which suggested to him that he was not receiving all case reports of reportable diseases. On Tuesday, April 4, 1911, he mailed a thousand letters to city and county health officers, county clerks, and city registrars, calling attention to the law signed by Governor Colquitt. Mr. Rosser's letter said in part,

> You may be aware that on March 23 [1911], the sanitary code for Texas became law ... This letter is sent to impress the significance of the enactment of the code, whose contents you doubtless know. Hitherto some doubt existed as to the constitutionality of the law. Now there can be no such question ... [T]he law is absolutely binding and carries provision for the imposition of a fine of from $10 to $1,000 for its violation.

Mr. Rosser continued,

> This department has no desire to be unnecessarily harsh, but it is determined that the provisions of the sanitary code, especially that part governing the making or reports of births and deaths, shall be fully obeyed. You will, I am assured, do your full duty and the changed status of the law will enable you to bring all physicians, undertakers, midwives, etc., to time. I believe I can rely upon your cooperation. Let them know that failure to report to you means a fine. We would like to avoid prosecutions if possible, but those who have hitherto laughed the law to scorn may find themselves differently situated now.[28]

On Friday, April 12, 1911, the Texas State Board of Health indicted its first alleged offender under the new law. The offender was the registrar of vital statistics at Mart (population three thousand in 1910), McLellan County, Texas.[29] The case was scheduled for trial in Waco, McLennan County, Texas. Mr. Rosser traveled a hundred miles from Austin to Waco for the trial, which the judge ordered postponed.[30]

The state vital statistics reports for the months of January, February, March, April, May, and June 1911 cited deaths due to meningitis (again, the type of meningitis was not always specified) as thirty-four, twenty-three, thirty-four, twenty-eight, twenty-two, and twenty-one, respectively (a total of 162 deaths).[31] The mortality rate for meningitis for the first six months of 1911 calculated to .42 *deaths per 10,000 Texan residents*. Thus, for two cold seasons in a row (1909–1910 and 1910–1911), the number of meningitis deaths (88 and 162 deaths, respectively, and mortality rates of .23 and .42 per 10,000 Texas residents, respectively) remained low.

After five months on the job, Mr. Rosser resigned (July 9, 1911).[32] Dr. Steiner replaced him with Mr. Robert Percy Babcock,[33] a bookkeeper and assistant hotel manager. Mr. Babcock reported deaths from meningitis for the months of July, August, and September 1911 as ten, twenty-nine, and sixteen, respectively.[31] Mr. Babcock admonished physicians, "[There is] still quite a large number of physicians in Texas who persist in refusing or failing to report births and deaths, notwithstanding the fact that there is a law now on the statute books imposing a fine of from $10 to $1,000 for such failure." He threatened physicians with "immediate steps ... to be taken by the department to see that this law is strictly complied with [so that] no one will be allowed to escape."[34] Meanwhile, Dr. Steiner reported on Saturday, July 8, 1911, that health conditions across Texas in general were never better and that, excepting for a few cases of typhoid fever and smallpox, Texas was free of contagious diseases.[35] The cluster of cerebrospinal meningitis cases two years earlier in McKinney, Texas, was a fading memory.

In March 1911, the Rockefeller Institute for Medical Research announced the end of its free distribution of Flexner antimeningitis serum and its intention to delegate to the state and municipal health departments and commercial establishments the routine preparation of antimeningitis serum for general use.[36] Dr. Park of the Research Laboratory of the New York City Board of Health assumed responsibility for producing and distributing antimeningitis serum to physicians outside of New York City until municipal and state health departments and commercial establishments could satisfy the physician demand for the antimeningitis serum.[37] Dr. Park's director of the special bureau of meningitis investigation of the Research Laboratory in 1911 was twenty-six-year-old Dr. Abraham Sophian.[38-39] On behalf of the Research Laboratory, he accepted Dr. Flexner's gift of the Rockefeller Institute's two horses used to generate antimeningitis serum.[40]

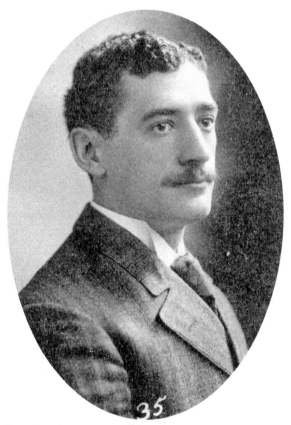

Dr. Abraham Sophian (1885–1957), 1906, age twenty-one years at graduation from Cornell University Medical College, New York City. The image is from the class composite held at the Weill Cornell Medicine Samuel J. Wood Library, New York City. The photo is courtesy of the Medical Center Archives of New York-Presbyterian/Weill Cornell.

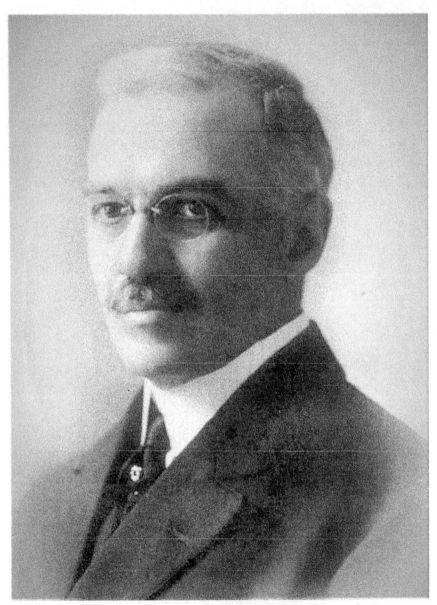

Dr. William Hallock Park (1863–1939), circa 1900.
The photographer is unknown. The image is held at the
National Library of Medicine, Bethesda, Maryland.

CHAPTER 2 NOTES

1   Thomas Mitchell Campbell (1856–1923) was born in Rusk, Cherokee County, Texas, to Thomas Duncan Campbell (1831–1894), a merchandiser and sheriff, and his second wife, Rachel Moore (1833–1864). Thomas M. Campbell attended Trinity University in San Antonio, Bexar County, Texas, for one year (1873–1874); studied law at night and entered the Texas bar in 1878; practiced law in Longview, Gregg County, Texas; served as general manager of the International-Great Northern Railroad (1892–1897); and resumed law practice. He entered Democratic Party politics and won two terms as governor of Texas (1907–1911). He oversaw the creation of many state agencies during his tenure, including the Texas State Board of Health. He married Fannie Irene Bruner (1856–1934) in 1878; they had five children. He died of pernicious anemia in Galveston at the age of sixty-seven years. See "Former Gov. Campbell Dies at Galveston," *Whitewright Sun* (Whitewright County, TX), April 5, 1923, 2; and Janet Schmelzer, "Thomas M. Campbell, Progressive Governor of Texas," *Red River Valley Historical Review* 3, no. 4 (Fall 1978): 52–63.

2   Dr. William McDuffie Brumby (1866–1959) was born in Delhi, Richland Parish, Louisiana, as one of the seven children of Dr. George McDuffie Brumby (1835–1898) and Rebecca Kincaid Gibbes (1837–1919). He attended the University of Alabama; earned his medical degree from Tulane University Medical Department in New Orleans, Orleans Parish, Louisiana, in 1889; and joined his father's medical practice in Delhi, Richland Parish, Louisiana, for seven years. In 1896, he moved to Houston, Harris County, Texas, and opened a medical practice. He subsequently served as the Houston city health officer (1902–1907); the Texas state health officer (1907–1911); and the president of the original Texas State Board of Health (1908–1911). In January 1911, he resigned from government service to work at the Equitable Life Insurance Company in San Antonio, Bexar County, Texas. He married his first wife, Thekla Meagher (1867–1915), in 1891; they had three children. He married his second wife, Lila Kirby Ralston (1880–1968), in 1915; they also had three children. He died of heart disease in Houston at the age of ninety-three years. A photo of Dr. Brumby is available at F. W. Gallagher, "William McDuffie Brumby," *Chest Journal* 7, no. 4 (April 1941): 130. See also W. M. Brumby, "Many and Varied Are Duties Added

to Those of Health Department," *Dallas Morning News*, October 1, 1910, 22; "Dr. W. M. Brumby, MD," in Ellis A. Davis and Edwin H. Grobe, *New Encyclopedia of Texas* (Dallas, TX: Texas Development Bureau, 1926), 2:1,391; and Patricia L. Jakobi, "Brumby, William McDuffie," *Handbook of Texas Online*, accessed October 17, 2017, https://tshaonline.org/handbook/online/articles/fbrcx.

3   The Texas state health system originated with the Quarantine Act of 1870, which authorized the Texas governor to appoint a "medical health officer for the State" and to build quarantine stations to fend off the frequent epidemics along the Gulf Coast and at the principal points of entry from other states. In 1891, the Texas State Quarantine Department consisted of the poorly funded quarantine and internal sanitation branches administered by the state health officer. In 1903, the Texas State Legislature renamed the Texas State Quarantine Department as the Texas Department of Public Health and Vital Statistics but made no appropriation for the latter function. See Robert Bernstein, "Texas Department of Health," *Handbook of Texas Online*, accessed December 13, 2017, https://tshaonline.org/handbook/online/articles/mdt40; K. E. Miller, *A Survey of the Public Health Problems and Needs in the State of Texas* (Washington, DC: US Public Health Service, 1937); Gerald M. Porter, "A History of State Organization for Public Health Administration in Texas, 1718–1927" (master's thesis, University of Chicago, 1942); and Howard E. Smith, *History of Public Health in Texas* (Austin, TX: Texas State Department of Public Health, 1974).

4   Bureau of Vital Statistics, Texas State Board of Health, *Annual Report of the Bureau of Vital Statistics for the Year 1917* (Austin, TX: Von Boeckmann-Jones Company, 1918), 7–19.

5   The act that established the Texas State of Board of Health is available at *General Laws of the State of Texas Passed by the Thirty-First Legislature at Its Regular Session Convened January 12, 1909, and Adjourned March 13, 1909, at Its First Called Session, Convened March 13, 1909, and Adjourned April 11, 1919, and at Its Second Called Session, Convened April 12, 1909, and Adjourned May 11, 1909* (Austin, TX: Von Boeckmann-Jones Company, 1909), 340–50.

6   The state legislatures of Texas, Arkansas, and New Mexico belatedly (compared with the rest of the continental states of the United States) established state boards of health in 1909, 1913, and 1919, respectively. See Ben Freedman, "The First State Board of Health

Laboratories in the United States," *Public Health Reports* 69, no. 9 (September 1954): 874.

7   See "State Board of Health Proposed by Brumby; He and Associates Complete Bill to Create Such; Would Merge Vital Statistics, Live Stock, Sanitary and Pure Food Departments, Changing Methods," *Dallas Morning News*, January 8, 1909, 6; and "Brumby Explains Health Bill," *Dallas Morning News*, January 12, 1909, 6.

8   The Texas Sanitary Code of 1910 is available at "Sanitary Code for Texas Adopted by the Texas State Board of Health and Approved by the Governor," *Texas State Journal of Medicine* 5, no. 10 (February 1910): 385–90.

9   "Sanitary Code Is Adopted; Will Have to Be Approved by Governor Before It Becomes Effective," *Dallas Morning News*, September 15, 1909, 11.

10 Bureau of Vital Statistics, Texas State Board of Health, *The Annual Report of the Bureau of Vital Statistics for the Year 1917* (Austin, TX: Von Boeckmann-Jones Company, 1918), 9–10.

11 Clyde Duff Smith (1874–1912) was born in Water Valley, Yalobusha County, Mississippi, as one of the two children of Andrew J. Smith (1840–1886), a store clerk, and Marietta "Etta" Duff (1849–1918). He married Raye Evans Smith (1878–1951) in 1895. They lived in Wichita Falls, Wichita County, Texas, before moving to Austin, where Clyde D. Smith served as the secretary of the Texas State Senate (1901–1909). He left that position to become the secretary and vital statistics registrar of the Texas State Board of Health (January 1910–January 1911). He then returned to his position as secretary of the Texas State Senate but died of illness in May 1912 at the age of thirty-seven years. His widow worked as a mail clerk at the Texas State Capitol for many years after his death. They had several children. See "Clyde D. Smith Appointed," *Dallas Morning News*, December 6, 1909, 7; "Becomes Secretary to Senate; Clyde Smith Will Resign as Vital Statistics Registrar," *Dallas Morning News*, January 6, 1911, 12; and "Simple Resolution by Senator Warren," in memoriam to the Honorable Clyde D. Smith, signed by state senators Warren, McNealus, and Speaker Terrell, *Senate Journal, Thirty-Third Legislature, Regular Session, Friday, January 17, 1913*, 70, accessed April 1, 2018, http://www.lrl.state.tx.us/collections/journals/journals.cfm.

12 Clyde Duff Smith exhibited his diplomatic interpersonal style in the following public statement: "There is no doubt but that, as the law

is better understood, the real necessity for a complete vital statistics record is being realized, not only by the fraternity of Texas, but by the public as well. A greater per cent of births and deaths is being reported than ever before and we hope for the time when we can feel assured that we are receiving comparatively all birth and death certificates. The public can assist us in accomplishing this end by insisting upon physicians, midwives and undertakers properly filling out birth and death certificates and filing with our registrars. They will then be sent to us. We will do the rest, by making a record of each one and then filing them in our new steel filing case, where they will remain for the benefit of the public now and in the future. If the public will do its part we will soon have as complete vital statistics record as could be desired. We again state that the cooperation the department is receiving is highly appreciated and we hope for a continuance." "4,506 Births and 2,126 Deaths during August; Report of Register [sic] of Vital Statistics; Tuberculosis Continues to Cause Heavy Percentage of the Total Death Roll in Texas," *Dallas Morning News*, September 27, 1910, 5.

13 "Texas Deaths: Fell Far Behind the Birth Rate, According to Statistics; Consumption in the Lead; Over Ten Per Cent of the Total Deaths in the State Was from that Cause—Pneumonia Is Second in the List," *Houston Post*, November 27, 1910, 5. See also "State Board of Health Annual Statistics Table, Shows 53,250 Births and 23,076 Deaths during Year," *Galveston Daily News*, November 28, 1910, 6.

14 "Demographics of Texas," *Wikipedia*, accessed August 18, 2018, https://en.wikipedia.org/wiki/Demographics_of_Texas.

15 Oscar Branch Colquitt (1861–1940) was born in Camilla, Mitchell County, Georgia, as one of the six children of Ann Eliza Burkhalter (1832–1879) and Thomas Jefferson Colquitt (1825–1886), a plantation and slave owner and a Confederate soldier during the American Civil War. Oscar Colquitt grew up on the family plantation until his father went bankrupt in 1878, whence the family moved to Texas to work as tenant farmers. Oscar attended Daingerfield [sic] Academy for one term, served a brief apprenticeship as a newspaperman, and founded the *Gazette* at Pittsburg, Texas. After selling the *Gazette*, he published the *Times-Star* of Terrell, Texas (1890–1897). He became active in the Texas Democratic Party and served in the Texas State Senate (1895–1897) and on the State Tax Commission. He was admitted to the bar in 1900. He was a member

of the State Railroad Commission (1903–1911). He reorganized the state transportation system, which led to his election as governor (1911–1915). He supported Germany early in World War I. After leaving office, he developed his oil and farming interests. He married Alice Fuller (1865–1949) in 1885; they had four children. Governor Colquitt died of influenza at the age of seventy-eight years. See George P. Huckaby, "Oscar Branch Colquitt," *Handbook of Texas Online*, accessed August 18, 2018, https://tshaonline.org/handbook/online/articles/fco32; "Colquitt, Oscar B.," in Nancy Capace, *Encyclopedia of Texas* (St. Clair Shores, MI: Somerset Publishers, 1999), 1:141–42; Dremont H. Hardy and Ingham S. Roberts, "Hon. Oscar B. Colquitt," *Historical Review of Southeast Texas* (Chicago, IL: Lewis Publishing Company, 1910), 2:740–42; and "Death Closes Career of Little Warrior; Colquitt's Burial Set at Austin; Governor 30 Years Ago to Be Laid to Rest in Suit He Wore When Inaugurated Executive," *Dallas Morning News*, March 9, 1940, 1.

16 Dencil R. Taylor, "The Political Speaking of Oscar Branch Colquitt, 1906–1913" (doctoral dissertation, Louisiana State University, Baton Rouge, 1979), 66; and Hugh Nugent Fitzgerald, *Governors I Have Known* (Austin, TX: Austin American-State, 1927), 31.

17 "Nominations by Colquitt: List Sent in Thursday Will Be Considered Today by Senate in Executive Session," *Dallas Morning News*, January 20, 1911, 2.

18 Dr. Ralph Steiner (1859–1926) was born in Austin, Travis County, Texas, as one of the four children of Dr. Josephus Murray Steiner (1823–1873) and Laura June Fisher (1835–1909). He earned his bachelor of arts degree in mathematics, geology, physics, and chemistry at the University of the South in Sewanee, Franklin County, Tennessee, in 1878 and his medical degree from the University of Maryland School of Medicine in Baltimore in 1883. He returned to Austin, Texas, and practiced general medicine and surgery for a decade. He applied for and won a consul position with the US Consul at Munich, Bavaria, Germany, during the second administration of US President Grover Cleveland (1893–1897). He did so, he said, to finance his living expenses while he studied ear, nose, and throat medicine in Europe. When he returned to Austin in 1897, he limited his practice to otolaryngology. After serving as the Texas state health officer and president of the Texas State Health Board (1911–1915), he resumed his private otolaryngology practice. He married Lily Bemond (1867–1927) in 1887; they had two children. He died after

a long illness at the age of sixty-seven years. See "Commencement at the University," *Maryland Medical Journal: Medicine and Surgery* 9 (May 1882–April 1883): 605; "Consul Steiner Resigned," *St. Louis Post-Dispatch*, October 22, 1896, 3; "Dr. Ralph Steiner Is Critically Ill," *Dallas Morning News*, May 1, 1926, 1; "Last Rites for Dr. R. Steiner," *Austin American* (Austin, TX), May 4, 1926, 3; "Dr. Steiner of Austin Is Dead," *Bryan Daily Eagle* (Bryan, TX), May 3, 1926, 1; "State Flag for Steiner," *Corpus Christi Times*, May 3, 1926, 3; and Arthur Wayne Hafner, *Directory of Deceased American Physicians, 1804–1929* (Chicago, IL: American Medical Association, c. 1993).

19 The six physicians appointed by Governor Colquitt to the Texas State Board of Health in January 1911 were Dr. Benjamin Franklin Calhoun (Beaumont, Jefferson County), Dr. Hugh Love McLaurin (Dallas, Dallas County), Dr. Adolph Herff (San Antonio, Bexar County), Dr. Benjamin Milton Worsham (El Paso, El Paso County), Dr. Ashley Wilson Fly (Galveston, Galveston County), and Dr. Khleher Heberden Beall (Fort Worth, Tarrant County). See "New State Board of Health," *Texas State Journal of Medicine* 6, no. 9 (January 1911): 225.

20 John Elijah Rosser (1882–1960) was born in Covington, Newton County, Georgia, as one of the three children of John Elijah Rosser Sr. (1852–1905) and Julia Pace (1848–1884). He earned his bachelor of philosophy degree at Emory College in Oxford, Newton County, Georgia, and afterward worked in many positions in various states. The University of Texas at Austin hired him as its faculty secretary and editor of a university publication (July 1909). He generated controversy at the university and left to write news stories for the *Houston Post* and the *Austin Statesman* for a year. Dr. Steiner then hired him as the secretary of the Texas State Board of Health and the state vital statistics registrar (January 11, 1909). He resigned from the position on July 9, 1911, for unknown reasons. He next managed the Southwest World Book Company for many years. He married Angie Ousley (1890–1950); they had two children. He died of a cerebrovascular accident and severe bilateral pulmonary emphysema at the age of seventy-seven years. See "University of Texas," *Houston Post*, July 11, 1909, 6; "Appoint Newspaper Man; John E. Rosser Named as State Registrar of Vital Statistics," *Galveston Daily News*, January 28, 1911, 4; "Place for John E. Rosser," *Dallas Morning News*, January 28, 1911, 13; and "Health Official Resigns; State

Registrar J. E. Rosser Succeeded by R. P. Babcock," *Dallas Morning News*, July 9, 1911, 1.

21   "Appoint Newspaper Man; John E. Rosser Named as State Registrar of Vital Statistics," *Galveston Daily News*, January 28, 1911, 4; and "Place for John E. Rosser," *Dallas Morning News*, January 28, 1911, 13.

22   See "Recommendations of State Board of Health," *Texas State Journal of Medicine* 6, no. 9 (January 1911): 227; and "Important Changes Are Recommended; Appointment of Chemist and Bacteriologist for Work of Pure Food Commission Is Urged," *Dallas Morning News*, February 8, 1911, 6.

23   See "Meeting of the Texas State Board of Health," *Texas State Journal of Medicine* 6, no. 11 (March 1911): 288.

24   "Sanitary Code Bill Passes Both Houses; Makes Health Regulations Capable of Enforcement; Provides for System of Vital Statistics and Corrects Weaknesses in Former Enactment," *Dallas Morning News*, March 11, 1911, 6; and "Texas Sanitary Code: Leniency Will No Longer Be Tolerated by Board of Health—Measure through Both Houses," *Galveston Daily News*, March 11, 1911, 3.

25   The section on vital statistics in the Texas Sanitary Code of 1911 provided that "the physician, surgeon, midwife, or parent shall report the birth of the child within five (5) days to the county or city registrar; that the undertaker shall file a death certificate for every death; and that all persons furnishing a coffin or box in which to bury the dead shall be deemed undertakers; that the city health officer or city clerk shall be the registrar for the incorporated city or town; that the county clerk shall be the registrar for the unincorporated portion of the county; that the registrar shall keep a record of the data shown on the certificates, and shall forward the original certificate to the State Health Department before the 10th of the month following; that all forms of certificates shall be prescribed by the State Registrar; that in case of rural deaths, where no undertaker is in attendance, that the physician shall file the certificates; and that sextons shall keep a record of all burials which occur in their respective cemeteries. The penalty for violation of any of these provisions is not less than ten ($10.00) dollars, nor more than one thousand ($1,000) dollars." Bureau of Vital Statistics, Texas State Board of Health, *Annual Report of the Bureau of Vital Statistics for the Year 1917* (Austin, TX: Von Boeckmann-Jones Company, 1918), 10.

26 "Gov. Colquitt Signs Bill," *Dallas Morning News*, March 24, 1911, 2.

27 "Deaths in February, Vital Statistics Report for Month Made Public," *Dallas Morning News*, March 27, 1911, 9.

28 "New Sanitary Code Will Be Enforced; Health Officers, Clerks, and Registrars Being Warned, State Registrar John Rosser Sends Out More than 1,000 Letters of Notification to Officials," *Dallas Morning News*, April 5, 1911, 7.

29 See "The First Prosecution under New Sanitary Code to Be Held at Waco," *Houston Post*, April 13, 1911, 3.

30 "Austin News Briefs," *Houston Post*, April 14, 1911, 3.

31 "Former Meningitis Statistics," *Dallas Morning News*, January 21, 1912, 6.

32 "Health Official Resigns; State Registrar J. E. Rosser Succeeded by R. P. Babcock," *Dallas Morning News*, July 9, 1911, 11.

33 Robert Percy Babcock (1881–1966) was born in Texas. He completed two years at an unnamed college before working as a bookkeeper, an assistant manager of an Austin hotel, and the secretary and vital statistics registrar of the Texas State Board of Health (1911–1914). Thereafter, he worked as a cashier at the US Internal Revenue Service and later worked many years as the deputy county clerk of Travis County, Texas. He married Alma Margaretha Heierman (1881–1953); they had one child. He died of a stroke and heart disease at the age of eighty-four years.

34 "Doctors Will Be Required to Report Vital Statistics," *El Paso Herald-Post*, September 19, 1911, 11.

35 "State's Health Conditions Good; Dr. Steiner So Reports after Visit to South Texas Towns," *Houston Post*, July 9, 1911, 8.

36 The two reasons for halting the manufacture and distribution of Flexner antimeningitis serum, according to the Rockefeller Institute for Medical Research, were 1) proof that the serum was efficacious, based on the human clinical trials conducted by Dr. Flexner with hundreds of physicians across the United States, and 2) the need to move the funds to other lines of investigation. See "Meningitis Serum Accepted; New Remedy Takes Place in List of Beneficial Agencies," *Dallas Morning News*, February 13, 1911, 2; "Antimeningitis Serum," *Texas State Journal of Medicine* 6, no. 11 (March 1911): 288; and Thomas Lynch, "Cerebrospinal Meningitis—Treatment," *Medical Herald* 31, no. 6 (June 1912): 296–98.

37 See Wade W. Oliver, *The Man Who Lived for Tomorrow: A Biography of William Hallock Park, MD* (New York: E. P. Dutton, 1941), 299–300.

38 Ibid., 297.

39 Dr. Abraham Sophian (1885–1957) was born in Kiev, Kiev Governorate, Russia, as the fifth of the six children of Morris Sophian (1849–1910), a carter, and Mathilda "Tillie" Pargomeschuk (or Pergamisherig) (1855–1920). At age five, he immigrated to New York City with his family. He attended public schools on the Lower East Side of Manhattan, earned his bachelor's degree from the College of the City of New York in 1902 at the age of seventeen years, and won by competitive examination a four-year state scholarship to attend Cornell University Medical College in New York City, from which he graduated in 1906 at the age of twenty-one years. He won by competitive examination a place on the medical house staff of New York City's Mount Sinai Hospital (January 1, 1907, to June 30, 1909) and won a George Blumenthal Jr. Fellowship, which he served in the pathology department of Mount Sinai Hospital (July 1, 1909, to June 30, 1910). Thereafter, he joined the Research Laboratory of the New York City Board of Health as the head of its special bureau of meningitis investigation (July 1, 1910). He wed Estelle Felix (1882–1970) on Wednesday, April 26, 1911 in Manhattan. On Wednesday, January 3, 1912, he boarded a train to Dallas, Texas, to assist in the control of the cerebrospinal meningitis epidemic there. See "Visiting Doctors Hear Dr. Sophian; Many from Other Texas Cities Attend Dinner by Physicians' Lunch Club; Treatment of Disease; Advises Administering Meningitis Serum on First Day— Outlines Precautions Advisable," *Dallas Morning News*, January 7, 1912, 8.

40 Phebe L. DuBois, "Differential Diagnosis and Treatment of Epidemic Cerebrospinal Meningitis," *Journal of the American Medical Association* 60, no. 11 (March 15, 1913): 820–22.

CHAPTER 3

MENINGITIS ASSAULTS DALLAS, OCTOBER 1911–JANUARY 1912

On Friday, September 1, 1911, Dr. Albert Ware Nash[1] succeeded Dr. Thomas B. Fisher[3] as the Dallas city health officer. During his farewell speech, Dr. Fisher prophetically advised Dr. Nash to pay "closer attention to the reports of vital statistics and contagious or infectious diseases."[3] Dr. Nash joined Dr. Henry Kern Leake,[4] the president of the Dallas Board of Health (a municipal advisory board), as members of the municipal administration of William "Willie" Meredith Holland, whom the people of Dallas elected as their mayor in April 1911.[5]

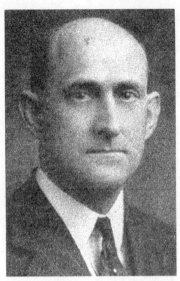

Dr. Albert Ware Nash (1883–1934) as a young man, from his obituary, "Deaths," *Texas State Journal of Medicine* 30, no. 2 (June 1934), 135. The photo is courtesy of Clair Duncan, director, TMA Knowledge Center, Texas Medical Association, January 12, 2018.

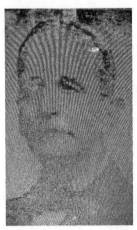

Dr. Henry Kern Leake (1847–1916), scanned from "Dr. H. K. Leake, Pioneer Texas Surgeon, Dead," *Dallas Morning News*, October 30, 1916, p. 5. The photographer is unknown.

On Saturday, September 2, 1911, Dr. Nash requested some "plain and suitable furniture" for the city health officer's quarters inside of the Dallas City Hospital, where he intended to live and work. Following his graduation from Vanderbilt University School of Medicine in Nashville, Davidson County, Tennessee, in 1906, he had served his internship at the Dallas City Hospital. He now intended to live there as the Dallas city health officer.[6] A year earlier, Dr. Nash's pregnant wife, Clara Julian Nash, had died of measles and premature birth.[1] The Dallas City Board of Commissioners approved Dr. Nash's request. He purchased the furniture and moved into the Dallas City Hospital.[6]

The Dallas City Hospital (henceforth, the City Hospital) was one of the six[7] hospitals (or sanitaria) in Dallas in 1911. It received municipal appropriations for the care of up to sixty-five patients at a time.[8] Because Dallas lacked a hospital for tubercular patients in 1911, the City Hospital housed them in tents and outdoor quarters on the hospital grounds. Most patients taken to the City Hospital in 1911 were indigent and in the latter stages of their diseases.

The City Hospital sat on seventeen acres of park land at Oak Lawn and Maple Avenues in the northern part of Dallas. Erected in 1894,[9] it consisted of five whitewashed wooden cottages interconnected by a wooden passageway. One-story buildings flanked the central two-story building of the hospital. The upper story of the central building was a private hospital for paying patients. The ground floor of the central building contained a parlor, Dr. Nash's office and bedroom, an operating room, a dispensary, a dining room, and a bathroom. The cellar of the central building contained a laundry room, furnace room, drying room, and fuel room. White female and male patients stayed in the cottages flanking the central building. African-American patients stayed in buildings behind the central building.[10]

In October 1911, Dr. Nash diagnosed and treated a patient with cerebrospinal meningitis. The patient died. The case startled and troubled him. Other physicians told Dr. Nash that he was mistaken about his diagnosis.[11] He did not believe that he was mistaken about his diagnosis. He soon learned from Dr. Steiner that cerebrospinal meningitis had killed twenty other people in Texas in October 1911. He also learned that Dr. Steiner had appointed

Dr. Samuel Newton Key[12] as the state bacteriologist (Thursday, November 2, 1911).[13]

On Sunday, November 12, 1911, Dr. Nash posted a letter to the 275 physicians practicing in Dallas seeking to register their names and addresses. His purpose was to improve compliance with the submission of vital statistics records and to orchestrate action on contagious diseases as necessary. In his letter, Dr. Nash described his difficulty in trying to locate some of the physicians, writing, "Almost daily this department has occasion to communicate with physicians of the city and sometimes it is very difficult to locate them; it is also a city ordinance that all physicians and midwives register with the City Health Officer."[14] Dr. Nash enclosed a stamped, addressed card for completion and return by each physician.

After posting his letters to Dallas physicians on Sunday, November 12, 1911, Dr. Nash traveled to Austin to attend Dr. Steiner's three-day conference of city and county health officers. Dr. Nash carried his own exhibits of his method of reporting and recording vital statistics in Dallas and the means used to assist physicians and others in supplying the information required by state law.[15] Health officers at the meeting presented papers whose titles included "The Evils Resulting from Prostitution," "Should Physicians Lecture to Pupils of Our High Schools, and on What Subject?" "Hookworm Disease," "Malta Fever," and "Shall the Sanitary Laws of Our State Continue to Be Only Partially Enforced?"[16] The number of attendees was light, but their interest was intense, noted one observer.[16]

At the end of November 1911, Dr. Nash counted nine reports of patients with cerebrospinal meningitis submitted by Dallas physicians; six of the afflicted patients died.[17] The population of Dallas in 1910 was 92,000 residents.[18] Using this population figure, the prevalence and mortality rates for cerebrospinal meningitis in Dallas for the month of November 1911 calculated to .98 *cerebrospinal meningitis cases per 10,000 Dallas residents* and *6.5 cerebrospinal meningitis deaths per 10,000 Dallas residents,* respectively. Using the same case and death count, the case fatality rate for the same time period calculated to *67 percent*.

The number of cases of cerebrospinal meningitis—ten (October and November 1911 combined)—was small, but Dr. Nash had a nagging feeling that he was witnessing an incipient cerebrospinal meningitis epidemic in Dallas. He acquired a supply of antimeningitis serum and learned to use it. By his side was his trusted friend and professional colleague Dr. George White Howard,[19] whom he appointed steward of the City Hospital on Sunday, November 26, 1911.[20-22]

On Monday, December 25, 1911, thirty-five-year-old Louis Spencer Flateau Jr,[23] a member of an old Texas family, died of cerebrospinal meningitis in his Dallas home only days after becoming ill. His death caused a stir in the city. The *Dallas Morning News* ran four stories about Mr. Flateau's illness, death, and burial.[24] Dr. Leake read the newspaper stories from his medical office in the Flateau Building in Dallas. On Wednesday, December 27, 1911, Dr. Steiner contemplated Mr. Flateau's death while traveling by train from Austin to Waco to speak on rural hygiene and hookworm infection before the State Teachers' Association convention.[25]

On Sunday, December 31, 1911, Dr. Nash counted seventy cases of cerebrospinal meningitis in Dallas sent to him by Dallas physicians for the month. Of the seventy patients, forty-five perished.[26] The prevalence of cerebrospinal meningitis in the city had risen from *.98 cerebrospinal meningitis cases per 10,000 Dallas residents* (October/November 1911 combined) to *7.6 cerebrospinal meningitis cases per 10,000 Dallas residents* (December 1911). The analogous mortality rate had fallen from *6.5 cerebrospinal meningitis deaths per 10,000 Dallas residents* (October/November 1911) to *4.9 cerebrospinal meningitis deaths per 10,000* (December 1911). The case fatality rate remained about the same at 64 percent.

Dr. Nash forwarded the Dallas cerebrospinal meningitis case and death counts to Mr. Babcock in Austin. He could not reply because he was attending the meeting of the American Public Health Association in Havana, Cuba.[27-28] Dr. Nash also relayed the data to Dr. Leake, who was working hard on finding the best place to build a new city hospital to replace the current City Hospital.[29-30]

In late December 1911, Dr. William Worthington Samuell,[31] a competent, thoughtful, and busy Dallas surgeon, became concerned about the growing number of cerebrospinal meningitis cases in Dallas requiring his care. Dr. Samuell knew how to perform the lumbar puncture procedure and infuse antimeningitis serum. He also kept careful track of his patients' outcomes following treatment with the antimeningitis serum. He quickly identified a discrepancy in his case fatality rate as compared with the one espoused by Dr. Flexner in New York City. Dr. Samuell remarked, "In New York, Dr. Flexner found that his serum was effective and perfected a cure in 90 per cent of the cases [i.e., a case fatality rate of 10 percent], where it has been tried. Here, the serum has not been near so effective, as the records show" a cure in 55 percent of cases (i.e., a case fatality rate of 45 percent).[17]

Dr. Samuell was not a bashful person. He sent a telegram to Dr. Flexner to request his opinion about the possible reasons for the observed discrepancy; he also wanted Dr. Flexner to come to Dallas to determine the reasons for the discrepancy. Dr. Flexner wired back, asking Dr. Samuell for the ages of the afflicted persons and the age range that showed the greatest mortality. Dr. Samuell responded that the age range of afflicted persons in Dallas was two to forty-five years and that the age range with the greatest mortality was twelve to forty-six years. Dr. Samuell added that Dallas was not the only city under siege; the city of Waco[32-33] also was fighting an exploding epidemic of cerebrospinal meningitis.[17]

On Sunday, December 31, 1911, a Rains County, Texas, judge wired Dr. Steiner in Austin to request his help in managing the cerebrospinal meningitis epidemic in his county. Dr. Steiner responded that he "considered these cases in all the districts well within the control of the health officers and that the state board could be of no material assistance."[34]

On Monday, January 1, 1912, Dallas schools were scheduled to reopen after the winter vacation. Dr. Nash, increasingly anxious about the evolving cerebrospinal meningitis situation in Dallas, called Dr. Steiner in Austin to ask his opinion about reopening the Dallas schools.[35] Dr. Steiner responded that cerebrospinal meningitis was wholly a local, not a pestilential or an epidemic, condition, and that simple isolation of the cases was enough to prevent the disease from spreading. Nevertheless, Dr. Nash's decision to keep the schools closed was a wise precaution. Also, on January 1, 1912, Dr. Steiner sent Dr. Key to Emory, Rains County, to assess the cerebrospinal meningitis situation there.[35]

On Tuesday, January 2, 1912, a group of Dallas physician leaders met at the Southland Hotel[36] purportedly to discuss the location of the new City Hospital. The physicians, however, quickly turned to a discussion of what most concerned them: the worsening cerebrospinal meningitis situation in Dallas.[37] Dr. Matthew Mann Smith[38] made a motion to form a committee headed by Dr. John Shade Turner,[39] the incoming president of the Texas State Medical Society. The committee's purpose was to represent the local medical profession in giving "conference, cooperation, and assistance" to the Dallas Board of Health regarding "the appearance of cerebrospinal meningitis in the community and the public anxiety attached to it."[37]

The ad hoc physician committee consisted of Dr. Turner, Dr. Edward Henry Cary (the dean of Baylor University College of Medicine in Dallas and an ophthalmologist),[40] Dr. Raleigh William Baird (a general practitioner),[41] Dr. Hugh Leslie Moore (president of the Dallas County Medical Society and a pediatrician),[42] Dr. M. M. Smith, and Dr. Charles McDaniel Rosser (a former Dallas city health officer and a founder of the University of Dallas Medical Department).[43] Dr. Turner contacted Dr. Leake to request permission "to sit in free conference" at the Dallas Board of Health meeting scheduled for eight o'clock that evening in Dr. Leake's office in the Flateau Building. Dr. Leake agreed to the request.[29]

The Dallas Board of Health convened as scheduled on the night of Tuesday, January 2, 1912. Dr. Nash spoke first, addressing his remarks to the members of the ad hoc committee of physicians present in Dr. Leake's office. He told them that he had received reports of eighty cases of cerebrospinal meningitis and fifty-two deaths from cerebrospinal meningitis since October 1, 1911, adding,

> I wish you [the ad hoc committee of physicians] would tell the people that in cases where cerebrospinal meningitis develops, that the health department has Flexner's serum on hand and has physicians who are competent to administer it. This rule of course applies to the poor of both races. Any person who is unable to purchase the serum may obtain it free of charge from the health department, and if they are not able to employ a physician, a city doctor will administer it.[21]

Dr. Turner spoke next, reading aloud a telegram from Dr. Flexner in which he suggested sending a physician representative from New York City to Dallas to assist the city in the control and scientific study of its ongoing cerebrospinal meningitis epidemic. Dr. Leake and Dr. Nash were taken aback by the turn of events, conferred, decided to accept Dr. Flexner's offer, and wired back to Dr. Flexner the following invitation:

> In response to your telegram proposing to send a representative to cooperate with the local profession, we have had a total of 81 cases in Dallas; others in surrounding territory. We understand the importance locally and generally of the scientific study of this disease and will be glad to have your representative.[28]

Dr. Flexner wired back to Dr. Leake and Dr. Nash that he was sending Dr. A. Sophian to Dallas. The latter was eager to understand the conditions in which the disease had developed in Texas and the percent mortality with and without the use of antimeningitis serum as a relieving agent.[17]

The next day, Wednesday, January 3, 1912, Dr. Turner, Dr. Leake, and other Dallas physicians reported that an ad hoc committee of local physicians had conferred with "the honorable Board of Health and City Health Officer, officio member of the board" to issue a "joint statement to the citizenship of Dallas and community anent [sic] the situation as we find it with reference to the prevalence of the disease cerebrospinal meningitis."[28] They pointed out that favorable climatic conditions during the winter and spring of recent years had prohibited the spread of epidemic cerebrospinal meningitis. By contrast, the current cold and wet season prevalent from 1911 to 1912 was acting favorably for the development of the microbe, resulting in a disease increase. The newspaper article then listed Dr. Flexner's lengthy rules for the correct treatment of cerebrospinal meningitis with antimeningitis serum available elsewhere.[44]

The physicians ended their joint statement with the following:

> In conclusion, noting the low mortality in those cases promptly diagnosed and properly treated, we beg to suggest alarm should not be indulged, but a more hopeful view should be taken by the people inasmuch as the more recent cases have been attended with fewer proportionate fatalities, justifying the expectation that with improved climatic conditions, the situation will continuously improve. We further wish to say that there is an abundance of authorized Flexner serum in this city for any immediate service.[28]

The following physicians signed their names: "Board of Health of Dallas, by Dr. H. K. Leake, President, Dr. A. W. Nash, City Health Officer, E. A. Aronson,[45] and J. M. Neel[46]; Physicians Committee, by Dr. John S. Turner, Dr. Edward H. Cary, Dr. R.W. Baird, Dr. H. Leslie Moore, Dr. C. M. Rosser, and Dr. M. M. Smith."[28]

On Wednesday, January 3, 1912, in Austin, Dr. Steiner received a request for help to manage the cerebrospinal meningitis epidemic in Clarksville (population 2,000 persons in 1910), Red River County, Texas. The requesting health official reported twelve to fourteen people stricken with the disease. Dr. Key was still in Emory, Rains County, working with local authorities on their cerebrospinal meningitis epidemic. Dr. Steiner instructed the Clarksville health officer to isolate and quarantine individual cases, close schools during the height of the affection, and administer antimeningitis serum. He assured the Clarksville health officer that the disease was not epidemic, not pestilential, and without danger of spreading between communities. It was caused entirely by local conditions, and until those conditions were definitely ascertained, the Texas State Board of Health could render no material assistance in the situation. He reiterated that he believed local authorities had the disease under control as far as protection in the respective cities was concerned.[47]

On that same day, Wednesday, January 3, 1912, in Dallas, Dr. Leake announced he had received a wire from Dr. Flexner. The telegram read, "Dr. A. Sophian leaves via New York Central ... and arrives at Dallas at [eight thirty in the evening] Friday [January 5, 1912]. He carries a supply of serum and is prepared to administer it and to assist generally in the study and control of the epidemic."[48]

The next day, Mayor Holland, after conferring with Dr. Nash, directed Dallas residents to clean and disinfect their premises, burn all trash and filth, and spread unslaked lime around damp places in their yards. In addition, he ordered the disinfection of all theaters and moving picture shows, street cars, jails, streets, and sidewalks. He told Dallas residents, "Full reports of all new [cerebrospinal meningitis] cases are being given the press. Nothing is being concealed. The streets and storms sewers are being thoroughly cleansed. The situation is well in hand and we feel that there is no occasion for alarm."[48]

Dr. Nash concurred with the mayor, opining,

> While there has never been a reason for undue alarm,
> there is still good cause for sanitary measures, for it
> is from unsanitary conditions that all of the diseases

get their footholds. Cleanliness and sunshine with plenty of good air will put almost any dangerous germ out of commission ... There is need of friendly rivalry among the people of the city as to who may be cleanest in clothing, surrounding, and physical self. There can be no objection to the extension of this to the conversation and the thoughts. Then there will be less fear of disease, that element that can cause death almost without disease.[48]

Dr. Nash then announced that Dr. Alfred Edward Thayer,[49] an academic pathologist with laboratories on the second floor of the Ramseur Science Hall of the Baylor University College of Medicine[50] (in Dallas in 1912), had agreed to examine "the pus or matter taken from the spinal column of patients believed to be suffering from meningitis." Such an examination, said Dr. Nash, "ought to be done in every case suspected, so that there may be a proper treatment and not the administration of the serum where it is unnecessary and cannot be beneficial."[48]

CHAPTER 3 NOTES

1 Dr. Albert Ware Nash (1883–1934) was born in Garland, Dallas County, Texas, as one of the thirteen children of Mary Frances Hobbs (1858–1918) and Judge Thomas Fletcher Nash (1850–1908). Judge Nash served on the Dallas County-of-Law Court of the Fourteenth District Court of Dallas County and as a member of the Texas State Legislature (1881–1885). Albert Ware Nash moved from Garland to Dallas, about fifteen miles to the southwest, at the age of nine; graduated from Dallas High School in 1902; and earned his medical degree from Vanderbilt University School of Medicine in Nashville, Davidson County, Tennessee, in 1906. He served as an intern and hospital steward at the City Hospital, Dallas (1906–1907) and as the Dallas assistant health officer (1907–1909) before entering private practice. He married Clara Julian (1888–1910) on July 7, 1909; she died on March 5, 1910. On September 1, 1911, he succeeded Dr. Thomas B. Fisher as the Dallas city health officer. Around a month later, he diagnosed the first case of meningitis in Dallas, which marked the beginning of the Texas cerebrospinal meningitis epidemic of 1911 to 1913. He served as the Dallas city health officer until 1915. The new Parkland Hospital, which replaced the City Hospital, was constructed during his administration as city health officer. He also helped to establish a nurses' school in connection with Parkland Hospital. He eventually left public health work to resume a medical practice. He served as president of the Dallas County Medical Society (1912–1913) and as a professor of therapeutics at the Baylor University College of Medicine (1909–1913), among other professional positions in the city. In 1913, he married Rose Emma Nielsen (1891–1934), the head day nurse at the City Hospital during the cerebrospinal meningitis epidemic of 1911 to 1912; they had two children. He suffered a heart attack in November 1932. In July 1933, he resumed his duties as medical director of the International Travelers Association in Dallas and opened a restricted medical office in his home. He died of a second heart attack two hours after his wife's death from a severe throat infection. She was forty-two and he was fifty years old. A double funeral was held for them. See "Dr. Fisher Retires from City's Service; Has Been City Health Officer for Five Years; Will Be Succeeded Today by Dr. A. W. Nash—Submits Some Recommendations," *Dallas Morning News*, September 1, 1911, 4; "Medical News, Texas," *Journal of*

the American Medical Association 57, no. 11 (September 9, 1911): 909; "Dr. Albert Ware Nash," in Ellis Arthur Davis and Edwin H. Grobe, *The Encyclopedia of Texas* (Dallas, TX: University of North Texas, 1922), 1:237; "Dallas Doctor and Wife Die within Two Hours Each Other," *Corsicana Semi-Weekly Light* (Corsicana, TX), February 13, 1934, 7; "Double Funeral Services Held," *Galveston Daily News*, March 15, 1934, 17; "Deaths," *Texas State Journal of Medicine* 30, no. 2 (June 1934): 135; and *Annual Announcement, Baylor University School of Medicine and School of Pharmacy, Dallas, Texas, 1910–1911* (Dallas, TX: Medical Department of Baylor University, 1910), 8.

2 See "Dr. Fisher Retires from City's Service; Has Been City Health Officer for Five Years; Will Be Succeeded Today by Dr. A. W. Nash— Submits Some Recommendations," *Dallas Morning News*, September 1, 1911, 4; and "City of Dallas Health Department Collection, Register and Researcher's Guide," *Texas Archival Resources Online*, Dallas Public Library, accessed June 29, 2017, http://www.lib.utexas. edu/taro/dalpub/08212/dpub-08212.html.

3 Dr. Thomas Barber (Barbour? Benton?) Fisher (1871–1960) was born on a farm in Dallas County, Texas, as one of the six children of Robinson Hunt Fisher (1836–1895) and Elisa Strain Ingles (1843–1897). The place of his medical education is unknown. He served as the Dallas county health officer (1906–1911) and the Dallas city health officer (1911–1915) before becoming a medical insurance company director. He married Suzanne Marseline Gahagan (1883–1963) in 1906; they had two children. He died of a stroke and colon cancer at the age of eighty-nine years. See "Early-Day Health Officer, Dr. Thomas Fisher, Dies," *Dallas Morning News*, November 23, 1960, 4.

4 Dr. Henry Kern Leake (1847–1916) was born in Yazoo City, Yazoo County, Mississippi, as one of the five children of Dr. William Josiah Leake (1815–1867) and Martha Letitia Hughes (1818–1874). Henry Leake grew up on his father's Mississippi plantation, received his early education through a private tutor, enlisted in the Confederate Army in 1861, and participated in the defense of Yazoo City against Union soldiers. He entered the Kentucky Military Institute in Lyndon, Jefferson County, Kentucky, in 1866 and graduated in 1870. He earned his medical degree from the University of Louisville Medical Department. He worked as a quarantine officer at Indianola (now a ghost town), Calhoun County, Texas, for four years before a terrific

hurricane famously leveled the town, including his own house, which drifted out to sea. In 1875, he moved to the then-small village of Dallas on the east bank of the Trinity River and opened a medical practice. After studying surgery in Europe in 1890, he returned to Dallas to open the first private sanitarium in the city. He became president of the Dallas Board of Health during the Mayor Stephen John Hay (1864–1916) administration (1907–1911). He married Lillie M. Montgomery (1849–1914) in 1869; they had eight children. Dr. Leake was known for his "gentility and the catholicity of his views." After his death from Bright's disease at the age of sixty-nine years, a colleague mentioned Dr. Leake's unusual deference toward the young physician from the Rockefeller Institute who came to Dallas during the meningitis epidemic [Dr. Sophian]. See "Dr. H. K. Leake, Pioneer Texas Surgeon, Dead; Became Seriously Ill a Few Days Ago, Following Acute Attack of Bright's Disease; Lived Here 41 Years; Opened First Private Sanitarium in Dallas, Founded Medical Journal and Highly Regarded," *Dallas Morning News*, October 30, 1916, 5; and "Funeral for Dr. H. K. Leake; Services Held at Home— Tribute Paid to Service of Pioneer Surgeon and Physician," *Dallas Morning News*, October 31, 1916, 14.

5   William "Willie" Meredith Holland (1875–1966) was born in Dallas, Dallas County, Texas, as the only child of William Colter Holland (1837–1918), a lawyer, and Sarah Jones Saffell (1839–1909). William M. Holland attended the University of Texas at Austin and earned his law degree from George Washington University Law School in Washington, DC (1898). He returned to practice law in Dallas. He served as a judge in the Dallas County Court-at-Law No. 1 (1907–1911) and as the mayor of Dallas (1911–1915), taking office at the age of thirty-six years. Among his achievements as mayor were guiding the city through the cerebrospinal meningitis epidemic of 1911 to 1913 and constructing Parkland Hospital. Following his service as mayor, he returned to law practice (1915–1960). He married Elnora Frances Beggs (1882–1960) in 1909; they had three children. He died of heart failure following prostatic surgery; he was ninety years old. See "Judge Holland Dies at 90," *Dallas Morning News*, March 12, 1966; "President Helped Elect Judge Holland," *Dallas Morning News*, March 12, 1966, 14; and Sam Acheson, "Hectic Term of Mayor Holland," *Dallas Morning News*, September 27, 1971, 2.

6   "Dr. Nash Assumes Duties; Becomes City Health Officer, Succeeding Dr. Fisher—Asks for New Furniture," *Dallas Morning News*, September 2, 1911, 5.

7   The six major hospitals in Dallas in 1911 were the City Hospital, St. Paul's Sanitarium, Texas Baptist Memorial Sanitarium, Leake Sanitarium, the County and City Union Hospital (known as Union Hospital), and Marsalis Sanitarium. St. Paul's Sanitarium, directed by the Sisters of Charity of Saint Vincent de Paul of the Roman Catholic Church, was the largest hospital in Dallas. Thirty-eight nurses tended to an average daily inpatient census of about 110 patients. Texas Baptist Memorial Sanitarium, directed by the Baptist General Convention of Texas, had an average daily inpatient census of about sixty patients, who received care from four graduate nurses and about fifty nurses in training. The Leake Sanitarium, founded by Dr. Henry Kern Leake, was a nonsectarian, private institution with a capacity of twenty-five patients, who received care from six nurses. The governments of Dallas City and Dallas County jointly operated Union Hospital as a contagious-diseases hospital. In 1911, it lacked any patients. One nurse lived there to take charge of any cases that arrived. Marsalis Sanitarium was a private institution established by Drs. J. H. Reuss and James H. Smart in 1905 for the general care of up to fifteen medical and surgical patients by five nurses. See "Health of People Given Attention; Death Rate Below the Average, but More Preventive Work Is Needed; Facilities in Hospitals; Some Charity Dispensed There, although Provisions Not Elaborate; City and State Regulations," *Dallas Morning News*, October 1, 1911, 14; Paula Bosse, "St. Paul's Sanitarium," *Flashback: Dallas*, accessed August 19, 2018, https://flashbackdallas.com/2015/08/23/st-pauls-sanitarium-1910/; and Paula Bosse, "The Marsalis House: One of Oak Cliff's 'Most Conspicuous Architectural Landmarks,'" *Flashback: Dallas*, accessed January 11, 2018, https://flashbackdallas.com/2014/05/30/marsalis-house/.

8   "Health of People Given Attention; Death Rate Below the Average, but More Preventive Work Is Needed; Facilities in Hospitals; Some Charity Dispensed There, although Provisions Not Elaborate; City and State Regulations," *Dallas Morning News*, October 1, 1911, 14.

9   The City Hospital on Oak Lawn and Maple Avenues in Dallas in 1911 was the city's third rendition of the hospital. The first Dallas City Hospital, built in 1881, was a single-room cottage with an attached lean-to, located at the corner of Wood and Houston Streets.

The second Dallas City Hospital was located in a remodeled school building at South Cross Street. The city also had a half interest in the Union Hospital erected in 1908 north of the city. The third City Hospital—the meningitis hospital of this book—was demolished in 1913 and replaced by the all-brick Parkland Hospital. See "In Hospital Facilities Dallas City and County Now Lead All Other Places," *Dallas Morning News*, October 1, 1910, 24; "Parkland Hospital Collection, 1889–2017," *University of Texas Southwestern Medical Center Library*, accessed June 30, 2017, http://library. utsouthwestern.edu/speccol/archives/FindingAid_Parkland_Coll. pdf; and John W. Boyd, *Parkland Hospital* (Charleston, SC: Arcadia, 2015).

10 "New City Hospital: How the Building Will Be Arranged; When It Will Be Completed," *Dallas Morning News*, November 30, 1893, 3.

11 "Flexner Serum Is Highly Effective; Treatment of Hospital Cases Reduces Percentage of Fatality to 0.94; Need Early Diagnosis; At Meningitis Sanitarium It Is Said Two or Three Deaths Result from Late Call," *Dallas Morning News*, January 12, 1912, 8.

12 Dr. Samuel Newton Key (1886–1956) was born in Georgetown, Williamson County, Texas, as the youngest of the four children of William Mercer Key (1850–1923), a lawyer and judge, and Rhoda Izora Scott (1854–1939). Samuel Key earned his bachelor's and medical degrees from the University of Texas at Austin and from the University of Texas Medical Branch at Galveston in 1903 and 1910, respectively. He served an internship at the Philadelphia General Hospital (1910–1911) before his appointment as the Texas state bacteriologist on November 2, 1911. He left the position on June 1, 1912, to pursue advanced medical work in New York City. He married Mary "Mae" Robertson (1896–1963); they had one child. Dr. Key died of a cerebrovascular stroke in Austin at the age of sixty-nine years. See W. J. Maxwell and John A. Lomax, *General Register of the Students and Former Students of the University of Texas, 1917* (Austin, TX: University of Texas Ex-Students' Association, 1917), 86; "Young Doctors Receive Diplomas of State University Medical Branch," *Houston Post*, June 1, 1910, 2; "Bacteriology Department and What It Accomplishes; Dr. Key Tells of Examination of Disinfectants; Speaks of Contaminated Water Supply, Diagnoses Made in the Laboratory," *Galveston Daily News*, February 26, 1912, 5; "The Travis County Medical Society," *Texas State Journal of Medicine* 7, no. 12 (February 9, 1912): 340; "State

Serum Factory Plans; Plan Can Not Be Put in Operation before Next Fall—Dr. Stimson, Supervisor of Plant, Here," *Austin American-Statesman*, March 7, 1912, 4; "Dr. Stimson on Ground; Is Man Who Will Inaugurate Serum Anti-Toxin Factory," *Houston Post*, March 7, 1912, 5; "State Bacteriologist Returns," *Galveston Daily News*, April 23, 1912, 9; "U. of T. Graduates Conspicuous," *Dallas Morning News*, May 12, 1912, 3; and "No title," *Houston Post*, May 2, 1912, 3.

13 See "State Bacteriologist Appointed," *Texas State Journal of Medicine* 7, no. 8 (December 1911): 227; and "S. N. Key Appointed State Chemist [*sic*]," *Dallas Morning News*, November 2, 1911, 9.

14 "Warns Doctors Law Requires Registration; City Health Officer Writes Letter to Physicians; Aims to Secure Better Vital Statistics Records and Action on Contagion and Infection," *Dallas Morning News*, November 12, 1911, 19.

15 "To Austin for Conference; City Health Officer Dr. Albert W. Nash to Attend Meeting of the City and County Men," *Dallas Morning News*, November 12, 1911, 19.

16 "State Health Officers Convene at Austin, Attendance Small but Interest Is Intense, Number of Technical Papers Are Read on Various Matters Concerning Department," *Dallas Morning News*, November 14, 1911, 6; and "Annual Conference of Health Officers," *Texas State Journal of Medicine* 7, no. 8 (December 1911): 228.

17 "Expert Visits Cases upon Reaching City; Dr. Sophian Has Begun Study of Local Meningitis Situation; Arrived in Dallas Last Night and Confers with Physicians—State Health Officer Here," *Dallas Morning News*, January 6, 1912, 5; and Rudolph H. von Ezdorf, "Cerebrospinal Meningitis in Texas," *Public Health Reports* 27, no. 8 (February 23, 1912): 270.

18 *Texas Almanac: City Population History of Selected Cities, 1850–2000*, accessed December 8, 2017, https://texasalmanac.com/sites/default/files/images/CityPopHist%20web.pdf.

19 George White Howard (1887–1962) was born in Dayton, Rhea County, Tennessee, as the eldest of the nine children of John Tate Howard (1859–1935), a clerk, and Perry Ann Darwin (1860–1911). The family moved to Abilene, Taylor and Jones Counties, Texas, in 1902, and to Merkel, Taylor County, Texas, in 1903. Dr. Howard's place of medical education is unknown. He was associated with the Dallas City Health Department for many years. He married Julia N. Wyatt (1889–1980); they had four children. Dr. Howard died of a

heart attack at the age of seventy-five years. See "Dallas Services for Dr. Howard," *Abilene Reporter-News* September 8, 1962, 12.

20 "No title," *Dallas Morning News*, December 30, 1910, 6.

21 "Dallas Has a Disease Scare; Dr. Nash Does Not Believe in Needless Alarm; Dr. Flexner Wired to; Famous Meningitis Expert Is Willing to Do All Possible to Help Situation—Opinions of Physicians," *Cleburne Morning Review* (Cleburne, TX), January 3, 1912, 5.

22 "Health Officer's Appointments," *Dallas Morning News*, November 26, 1911, 6.

23 Louis Spencer Flateau Jr. (1876–1911) was born in Pittsburg, Camp County, Texas, as one of the nine children of Ella Letitia Pitts (1855–1933) and Captain Louis Spencer Flateau (Flatau) Sr. (1843–1920), an inventor with many patents, a veteran of the Confederate Army, a steamboat pilot on the Red and Mississippi Rivers, and an officer with Flatau's [*sic*] Roofing and Fire Proof Paint in St. Louis, Missouri. Louis S. Flateau Jr. was active in the Texas militia and was one of the organizers and the first captain of the Dallas Artillery Company. Later, he was promoted to major and, when he retired, commanded the artillery division of the entire Texas National Guard. He married Ruth Bryan (born in 1882) in Los Angeles in 1902; they had no children. See "L. S. Flateau Jr. Passes Away; Succumbs to Attack of Meningitis Early This Morning—Was Member of Prominent Old Family," *Dallas Morning News*, December 25, 1911, 11; and (about his father) "Pioneer Texan Dies after Long Illness in St. Louis Hospital," *Galveston Daily News*, July 15, 1920, 5.

24 "L. S. Flateau Seriously Ill, Prominent Dallas Man Suffering with Meningitis and a St. Louis Specialist Is Summoned," *Dallas Morning News*, December 24, 1911, 4; "L. S. Flateau Jr. Passes Away, Succumbs to Attack of Meningitis Early This Morning—Was Member of Prominent Old Family," *Dallas Morning News*, December 25, 1911, 11; "Major Flateau Funeral Today, Services Will Be Held at Home on Maple Avenue at 10:30 A.M.; Pallbearers Are Named," *Dallas Morning News*, December 26, 1911, 5; and "Friends Pay Tribute to Major L. S. Flateau," *Dallas Morning News*, December 27, 1911, 5.

25 "Steiner Goes to Waco," *Dallas Morning News*, December 29, 1911, 9.

26 Rudolph H. von Ezdorf, "Cerebrospinal Meningitis in Texas," *Public Health Reports* 27, no. 8 (February 23, 1912): 270.

27 "Minutes of the Thirty-Ninth Annual Meeting of the American Public Health Association, Havana, Cuba, December 5–9, 1911," *Public Health Papers and Report 37, Presented at the Thirty-Ninth Annual Meeting of the American Public Health Association, Havana, Cuba* (Concord, NH: Rumford Printing Company, 1913), 233–62.

28 "Registrar Babcock Goes to Cuba," *Fort Worth Star-Telegram*, December 1, 1911, 19.

29 "Physicians Appoint Special Committees to Present Hospital Removal to Other Organizations," *Dallas Morning News*, January 3, 1912, 4.

30 "Dr. Leake Gives His Views; Explains Why He Believes City Hospital Should Be Centrally Located," *Dallas Morning News*, December 30, 1911, 5.

31 Dr. William Worthington Samuell (1878–1937) was born in Georgetown, Harlan County, Kentucky, as one of the three sons of Hazael [*sic*] Offutt Samuell (1844–1922), a farmer, and Sarah "Sallie" Worthington (1845–1914). One-year-old William moved with his family to Dallas County, Texas, in 1879. He received his early formal education in the Dallas public schools; earned his bachelor's degree from the University of Texas at Austin (1897); received his medical degree from Tulane University Medical Department in New Orleans, Louisiana (1900); and served an internship at Charity Hospital in the same city (1900–1901). He then sailed for Europe on November 6, 1901, to pursue postgraduate medical studies. On his return, he lived in Mississippi before moving back to Dallas to open a surgical practice. In 1911, he purchased an ambulance for the city of Dallas. He established the Samuell Clinic in Dallas in 1913. He was considered one of the busiest surgeons in the United States. When he died of a heart attack at the age of fifty-nine years, the procession of mourners stretched two miles to the cemetery. He married Addie M. Keating (1889–1977); they had no children. See "Death Claims W. W. Samuell, Famed Surgeon; Founder of Dallas Clinic Dies of Sudden Heart Attack; Funeral to Be Held Tuesday Morning; Known for Speed; Associates Estimated He Operated More Cases Than Any in Country," *Dallas Morning News*, December 13, 1937, 1; "A Dallas Boy," *Dallas Morning News*, May 10, 1900, 10; "Dallas Will Have a New Sanitarium; Handsome Five-Story Edifice to Cost $75,000, Will Be Built by Dr. W. W. Samuell," *Dallas Morning*

News, April 6, 1913, 15; and Sam Acheson, "Hectic Term of Mayor Holland," *Dallas Morning News*, September 27, 1971 [*sic*], 2.

32 The Waco case and death counts for cerebrospinal meningitis between Friday, December 14, 1911, and Wednesday, January 10, 1912, were ninety and thirty-two, respectively. Based on these case and death counts, the prevalence, mortality, and case fatality rates for Waco (population of 26,000 in 1910, see note #33 below) between December 14, 1911, and January 10, 1912, calculated to *34.6 cerebrospinal meningitis cases per 10,000 Waco residents*; *12.3 cerebrospinal meningitis deaths per 10,000 Waco residents*; and *36 percent*, respectively. "Waco Meningitis Bulletin," *Dallas Morning News*, January 11, 1912, 8.

33 The population of Waco, Texas, in 1910 was taken from *Texas Almanac: City Population History of Selected Cities, 1850–2000*, accessed December 8, 2017, https://texasalmanac.com/sites/default/files/images/CityPopHist%20web.pdf.

34 "Meningitis in Rains County," *Galveston Daily News*, December 31, 1911, 22.

35 "Opinion of Dr. Steiner," *Dallas Morning News*, January 2, 1912, 14; "Many Deaths from Meningitis," *Dallas Morning News*, January 1, 1912, 20; "Schools Suspended Account Meningitis," *Bryan Daily Eagle*, January 2, 1912, 2; and "Investigations at Emory," *Dallas Morning News*, January 3, 1912, 5.

36 The Southland Hotel, located at Main and Murphy Streets, was the first skyscraper in Dallas to use steel-framed construction to improve its resistance to fire. It had a drinking fountain that dispensed cold water through a figure of Venus and was the nation's second hotel with running ice water in every room. See Sam Childers, *Historic Dallas Hotels* (Charleston, SC: Arcadia Publishers, 2010), 27.

37 "Physicians Appoint Special Committees to Present Hospital Removal to Other Organizations," *Dallas Morning News*, January 3, 1912, 5.

38 Dr. Matthew Mann Smith (1864–1924) was born in Bluff Springs, Travis County, Texas, as one of the eleven children of Felix Ezell Smith (1831–1891), a farmer, and Mary Sophronia Mann (1838–1916). Matthew Mann Smith earned his bachelor (1888) and master (1889) of science degrees from the University of Texas in nearby Austin and his medical degree from the Jefferson Medical College of Thomas Jefferson University in Philadelphia in 1891. He served as the Austin city physician (1891–1895) and moved to Dallas in

1907, where he served as physician to the State Institute for the Deaf. For many years, he published the *Texas Medical News*. He married Eleanor Lee Anderson (1871–1957) in 1894; they had two children. Dr. M. M. Smith died after a long illness at the age of fifty-nine years. See "Medical Director of Fraternal Order Dies," *Dallas Morning News*, January 11, 1924, 13; "Matthew Mann Smith," in W. J. Maxwell and John A. Lomax, *General Register of the Students and Former Students of the University of Texas, 1917* (Austin, TX: University of Texas Ex-Students' Association, 1917), 16; and "Matthew Mann Smith," in W. J. Maxwell, *General Alumni Catalogue of Jefferson Medical College Alumni, 1890–1899* (Philadelphia, PA: Jefferson Medical College, 1917), 149–50.

39 Dr. John Shade Turner (1866–1936) was born in Americus, Sumter County, Georgia, as the eldest of the five children of Green Brantley Turner (1839–1927), a farmer, and Martha "Mattie" Jane Scott (1840–1909). The family moved to Texas the same year John Shade Turner was born, settling at Cleburne, Johnson County, Texas. He earned his medical degree from the University of Louisville Medical Department; practiced medicine privately for eight years; served as the assistant superintendent of the State Hospital for the Insane at San Antonio (1897–1900); served as the superintendent of the North Texas State Hospital for the Insane at Terrell, Kaufman County, Texas (1900–1907); and consulted on mental and nervous diseases for two years (1907–1909). In 1909, he moved to Dallas to serve as a medical director of the Southland Life Insurance Company. He was elected president of the Texas State Medical Association (1912–1913) and remained a member of the Texas State Medical Association Board of Trustees for twenty more years (1913–1933). He married Mattie Hightower in 1885; they had five children. He died from a heart attack at his vacation home in the Ozark Mountains at the age of seventy years. See "Doctor Who Moved to Hotel to Fight Meningitis Scourge Dies after Bathtub Accident," *Dallas Morning News*, August 30, 1936, 10; and "Gifts Presented to Foes of Meningitis," *Dallas Morning News*, February 2, 1912, 2.

40 Dr. Edward Henry Cary (1872–1953) was born in Union Springs, Bullock County, Alabama, as the youngest of the four children of Joseph Milton Cary (1833–1872), a farmer, and Lucy Jeanette Powell (1842–1924). He had eye weakness as a child. He studied at Union Springs Academy in Union, Alabama, before attending high school in New York City. He entered Bellevue Hospital Medical

College (1895), earning his medical degree there in 1898. He served a one-year internship at Bellevue Hospital and an additional year as house physician at the New York Eye and Ear Infirmary. In 1901, he returned to Dallas to practice ophthalmology. In 1902, he became dean of the University of Dallas Medical Department and led the movement for the medical department of the University of Dallas to become the medical department of Baylor University (1904). He thereafter became dean of the Baylor University College of Medicine until 1929, when he became dean emeritus. From 1909 to 1929, he was chairman of the staff of the Baylor University Hospital. In 1939, he and a group of Dallas businessmen organized the Southwestern Medical Foundation, which, on May 5, 1943, established the Southwestern Medical College, now known as Southwestern Medical School of the University of Texas. He organized the Baylor Medical Unit that served in France during World War I. He married Georgie Fonda Schneider in 1911; they had five children. He died of heart failure at the age of eighty-one years. See "Dr. Edward H. Cary," in Ellis A. Davis and Edwin H. Grobe, *New Encyclopedia of Texas* (Dallas, TX: Texas Development Bureau, 1926), 2:1368; "Edward H. Cary," *Dallas Morning News*, December 12, 1953, 2; John S. Chapman, *The University of Texas Southwestern Medical School: Medical Education in Dallas, 1900–1975* (Dallas, TX: Southern Methodist University Press, 1976); Booth Mooney, *More Than Armies: The Story of Edward H. Cary, MD* (Dallas, TX: Mathis, Van Nort Company, 1948); John S. Fordtran, "Medicine in Dallas 100 Years Ago," *Proceedings of Baylor University Medical Center* 13, no.1 (January 2000): 34–44; and "Medical Colleges of the United States, Dallas," *Journal of the American Medical Association* 59, no. 8 (August 24, 1912): 632.

41 Dr. Raleigh William Baird (1870–1941) was born in Shreveport, Caddo Parish, Louisiana, as one of the twelve children of William Leroy Baird (1796–1883), a farmer who fought in the War of 1812, and Mary Ann Law (1827–1880). Raleigh Baird earned his bachelor's degree at Southwestern University in Georgetown, Williamson County, Texas (1893) and his medical degree at Bellevue Hospital Medical College (1896). After serving on the house staff of Bellevue Hospital (1896–1898), he moved to Dallas and opened a medical practice (1900). In 1915, he founded the Dallas Medical and Surgical Clinic, serving as its president from 1915 until his death. He married Lavinia "Linnie" Starley Bishop (1875–1948) in 1900; they had five

children. See *Alumni of the Medical Schools, New York University Alumni Catalogue, 1833–1907* (New York: General Alumni Society, 1908), 509; and "Head of Dallas Clinic Dies at His Home, Rites Slated for 2 P.M.," *Dallas Morning News*, July 14, 1941, 9.

42 Dr. Hugh Leslie Moore (1874–1950) was born in Tompkinsville, Monroe County, Kentucky, as the youngest of the six children of Dr. Samuel William Moore (1830–1913) and Sarah "Sally" Rebecca Bedford (1841–1917). The family moved to Van Alstyne, Grayson County, Texas, in the 1880s, where Dr. Samuel W. Moore served as mayor in 1890. Hugh Leslie Moore earned his bachelor's degree from Columbia College (in existence 1889–1899 in Van Alstyne, Texas) in 1894 and his medical degree from Bellevue Hospital Medical College in New York City (1897). He interned at Bellevue Hospital and studied in London and Boston before joining his oldest brother, Dr. Stephen Douglas Moore, in private practice in Van Alstyne. In 1908, Dr. Hugh Leslie Moore moved to Dallas to become the first Texas physician to specialize in the diseases of children. He served on the staffs of Bradford Memorial Hospital for Babies, Parkland Hospital, and Children's Medical Center. He was president of the Dallas County Medical Society in 1912. He married Lydia Ann Rebecca Bowen (1880–1975); they had two children. See *Alumni of the Medical Schools, New York University Alumni Catalogue, 1833–1907* (New York: General Alumni Society, 1908), 496; and "Dr. Hugh Leslie Moore's Services Scheduled Today," *Dallas Morning News*, January 21, 1950, 10.

43 Dr. Charles McDaniel Rosser (1862–1945) was born in Cuthbert, Randolph County, Georgia, as one of the eight children of Dr. Moses Franklin Rosser (1824–1897), a Methodist minister, and Julia Amelia Smith (1832–1917). The family moved to Texas in 1865. Charles graduated from East Texas Academic Institute in Leesburg, Camp County, Texas; taught school; read medicine under the direction of Dr. Edwin P. Becton of Sulphur Springs, Hopkins County, Texas; and earned his medical degree from the University of Louisville Medical Department (1888). He moved to Dallas in March 1889, edited the *Courier Record of Medicine*, and served as the Dallas city health officer (1891–1892). He was the surgeon of the Houston and Texas Central and Texas Trunk Railroads and a medical examiner for various life insurance companies. He helped found the University of Dallas Medical Department in 1900 and served as president of the Texas State Medical Association. He married

Elma Curtice (1867–1944) in 1890; they had two children. See "Dr. Chas. M. Rosser," in Ellis A. Davis and Edwin H. Grobe, *New Encyclopedia of Texas* (Dallas, TX: Texas Development Bureau, 1926), 2:1371; *Memorial and Biographical History of Ellis County, Texas* (Chicago, IL: Lewis Publishing Company, 1892), 668–69; John S. Fordtran, "Medicine in Dallas 100 Years Ago," *Proceedings of Baylor University Medical Center* 13, no.1 (January 2000): 34–44; "Well-Known Physician, Author Dies," *Dallas Morning News*, January 28, 1945, 1, 12; and Joan Jenkins Perez, "Charles McDaniel Rosser," *Handbook of Texas Online*, accessed August 19, 2018, https://tshaonline.org/handbook/online/articles/fro88.

44 An excerpt from Dr. Flexner's rules for administering antimeningitis serum in the treatment of cerebrospinal meningitis follows: "1. When lumbar puncture is performed in a suspicious case, be prepared to inject the serum. If the cerebrospinal fluid withdrawn is cloudy, make the injection of the serum immediately and without waiting for a bacteriological examination. The next doses of the serum are to be given only if diplococcus intracellularis has been demonstrated. 2. Always withdraw as much cerebrospinal fluid as possible at each puncture and inject full doses of the serum. Thirty cubic centimeters of serum should be injected in every instance in which this quantity of fluid or less has been removed, unless a distinctly abnormal sense of resistance in the spinal cord is encountered after as much serum has been injected as fluid has been removed. When the amount of fluid withdrawn exceeds 30 cubic centimeters, introduce a large quantity of serum—up to 45 cubic centimeters, or even more." For the rest of the rules, see "Physicians Appoint Special Committees to Present Hospital Removal to Other Organizations," *Dallas Morning News*, January 3, 1912, 4; and Charles Hunter Dunn, "The Serum Treatment of Epidemic Cerebrospinal Meningitis," *Journal of the American Medical Association* 51, no. 1 (July 4, 1908): 15–21.

45 Dr. Emile A. Aronson (1863–1942) was born in Mitau (near Riga), Latvia, as one of the three sons of Herman Aronson (1831–1893) and Annette Levit. He studied medicine in several European universities and immigrated to the United States in 1890. He arrived in Dallas at an unknown time to start a practice in general medicine. He served as the vice president of the Dallas County Medical Society and vice president of the Alexander Kohut Lodge No. 247, Order of B'rith Abraham, a Hebrew organization. He married Hattie Loeb (1869–1951); they had one child. He died of diabetes and renal insufficiency

at the age of seventy-nine years. See "E. Aronson, Pioneer Dallas Physician, Dies," *Dallas Morning News*, July 15, 1942, 7.

46 Dr. John M. Neel (1863–1921) was born in Morgantown, Butler County, Kentucky, as one of the eight children of Margaret Jane Brown (1838–1902) and James F. Neel (1832–1867), a farmer. He earned his medical degree from Memphis (Tennessee) Hospital Medical College in 1888 and moved to Texas, first settling in Windom, Fannin County, and then moving to Bonham, Fannin County. He once held the position of Fannin county health officer. He moved to Dallas in 1908, where he served as president of the Dallas County Medical Association. He married Francis W. Wood (1871–1940) in 1888; their two children died in infancy. See "Dr. John M. Neel, Local Physician, Dies Saturday," *Dallas Morning News*, March 20, 1921, 4; and "Deaths," *Journal of the American Medical Association* 76, no. 18 (April 30, 1921): 1,262.

47 "Situation at Clarksville," *Dallas Morning News*, January 4, 1912, 14.

48 "Mayor Asks Citizens to Cleanse Premises; Dr. A. Sophian, New York, Will Study Dallas Conditions; Four Deaths of Meningitis Reported to Health Officer, One Being a White Person," *Dallas Morning News*, January 4, 1912, 14; and "Believe Meningitis Situation Improved; Four Deaths and Five New Cases in Dallas Thursday; City Is Disinfecting Streets and Offers to Make Free Pathological Examination for Patients," *Dallas Morning News*, January 5, 1912, 3.

49 Dr. Alfred Edward Thayer (1863–1953) was born in Yonkers, Westchester County, New York, as the youngest of the four children of Stephen Howard Thayer Sr. (1811–1890), a lawyer, and Elizabeth Russell Cox (born in 1829). Dr. Thayer attended Barton Academy in Mobile, Mobile County, Alabama; studied for three years at Williams College (1878–1881) in Williamstown, Berkshire County, Massachusetts; earned his medical degree from the College of Physicians and Surgeons of New York City (1884); served a residency at the New York and St. Luke's Hospital (1884–1886); traveled studied pathology in Europe; completed a fellowship in pathology at Johns Hopkins University (1889–1890); taught anatomy at Yale College (1890–1891); and became a professor of pathology and bacteriology at West Virginia University (1899–1900). He left West Virginia University to join the fledgling Cornell University Medical College in New York City, where he served as an assistant

instructor in gross [sic] pathology (1900–1903). During that time, he also served as a vital statistician with the New York City Health Department and an acting assistant surgeon in the United States Marine Hospital Service. In 1902, while at Cornell University Medical College, he published *Compend of Special Pathology* (Philadelphia, PA: P. Blakiston's Son and Company, 1902). It is likely that Dr. Thayer taught Abraham Sophian during Abraham's first year of medical school at Cornell University Medical College (1902–1903). Dr. Thayer left New York City in 1903 to join the pathology department at the University of Texas Medical Branch at Galveston (1903–1907), where he published *Compend of Pathology: General and Special; A Students' Manual in One Volume* (Philadelphia, PA: P. Blakiston's Son and Company, 1906). He worked to find the cause of yellow fever and believed, erroneously, that he had identified a bacterial cause. He resigned from the University of Texas Medical Branch in 1907 because of his wife's health and moved to Florida before joining the pathology department at the Baylor University College of Medicine in Dallas (1908–1912). On July 1, 1912, he left Dallas for Mobile, Mobile County, Alabama, to chair the pathology department at the University of Alabama Medical Department. He spent the remainder of his career at the University of Alabama in Mobile. His first wife was May Cahoone Kinney (1869–1909). His second wife was Elizabeth Carrie Starr (1893–1977); he had no children. He died at the age of ninety years near Mobile, Alabama. See "The University," *Houston Post*, October 4, 1903, 2; "One of Medical Faculty Quits," *Houston Post*, August 13, 1907, 7; *Cactus, University of Texas Yearbook, 1906* (Austin, TX: von Boeckmann–Jones Company, 1906), 329; "University Notes," *Wheeling Daily Intelligencer* (Wheeling, West Virginia), November 20, 1899, 4; George J. Rice, G. Weldon Tilley, and Peter A. Dysert, "A History of Pathology and Laboratory Medicine at Baylor University Medical Center," *Proceedings of Baylor University Medical Center* 17, no. 1 (January 2004): 42–55; "Medical News, Alabama," *Journal of the American Medical Association* 68, no. 26 (June 29, 1912): 2,037; Marilyn Miller Baker, *The History of Pathology in Texas* (Austin, TX: Texas Society of Pathologists, 1996); and Walter Henrik Moursund, *A History of Baylor University, College of Medicine, 1900–1953* (Houston, TX: Gulf Printing Company, 1956), 50, 205.

50 In 1903, the University of Dallas Medical Department associated with Baylor University in Waco and changed its name to the Baylor

University College of Medicine. Baylor University was located in Waco, while Baylor University College of Medicine was located in the Ramseur Science Hall in Dallas in 1912. See Walter Henrik Moursund, *A History of Baylor University, College of Medicine, 1900–1953* (Houston, TX: Gulf Printing Company, 1956).

CHAPTER 4

HELP FROM A NEW YORK CITY MENINGITIS EXPERT, JANUARY 1912

D r. Abraham Sophian arrived at the Texas and Pacific Railway Depot in Dallas, Texas, at eight thirty o'clock on the cold, rainy evening of Friday, January 5, 1912.[1] Dr. Leake, Dr. Nash, Dr. Neel, Dr. Rosser, Dr. John Oliver McReynolds,[2] Dr. Turner, Dr. Fisher, Dr. William Alexander Boyce,[3] Dr. Manton Marble Carrick,[4] and Dr. Cary met him at the train station. They observed a tall, thin, long-limbed, mustachioed man wearing a dark bowler hat, a long dark wool coat, and dark brown boots. He was affable but little inclined to talk and eager to begin work.[5] They congratulated him on his arrival exactly on time and promised the cooperation of Dallas physicians in his study of the ongoing cerebrospinal meningitis epidemic. Dr. Steiner had not arrived in Dallas from his office in the Texas State Capitol in Austin. Earlier that day, he had announced that he would be traveling to Dallas to make his own assessment of the Dallas cerebrospinal meningitis situation.[5]

The group of Dallas physicians accompanied Dr. Sophian from the train station to the Oriental Hotel[6] and crowded into his hotel room to hold a brief meeting. Dr. Nash reviewed the

Dallas meningitis case and death counts, current as of that evening (Friday, January 5, 1912), as follows:

October 1911—one case, one death,

November 1911—nine cases, six deaths,

December 1911—seventy-one cases, twenty-seven deaths, and

January 1–5 (inclusive), 1912—forty-eight cases, nineteen deaths.

The total number of cases since the onset of the cerebrospinal meningitis epidemic in October 1911 was 129, with 53 deaths. Dr. Nash stopped talking, turned to look at Dr. Sophian, and waited. Dr. Sophian spoke plainly and openly. He confirmed "his readiness for immediate work and his intention of remaining in the city for definite results in the abating of the disease." He explained,

> The germ of meningitis, as other germs, we have with us always. Climatic conditions which decrease the vitality of the body make the physical man more easily accessible to its attack ... The disease is mildly contagious, rather than decidedly infectious, and the only danger is from contact with persons who have the disease, or persons who have been in contact with such persons, and not fumigated. Healthy persons may take the germ to a body whose condition invites the work of the germ. It is not an air disease, and danger is not to be anticipated from the blowing around of the germ.[1]

Dr. Sophian praised Dr. Nash's decision to close the Dallas public schools for at least another week and cautioned people against going to any places "where crowds are herded together." He said that the six Dallas hospitals "[could and should] take the cases of meningitis as fearlessly as they took cases of typhoid fever" and that the "use of the sprays and disinfectants and the washing of the streets and sidewalks" was good policy generally. He complimented the Dallas Board of Health for recommending sanitary measures throughout the city, adding, "There was a need for "great precaution and use of the ordinary means of sanitation and cleanliness." Dr. Sophian added, "People having good homes should stay in them as much as possible, avoiding crowds, as it was from persons the germs are accumulated." Furthermore, he said there was no cause for a general alarm over the Dallas cerebrospinal meningitis epidemic, which was not worse than in other cities and towns of the state.[1]

Dr. Sophian expressed his gratitude for the offer made by pathologists at both Southwestern University Medical Department[7] and Baylor University College of Medicine to provide laboratory support in the care of cerebrospinal meningitis patients in Dallas. These services included microscopical analysis of cerebrospinal and other fluids obtained from afflicted patients, culture of the cerebrospinal and other fluids to verify the microscopical diagnoses, and possibly using cultures to produce biological products.[1]

Dr. Sophian advised against the intraspinal administration of antimeningitis serum by persons unfamiliar with the technique and announced his intention to conduct demonstrations on the technique for all physicians who desired training in that skill.[1] He said that the antimeningitis serum could reduce the lethality [case fatality rate] of the disease from 80 percent to 20 to 30 percent of afflicted individuals.[8] Dr. Sophian then advised the group of physicians in his hotel room to have themselves vaccinated against the disease.[1] By *vaccinated* at this time, he meant receipt of a subcutaneous injection of ten cubic centimeters of antimeningitis serum, which, he said, provided temporary protection against contracting cerebrospinal meningitis from afflicted patients.[9]

Instead of going to bed after the brief meeting, Dr. Sophian, Dr. Nash, Dr. Leake, and a few other physicians visited a sixty-year-old cerebrospinal meningitis patient in her Dallas residence. Dr. Sophian set up and operated a blood pressure measurement device attached to the woman's arm. When Dr. Sophian was ready, the patient's physician performed a lumbar puncture procedure and withdrew forty cubic centimeters of cerebrospinal fluid. The physician then began pushing about forty cubic centimeters of antimeningitis serum through the barrel of the syringe attached to the needle entering the spinal canal. Dr. Sophian soon announced that the patient's systolic blood pressure had dropped from 105 to 75 millimeters of mercury.

The Dallas physicians surrounding the patient's bed gasped, as they never before had monitored blood pressure during an intraspinal serum infusion and were unaware of the potential effects of this procedure on a patient's blood pressure. Previously, they had attributed a patient's troubles during or after a treatment with intraspinal antimeningitis serum to the patient's underlying disease process, not to the lumbar puncture procedure. Dr. Sophian counseled that blood pressure monitoring improved the safety of the lumbar puncture procedure by providing valuable readings useable by the physician to control both the rate and amount of antimeningitis serum infusion. After the demonstration, Dr. Leake and Dr. Nash escorted Dr. Sophian back to the Oriental Hotel and made plans to meet with him again in the morning.

At seven thirty o'clock on Saturday morning, January 6, 1912, Dr. Sophian, Dr. Leake, and Dr. Nash revisited the patient whose blood pressure had dropped during the previous night's infusion of antimeningitis serum. She was much improved. Dr. Sophian, Dr. Leake, Dr. Nash, and a few other physicians then visited other afflicted patients in their homes, including one woman whose physician infused eighty cubic centimeters of antimeningitis serum. Her blood pressure, monitored by Dr. Sophian, dropped so rapidly that her physician thought she had died. She was not dead, but Dr. Sophian again cautioned the physician to slow down the rate of antimeningitis serum infusion, to consider using a smaller volume of antimeningitis serum, and to use the blood pressure device measurements as a guide to regulate the procedure.[10]

At the end of the rounds made to patients' residences that Saturday morning, January 6, 1912, Dr. Sophian returned to the Oriental Hotel to present two talks—one to the Dallas Medical Lunch Club[10] at one o'clock in the afternoon and the other to the Dallas County Medical

Society in the evening.[11] One hundred fifty physicians attended the Dallas Medical Lunch Club meeting in the ladies' ordinary[12] room of the Oriental Hotel. Dr. Steiner was among the physicians. He attended the session on the condition that no one should call upon him, emphasizing that he was at the meeting to investigate and observe, not to speak.[11] Mayor Holland also was in the audience. The attendance of out-of-town physicians so exceeded expectations that many physicians ate their lunch in the hotel hallway.[11]

At the meeting, Dr. Clay Johnson[13] of Fort Worth motioned for a vote of thanks to the group of Dallas physicians who were responsible for bringing Dr. Sophian to Dallas. Dr. Sophian, they noted, as a representative of Dr. Flexner, came without expense to the city of Dallas to study the cerebrospinal meningitis situation, visit patients, and instruct physicians in the technique of intraspinal antimeningitis serum administration.[11]

Mayor Holland expressed "his pleasure at the presence of so many doctors from so many places." He added, "Dr. Sophian has already said to me that his treatment is such in Dallas and the people have been so kind, that it would take but little urging for him to desert Little New York and to make his home in Big Dallas."[11]

Dr. Nash announced that Dr. Sophian would be conducting a clinic to demonstrate the technique for administering intraspinal antimeningitis serum in the basement of St. Paul's Sanitarium[14] at three-thirty that same afternoon (Saturday, January 6, 1912). Dr. Nash urged all interested physicians to attend. He further explained that he had intended to send small groups of physicians to observe Dr. Sophian's technique in the residences of cerebrospinal meningitis patients. However, the patients whom Dr. Sophian already had visited had become so overwhelmed by the presence of so many physicians that Dr. Nash had decided not to carry forward that method of physician education.[11]

Mr. Alexander Sanger,[15] representing the Dallas Chamber of Commerce, next said, "We are appreciative of the Rockefeller Institute and the backing that has sent this man [referring to Dr. Sophian] to study in our city and to aid in the advancement of science as related to this disease. He deserves success and for his own good and for ours, we hope he will succeed. We are all ready to do what we can to aid his research." Mr. Sanger continued, "With such representatives as we have here, and they tell me it is like a meeting of the State Medical Association, the benefit from the expert's visit will be far and wide. When he knows us better, he will admit that both the city and the state health boards are in good hands. He can help us and we will help him."[11]

Dr. Leake then introduced Dr. Sophian, saying, "It is splendid to see so many representative doctors from all over North Texas who have come to see and hear this man. For all his quiet and modest bearing, he is a distinguished man and not a faker." Dr. Leake spoke about Dr. Sophian's professional background.

> [Dr. Sophian] is a graduate of the College of the City of New York, of Cornell University Medical College, intern and house surgeon for Mount Sinai Hospital [New York City], one of the most famous in the country, successor to Dr. Flexner, as City Pathologist for New York City and co-laborer with Dr. Flexner in the investigations and excellent work of the Rockefeller Institute ... This young man has come here in the interest of science and of medicine and deserves your welcome and your cooperation, for it is upon such work as this that much of the happiness and health of the people depends. It is to be hoped, and I believe it will be realized, that you will assist in every possible way in his work.[11]

Dr. Sophian acknowledged the audience's warm reception. He had to be encouraged to speak a little louder, though "the house was very quiet for his words." He started again, saying, "Work is far more pleasing to me than talk. My end of medical practice is the working end. I have heard much of Southern hospitality, but what I heard is not to be compared with what I have experienced since I got to Dallas. I hope by tonight to have my message more systematized than I can give you now."[11] He continued,

Just a few words about the medical and the
biological aspects and the general motive of the
disease, meningitis: first, the susceptibility, then
the organization of the germ. Though the germs
are probably present all the time, there are months
on months without an epidemic of the disease ...
Meningitis and other cerebral diseases are affected by
weather and by physical condition and it is necessary
to impress this upon the people. The control of the
epidemic depends upon the cooperation of the people,
who must accommodate themselves by clothing
and other carefulness to the changes of climatic
conditions, adopting proper hygienic measures.[11]

Dr. Sophian added that the investigation that lay ahead
was particularly concerned with curing persons infected with
cerebrospinal meningitis and the development of measures to prevent
the spread of the meningococcus among the people. He explained,

Those who are sick may infect the well, so that healthy
persons may carry the germ in the nose and throat, and
while not themselves affected by them, may turn them
over, unwittingly, to others whose physical conditions
and low vitality invite the development of the disease.
Thus, the effect may be upon the entire community or
spread even further ... Sudden changes in the seasons
or the climatic conditions or in the vitality of persons
tend to increase the liability to contagion. But, dealing
first with the healthy, it is advisable to have strict
quarantine of the cases of disease, concentrating the
cases, if possible, for care and treatment. It is then
advisable to prevent the healthy from carrying the
germs to those liable to infection.[11]

Dr. Sophian asked the audience, "Who is a carrier?" He
answered his own question: "It is hard to determine. If this

could be ascertained, it could lead to the immediate control of the epidemic. It is necessary to learn, as well as we can, who are carriers, for the protection of the well. For safety, therefore, it is best to treat every person as if he is a carrier, to attempt the proper preventing treatment upon everyone." He encouraged spraying the nose and mouth with an antiseptic and taking an oral dose of urotropin.[9,16] He reemphasized the need for active community treatment to prevent the spread of cerebrospinal meningitis. This approach, he noted, was similar to the approach used to prevent typhoid fever—that is, with a typhoid vaccine.[17]

Next, Dr. Sophian spoke briefly about the intraspinal technique of administering antimeningitis serum. "Care must be exercised and only competent hands should administer" the antimeningitis serum into the spinal canal. The antimeningitis serum should be administered as early as possible in the clinical course of the disease—the first day, if possible. Early administration of the antimeningitis serum depends on 1) cultivating an early suspicion of a developing case of cerebrospinal meningitis and 2) performing a lumbar puncture procedure to confirm the diagnosis. Dr. Sophian added, "The lumbar puncture should be made and spinal fluid extracted for immediate pathological examination. Better to err on the wrong side than to lose a chance of doing a good thing for the patient. The lumbar puncture will do no harm, in any case."[11]

Dr. Sophian cautioned against administering too much intraspinal antimeningitis serum too rapidly, which produced "many bad results." A better way of judging the amount of cerebrospinal fluid to withdraw, the amount of antimeningitis serum to infuse, and the rates of each was to monitor the patient's blood pressure. Dr. Sophian noted, "The removal of the fluid will cause a drop in the [blood] pressure ... Sometimes [the drop] is from 5 to 10 [millimeters of mercury]. Removal of large quantities may cause a change of 20 to 30 [millimeters of mercury]."[11]

Dr. Sophian noted that the antimeningitis serum should be of body warmth and could be infused by using either gravity pressure or a syringe. Ordinarily, the gravity method was the safest and best way because of the ever-present danger of adversely affecting the patient's blood pressure and heart functioning by manually pushing the serum through the barrel of a syringe into the inflamed meninges. The advantage of the gravity method was its amenability to regulating the rate of infusion, including stopping it altogether if needed. He acknowledged that in some instances, the syringe was necessary, as the gravity pressure could be insufficient to transfer the serum into the canal.[11]

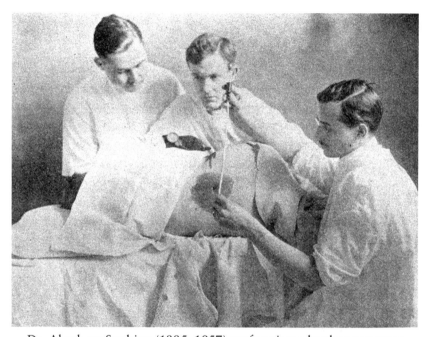

Dr. Abraham Sophian (1885–1957) performing a lumbar puncture procedure and infusion by gravity of Flexner antimeningitis serum, circa 1912–1913. The original caption accompanying the image is: "This picture illustrates the operation of lumbar puncture and the technique in injecting the antimeningitis serum. The patient is lying on his left side over the right flexing the hips on his abdomen and bending his head forward. The skin at the site of the operation has been painted with tincture of iodine. The site of the operation is draped off with sterile towels. The needle has been inserted at the level of the crest of the ileum, which is marked with tincture of iodine. The assistant at the head of the patient is taking blood pressure observations. The serum is being injected by gravity." The photographer is unknown. The image was scanned from Abraham Sophian, *Epidemic Cerebrospinal Meningitis* (St. Louis, MO: C. V. Mosby, 1913), 171.

In conclusion, Dr. Sophian said, "It is splendid to see so many of you here from so wide a territory. Already this serum is better known to you than to many in New York. There it is hard to introduce a thing. It is hard to get the practitioners together. You will be administering and getting results long before many of the New York physicians will have heard of the method."[11]

Following his talk to the Dallas Medical Lunch Club, Dr. Sophian conducted his intraspinal antimeningitis serum clinic in the basement of St. Paul's Sanitarium. Dr. Nash earlier had arranged for the transport from the City Hospital to St. Paul's Sanitarium of two African-American cerebrospinal meningitis patients under his care at the City Hospital.[18] A large number of physicians attended the clinic. An unknown number of them volunteered to receive a subcutaneous dose of antimeningitis serum as a preventive.[18] Dr. Nash removed the two patients from the premises immediately following the end of the clinic and disinfected the room in response to the urgent request of the Sisters of Charity of Saint Vincent de Paul, who administered the hospital.[19] The latter balked at allowing another cerebrospinal meningitis patient into their hospital, citing existing inpatients' concerns and the possibility of driving away people who needed hospitalization but would not seek it at St. Paul's Hospital because of the presence of cerebrospinal meningitis inpatients.[20] Administrators of the other private hospitals in Dallas responded in like manner.

The same afternoon as Dr. Sophian's clinic, Mayor Holland convened a meeting of Dr. Leake, Dr. Nash, and Dr. Sophian to discuss a solution to the private hospitals' concerns over the admission of cerebrospinal meningitis patients. Mayor Holland proposed using the City Hospital's sixty-five beds exclusively for the care of cerebrospinal meningitis patients. Dr. Nash and Dr. Sophian were enthusiastic about the proposal. Dr. Nash would transfer all the existing patients at the City Hospital to the forty-bed Union Hospital north of Dallas. Although built as a contagious-diseases hospital, Union Hospital had contained no such patients for six months. In addition, it had been disinfected. Mayor Holland noted that, for the foreseeable future, the Dallas municipal government would reimburse the Dallas private hospitals for the admission and care of all new *non*-cerebrospinal meningitis patients who ordinarily would have received their care at the City Hospital.[20]

At the same meeting on Saturday, January 7, 1912, Mayor Holland and Dr. Leake asked Dr. Sophian to develop a set of precautionary and sanitary rules to control the spread of meningitis in Dallas. They planned to publish the list in the following day's (Sunday) edition of the *Dallas Morning News*. Dr. Sophian crafted the following ten rules, using his own words:

1. Have no dread of the disease, further than that which induces care in the condition of the health of the person, cleanliness of the body and of the premises.
2. Washing of streets and use of the disinfectant upon them are good general measures at any time. They are not particularly applicable to the prevention of meningitis.
3. Spray or gargle of the throat and nose with mild antiseptic agents are commended.
4. Isolation of the cases, quarantine as far as possible, and concentration to a treating place for care and separation from the well.
5. Care of the persons of healthy people, so that they may not become carriers of the germ to others whose condition incites the inroad of the disease.
6. Stay at home as much as possible, if home is a comfortable place. Avoid crowds, refrain from visiting unnecessarily the places where many persons gather, places of amusement, shows, and loitering places.
7. Use those sanitary measures for cleanliness, good at any time.
8. Use warm clothing when exposed to cold. Adapt the body, by use of proper agents, to changes in climatic conditions and to the rise and fall of the bodily vitality.

9. Where meningitis is suspected, have prompt diagnosis and pathological test. Disease does not necessarily mean death.
10. Be cheerful. Avoid gloomy talk of disease, even this disease. A bright disposition is good everywhere.[21]

At eight- o'clock on the evening of Saturday, January 6, 1912, Dr. Sophian spoke in the Oriental Hotel's ballroom to more than four hundred doctors of the Dallas County Medical Society.[22] Dr. John Caleb Erwin, the physician who had cared for the five McCallum family members afflicted with cerebrospinal meningitis in McKinney, Texas, in 1909 (see chapter 1), was in the audience. Dr. Sophian generally repeated the speech that he had given to the Dallas Medical Lunch Club earlier that day but provided additional details about a meningococcal vaccine as a means for stemming the spread of a cerebrospinal meningitis epidemic.

Dr. Sophian explained, "The ideal method [of controlling a cerebrospinal meningitis epidemic] is to produce immunes. The old menace to armies was typhoid fever.[23] By immunitization [sic], this danger has been eliminated." Two or three injections of a relatively small dose of vaccine some ten days apart would "prevent the development of a large case later." He acknowledged, "There will be slight temporary discomfort, maybe temporary disability, but the patient or person treated will be made immune." Dr. Sophian said that Texas had the chance to be the first to produce persons immune to cerebrospinal meningitis. He added, "I hope she will rise to the opportunity." While the experimental vaccine was under consideration, Dr. Sophian encouraged the contacts of cerebrospinal meningitis patients to receive a subcutaneous inoculation of a small dose of antimeningitis serum. He believed that "one small dose of serum will immunitize for a [at least a] few days." These inoculations, he added, could be repeated.[22]

Dr. Sophian's address aroused and evoked many questions from the audience. He listened to each question, took notes, moved to the next questioner, took notes on that questioner's question, and then answered all the questions at one time in a short final speech. He gave the following responses to the questions that he received: The efficacy of intraspinal antimeningitis serum was a certain matter and had been used successfully in thousands of cases. A physician who diagnosed a case early and administered the serum properly almost certainly would improve his patient's outcome. Physicians who administered the serum incorrectly could cause much harm to their patients. Urotropin was a useful precaution against the disease. Anesthetic use during a lumbar puncture procedure was not a good idea. The period of incubation of the disease was a variable, unknown quantity. A healthy meningococcal carrier might carry the germs for a long time and then contract the disease or give it to others.[22]

Dr. Sophian continued: Humans were almost the only carriers of meningococcal germs. Fresh air and sunshine quickly destroyed the germs. A person rarely contracted meningitis a second time after recovering from a first attack. Patients should not rush their convalescence after such sickness, even if they appeared and felt much better. Atmospheric conditions seemed to be the largest factor in meningitis epidemics. Administering antimeningitis serum to a person who did not have meningitis would cause no harm. The arrival of a large supply of antimeningitis serum (110 liters— enough for 3,500 doses[24]) from the Research Laboratory in New York City to Dallas was imminent. This amount was sufficient to supply the needs of Dallas and all other places in Texas where there was cerebrospinal meningitis.[22]

Dr. Cary thanked Dr. Sophian for his excellent talk and his efforts to improve conditions in Dallas and thanked Dr. Flexner (in absentia) for sending Dr. Sophian to Dallas. Dr. Turner, Dr. Thayer, Dr. John Spencer Davis,[25] and Dr. John Caleb Erwin (of McKinney, Texas) each briefly spoke. Dr. Erwin declared that there was "no question of the effectiveness of the serum, if administered early." He shared his experience during the 1909 cerebrospinal meningitis outbreak in McKinney, where the mortality was 100 percent before he used the antimeningitis serum and 20 percent after he used it. He said there had been no bad aftereffects from the administration of the antimeningitis serum in any of his cerebrospinal meningitis patients.[22]

On Sunday, January 7, 1912, Dr. Sophian and members of the Dallas Board of Health visited homebound patients with cerebrospinal meningitis all day. Dr. Leake issued a long statement that evening, saying, "It is very important in the present situation that the citizens of Dallas read carefully the rules laid down by Dr. Sophian as published in Sunday morning's *Dallas News* [*sic*], and observe these rules closely. This will be the most efficient way of stamping out the epidemic and at the present is the only known way of doing so."[26] Dr. Leake added,

> It has been decided by the [Dallas] Board of Health that it will be impossible for Dr. Sophian to see all of the cases in the city. He will not be able to see even all of the charity cases, so that it has been determined to appoint several physicians [Drs. Neel, Turner, and Carrick, the "diagnosticians"] to assist him. These physicians will be sent out to see many of these cases in order to make the diagnosis before the patients are transferred to Parkland Hospital [the City Hospital], which has been set aside solely for the treatment of meningitis cases.[26]

By concentrating all cerebrospinal meningitis patients in a single treatment center, said Dr. Leake, Dr. Sophian's work would be facilitated by accurately diagnosing and treating a larger number of patients.[26] Dr. Leake added that Dr. Sophian had traveled to Dallas at the "instance of the Rockefeller Institute to prosecute his investigations of the disease." The institute had provided for ten to fifteen days in Texas, making no provision for Dr. Sophian to stay longer than that. He was in the employ of that institute, said Dr. Leake, and for Dallas to retain his services after the time limit set would require Dr. Sophian to temporarily sever his connection with the institute. The Dallas Board of Health and the mayor wanted him to remain in Dallas as long as they thought his services were necessary—a month, six weeks, or two months. Dr.

Leake proclaimed, "Tonight, arrangements with that end in view were perfected."[26]

Dr. Leake further explained that, as of Monday, January 8, 1912, the City Hospital had been cleared of all other cases and transformed into a hospital exclusively for the care of cerebrospinal meningitis patients. As fast as the cases developed, he noted, they would be moved into this hospital, which had been fumigated, disinfected, and placed in first-class order for the purpose, including provisions for proper heating by steam and additional stoves. He also had secured nurses for the hospital. Dr. Leake denied that any legal steps had been taken to force people to go to the hospital, saying, "I don't think the situation demands that now. We are not having the trouble we expected in moving the patients. As soon as they are told that it is better for them to be there and that the expert cannot go to many cases, and, in some instances, will not treat them at their homes at all, they are ready to move."[26]

Dr. Leake concluded, "We are placarding the houses and quarantining them. Fumigation is just as thorough as we can make it. We find it almost impossible to quarantine as thoroughly as we would like to. Too much stress cannot be laid on the injunction to the people not to visit houses that have been quarantined and upon the inmates of those houses not to leave."[26]

That same Sunday evening, January 7, 1912, Dr. Sophian issued a public correction about his employment. The Research Laboratory of the New York City Health Department, not the Rockefeller Institute for Medical Research, employed him. Furthermore, the Research Laboratory, not the Rockefeller Institute, had sent him to Dallas.[26]

On Sunday, January 7, 1912, Dr. Steiner, now back in Austin, mailed to all the city and county health officers in Texas a circular articulating the Texas State Board of Health's new rules governing the statewide cerebrospinal meningitis situation. The circular instructed health officers and physicians to isolate and place in absolute quarantine all cases of cerebrospinal meningitis; close public schools and discourage public gatherings on appearance of the disease in a community; clean and disinfect sidewalks, streets, and alleys, as carriers conveyed the disease by means of the nose and throat secretions; enforce the anti-spitting ordinance; advise the use of an antiseptic spray in the nose and throat; and disinfect all streetcars and public conveyances.[27]

Also, on Sunday, January 7, 1912, Dr. Steiner scheduled a meeting of the Texas State Board of Health for Wednesday, January 10, 1912, to be held not in Austin but at the Oriental Hotel in Dallas. The purpose of this meeting was to "carefully review the entire meningitis situation in the state and suggest measures for its extermination."[28] He also reported that Dr. Key had returned from Emory, Rains County, Texas, with live meningococci to use in experiments in the state pure food department laboratory in a room in the Texas State Capitol building in Austin. The *Dallas Morning News* confirmed that Dr. Key was maintaining a "regular germ culture, where he is making a special study of meningitis, typhoid, and other germs."[28]

On Monday evening, January 8, 1912, Dr. Leake issued another statement to advise that "all people who can, ought to be 'vaccinated' against meningitis." This treatment, explained Dr. Leake, consisted of an injection of subcutaneous antimeningitis serum, which a family's physician could administer. Dr. Sophian, Dr. Nash, and other physicians at the City Hospital already had received a subcutaneous injection of antimeningitis serum. The treatment was not expensive, was not very painful, and left no evil after-effects. "While such 'vaccination' did not give absolute immunity, so far as was known, it was thought that should a person so immunized contract the disease, it would be much milder and respond to treatment more readily than otherwise." The procedure consisted of the injection of a small amount of the antimeningitis serum underneath the skin in a manner similar to inoculation with diphtheria antitoxin.[29]

On Monday and Tuesday, January 8 and 9, 1912, Dr. Nash and Dr. Sophian admitted fifteen cerebrospinal meningitis patients to the City Hospital. Dr. Turner, Dr. Carrick, and Dr. Neel meanwhile established a cerebrospinal meningitis headquarters in rooms eight and ten of the Oriental Hotel to receive reports by telephone of persons possibly infected with cerebrospinal meningitis in Dallas. These three physicians visited the potential victims and transferred probable cases to the City Hospital. Soon overwhelmed with the number of requests, the three physicians urged people with family physicians to call them first and instruct them to call headquarters for possible cases of cerebrospinal meningitis.[29] The three physicians would then take over.

Dr. Nash announced on Wednesday, January 10, 1912, that the City Hospital held nineteen patients with confirmed cerebrospinal meningitis. Furthermore, he had received a shipment of fifty liters of antimeningitis serum, sufficient for 1,000 injections, to add to the supply already on hand. He expected another shipment from the Research Laboratory in New York City on Thursday night, January 11, 1912.[30] Dr. Nash also said,

> I feel confident that the situation is considerably improved and that we have it well in hand. The cases of meningitis are coming to the hospital nicely and we are in position to take care of those who come. So far, we have not lost a case that came to the hospital. It is unlikely that we can save everyone who comes, but so far, we have not had a death in the hospital from meningitis ... The City Hospital now has only meningitis cases and the entire hospital will be used for treatment of this disease exclusively. We have a full corps of doctors [the hospital steward[31] and six hospital interns[32]] and nurses [two head nurses and many ward nurses[33]] in attendance and Dr. Sophian and I will be here all the time to give attention to the meningitis patients.[30]

Dr. Nash then clarified Dr. Leake's earlier statement on vaccination as follows:

> Please let it be understood that the treatment Dr. Sophian and I took was not vaccination. The

injection of the serum was merely an immunizing dose and was not in any sense a vaccination. We merely injected a small amount of the serum under the skin, not into the spinal column. While we cannot say positively what results will be accomplished, we hope that the treatment will protect us against taking the disease.[30]

On Wednesday, January 10, 1912, Dr. Steiner convened his meeting of the Texas State Board of Health in the Oriental Hotel in Dallas.[34] Four board members—Dr. Hugh Love McLaurin[35] of Dallas, Dr. Benjamin Milton Worsham[36] of El Paso, Dr. Sidney Mainer Lister[37] of Houston, and Dr. Beall of Fort Worth—attended the meeting. The fifth board member, Dr. Ashley Wilson Fly[38] of Galveston, was absent.

The board passed a resolution complimenting the Dallas Board of Health on the efficient manner in which it and the physicians of Dallas were handling the cerebrospinal meningitis situation in their city. In addition, the board reported receiving authorization to secure a supply of the approved New York Board of Health antimeningitis serum for distribution throughout the state. Furthermore, the board advised health officials to invite and encourage the cooperation of African-American physicians,[39] including Dr. Benjamin Rufus Bluitt and Dr. David W. Shields,[40] in treating African-American afflicted with cerebrospinal meningitis. The board also urged county attorneys to prosecute all unauthorized persons prescribing for sick people and anyone delaying a proper diagnosis and treatment of cerebrospinal meningitis; advised closing public schools and discouraging public gatherings when the disease appeared in a community; and emphasized the importance of the use of antiseptic nose and throat sprays.[34]

After meeting at the Oriental Hotel, the members of the Texas State Board of Health attended a clinic held for them by Dr. Sophian and Dr. Nash at the City Hospital. Soon after his return to Dallas, Dr. Steiner remarked, "Dallas is the only place where the disease seems to be at a standstill."[41] Austin had its own issues relating to the cerebrospinal meningitis epidemic, even though no cases had yet appeared there. Fifty families (mostly women and children) from points in North Texas had migrated to Austin to seek a temporary residence and a second large group of families passing through Austin was on its way to San Antonio, where the disease also had not yet appeared.[42]

On Wednesday, January 10, 1912, the Associated Press, a not-for-profit news agency headquartered in New York City, published a story that alleged that Dr. Sophian had opted to remain in Dallas to help combat cerebrospinal meningitis even after learning that his mother was dying in New York City. Many of the newspapers throughout the United States that were linked to the Associated Press published the story.[43] Dr. Sophian was so busy caring for the influx of cerebrospinal meningitis patients to the City Hospital that he remained mute to the story.

On Friday, January 12, 1912, at noon in the Oriental Hotel, Drs. Sophian and Nash provided a cerebrospinal meningitis update for over one hundred attendees of the Dallas Medical Lunch Club.[44] Dr. Sophian described the imminent new program to establish and maintain an improved quarantine for persons who had been exposed to cerebrospinal meningitis. Beginning Saturday, January 13, 1912, a team of fourth-year medical students would visit all the residences where cerebrospinal meningitis had appeared. Each medical student would carry with him a satchel containing supplies, including microscope slides, sterile swabs in tubes, a flask of sheep's serum glucose broth, a flask of alcohol, an alcohol lamp, Petri dishes with adhesive straps, and a notebook.

The purpose of the medical-student visits was to obtain nose and throat specimens to conduct tests for the presence of meningococci. The medical students were trained to swab the noses and throats of the contacts, make smears of the specimen on glass slides, inoculate the culture tubes of sheep's serum glucose broth with the ends of the swabs, and return the culture tubes to Dr. Thayer in the Ramseur Science Hall of Baylor University College of Medicine in Dallas. The exposed persons were to be quarantined in their residences until the tests of their nasal and throat secretions, performed in Dr. Thayer's laboratory, were negative, proving that each exposed person was not a healthy carrier of the cerebrospinal meningitis germ.[44]

Dr. Sophian next stressed that contacts of cerebrospinal meningitis victims should be immunized with a dose of subcutaneous antimeningitis serum, adding,

> I think that I warded off one case of meningitis this way. The patient had all of the symptoms, but after being immunized did not develop the disease. Ten cubic centimeters is usually enough for this kind of dose.[45] There is practically no danger in the treatment. When one takes the treatment, there is liable to be serum sickness,[46] but this is of no great consequence.[45]

Dr. Sophian did not advise the use generally of subcutaneous antimeningitis serum in the population, as there was an insufficient amount of antimeningitis serum available to immunize the 92,000 residents of Dallas. Dr. Sophian concluded, "Dr. Nash and I have decided to conserve, in so far as is possible, the serum where a large quantity is likely to be needed. I would advise the use for immunization where there has been direct exposure to a bad case of meningitis, but I would not advise the use generally."[45]

When an audience member asked Dr. Sophian whether or not meningitis was contagious, Dr. Sophian replied, "It is infectious. Personally, I have never been able to get the difference between infectious and contagious." In reply to a question about placarding houses, he said, "The health department is requiring all houses where meningitis develops to be placarded and given circulars for the care of the premises and persons thereon. This issuance of directions is the next best thing to putting a man outside of the house to enforce absolute quarantine ... Unless conditions become very bad, it would hardly be practical to put guards out."[45]

Dr. Thomas J. Crowe,[47] a homeopathic[48] physician and a member of the Texas State Board of Medical Examiners, next presented Dr. Sophian with a Texas state medical license that qualified him to practice medicine and surgery in the state of Texas.[49] Dr. Crowe then launched into the following, unexpected invective:

> It isn't often that the State of Texas is forced to call in outside aid to take care of any health situation that arises, because we have about as good physicians here as are to be found anywhere. However, it seems that this is one instance in which we have got into trouble. The Dallas physicians have in this meningitis situation jumped from one extreme to the other; from the extreme of indifference to a condition of frenzied panic.[44]

Dr. Crowe continued,

> Meningitis has been in Dallas since Oct. 1, but there was very little said about it and very little attention paid until a prominent person died [Mr. Flateau?]. Then there came a frenzy of interest. Where the infection comes from we know nothing. The disease springs up in a night, appearing here and there, at widely separated places and from no apparent cause. What we should have done was to have been more careful from the start. We should have given more attention to conditions early in the appearance of the disease here.[44]

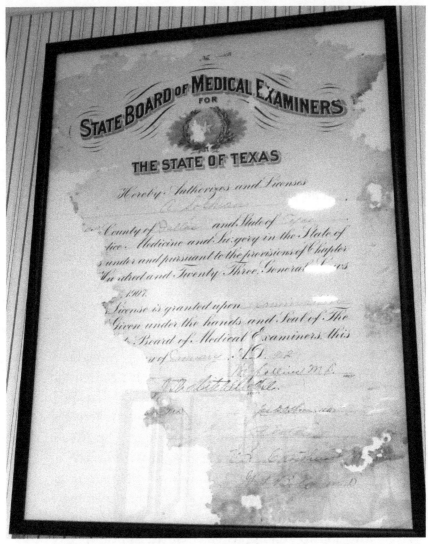

Dr. Abraham Sophian's Texas medical license from the Texas State Board of Medical Examiners, January, 1912. The document is in the Dr. Abraham Sophian Archive. Photographer: M. R. O'Leary, 2018.

Dr. Crowe's remarks riled Dr. Nash, who remonstrated,

> If one will take the trouble to read the health code of Texas—I have read it a whole lot—they will find that spinal meningitis is not a quarantinable disease.

However, in emergencies, we can take steps that are necessary to control the disease. No man can take radical steps, such as have been necessary here, without being backed up by not only the physicians, but the citizens of Dallas.

Dr. Nash continued,

I have known of every case of meningitis that has been in Dallas. I diagnosed the first case that appeared here. Certain people tried to sit down on me and said that I was radical; that I was mistaken about my diagnosis. It's a whole lot easier to sit on the housetop and tell how a trench ought to be dug than to get down in the trenches and dig. While Dr. Sophian and I are working 20 hours a day to try and stamp out meningitis, a few others are getting around and doing the shouting. I think, though, that the people know who is doing the real work. We are doing the best we can. Realizing that I'm a comparatively young man, I conferred a week ago with older heads about this situation. They told me that we didn't have so much meningitis here.[44]

Dr. Nash added,

Personally, I don't see anything in present conditions to bring about a panicky feeling. The records of the health department, showing every case of meningitis that has been in Dallas, are open to the public. The newspapers have printed the facts in regard to the situation. Some of the papers have seen fit to comment on these facts, but they alone are responsible for such comments.

He concluded,

> Let physicians urge on patients who haven't the best
> of comforts and conveniences in their homes to go
> to the City Hospital; then, the house where the case
> originates can be thoroughly disinfected, so other
> members of the family can go back there without
> fear of contracting the disease and the patient
> personally will get better treatment. The physicians
> of the city are cooperating wonderfully in this work
> and I feel that I can work better because of this
> knowledge that they are back of us.[44]

On the same Friday, January 12, 1912, that Dr. Sophian and
Dr. Nash were speaking to the Dallas Medical Lunch Club, the
Dallas Morning News published an article[50] about another person's
opinion of the cerebrospinal meningitis epidemic in Dallas. His
name was Erskine Horton Roach.[51] He was a Dallas resident, the
manager of a wholesale grocery business, and a major in the US
Army. It is unknown whether Major Roach and Dr. Crowe were
friends. Major Roach lectured,

It is about time call the meningitis epidemic off, if not to the
interest of business and the general comfort of the people, at least
on the score of common sense. According to the published statistics,
we have had about 185 cases of meningitis in the city in four
months, and we have forty or fifty cases at this time. According to
Webster's dictionary, epidemic means "common to, or affecting at
the same time a large number in a community; spreading widely,
attacking many persons at the same time, generally prevailing;
affecting a great many as an epidemic disease." Many is defined
by Webster as "a large or considerable number."

He continued,

> Now, I submit that 185 cases of any kind of disease,
> in the course of four months in a community of

100,000, do not come up to the lexicographer's idea of an epidemic. But whether they do or do not, the death rate has never been during the four months, nor is it now, greater than normal. And, I believe, physicians are agreed that the death rate is higher among meningitis patients than among those affected with any other disease. There are no doubt, in the city, more than fifty persons down with any of several diseases, but we do not hear that any of these are epidemic.

He added,

The exaggerated reports which have been authoritatively sent out are hurting the city. A New York man who arrived in Dallas today was very much surprised to find business going on in the normal way, and the people freely mingling and no evidences of a panic. He said that on the way from New York he heard and read so much about the terrible epidemic of meningitis at Dallas that, if his business had not been so urgent, he would have turned back at St. Louis.

Major Roach concluded,

Meningitis is no doubt a terrible disease, and it is well to take every precaution against the spread of it. But it is not a precaution needlessly to fill the people with panic fear, and to proclaim the existence of the disease in epidemic form when the facts do not support the proclamation. It is understood all over the world that meningitis is epidemic in Dallas. Do the facts warrant this?[50]

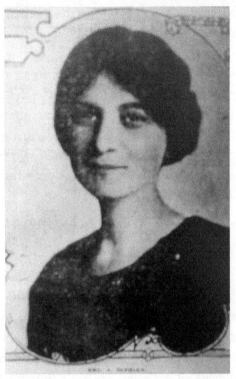

Estelle Felix Sophian (misspelled Sophien in the caption) (1882–
1972), April 1912. The image was scanned from the *Kansas City
Post*, April 16, 1912, p. 1. The photographer is unknown.

The next day (Saturday, January 13, 1912), the *New York
Times* added the following to the negative broadside on Dallas
and Texas:

> Reports sent to Northern and Eastern newspapers
> have exaggerated the meningitis situation in Dallas
> and Texas. There have not been more than 500
> authenticated cases in Texas. Of this number 190
> have been officially reported in Dallas, about 100
> in Fort Worth and 97 in Waco. The other cases are
> scattered over the State.[52]

[Note that the prevalence rates for cerebrospinal meningitis in the three aforementioned cities for this time period calculated to *20.7 cases per 10,000 Dallas residents*; *13.7 cases per 10,000 Fort Worth residents* (Fort Worth's population was 73,000 in 1910[53]); and *38.3 cases per 10,000 Waco residents* for October, November, and December 1911, and about half of January 1912 combined.]

The same day (Saturday, January 13, 1912) that the *New York Times* admonished Texans for overreacting to their cerebrospinal meningitis epidemic, Dr. Sophian's wife, Estelle Felix Sophian,[54] who had remained in New York City while her husband was in Texas, contacted the Associated Press about Dr. Sophian's alleged dying mother. Estelle said that her own mother, not Dr. Sophian's mother, had been ill for seven months and finally had died. Furthermore, before leaving for Texas, Dr. Sophian had arranged for the care of his ill mother-in-law by an eminent physician in New York City. Under the circumstances, said Estelle, she and the rest of the Felix and Sophian families did not wish Dr. Sophian to leave his work in Dallas. The Associated Press published the correction.[55]

The same evening, Saturday, January 13, 1912, Dr. Sophian "partially collapsed" from overwork and loss of sleep. He slept for a day and returned to the City Hospital at noon on Sunday, January 14, 1912.[56] Dr. Nash, who also was exhausted, performed double duty until Dr. Sophian was able to return to work.[57] On Sunday, January 14, 1912, C. W. Hartman, the manager of the Studebaker Corporation of Texas, placed a Studebaker Flanders 20 touring car at the disposal of Dr. Sophian to facilitate his travel between the Oriental Hotel and the City Hospital.[58]

On Monday, January 15, 1912, Dr. Steiner announced from Austin that the cerebrospinal meningitis situation across Texas was improved. He lamented that he could not provide the actual data to support his pronouncement, because many county and city health officers were not filing their vital statistics reports with the state registrar in a timely manner.[59]

On Tuesday, January 16, 1912, as Dr. Sophian toiled at the City Hospital, Dr. Park publicly reproved the staff members of the Rockefeller Institute for Medical Research for fostering the impression that their organization had been responsible for sending Dr. Sophian to Dallas.[60] The following is an excerpt from the letter written by Dr. Park and published in the *New York Post*:

> As a matter of fact, I think the Rockefeller Institute perfectly justified in getting all the credit and publicity that it can ... But at the same time, I am an employee of the department of health of New York City, and New York City spends a lot of money on our department, and expects that we, too, shall accomplish results as a recompense ... Only the other day, I went before the board of estimate to ask for an increased appropriation, and the question asked me at once was: "What have you accomplished with your laboratory work to deserve such an increase?" Now, what sort of position am I in to answer that question, if the Rockefeller Institute [for Dr. Sophian's work in Dallas] is getting all the credit that ought to go to the city's Research Laboratories?[60]

Dr. Park added,

> It is a matter of plain, simple truth that Dr. Sophian is a paid employee of the city and a subordinate of my staff, in charge of the special bureau of meningitis investigation. The city gave him a leave of absence to go to Texas at the request of the Dallas municipality, and we fully expected to pay his salary and expenses, although the Dallas authorities have since announced their readiness to do that. The

Rockefeller Institute has had nothing to do with the conduct of his successful campaign, except to offer him advice through Dr. Flexner, advice which has often been contrary to that which I wired him, and which has made his position somewhat embarrassing.[60]

The next day (Wednesday, January 17, 1912), Dr. Steiner learned that Dr. Rudolph H. von Ezdorf,[61] a passed assistant surgeon[62] of the US Marine Hospital Service in Washington, was making his way to Texas to "confer with the State health authorities of Texas and to investigate the prevalence of [cerebrospinal meningitis]." Dr. Steiner took credit for requesting the visit.[63] Dr. von Ezdorf's expected arrival in Austin was Saturday, January 20, 1912.[64]

On the evening of Wednesday, January 17, 1912, Dr. Sophian and Dr. Nash discontinued the physician clinics at the City Hospital, explaining,

It has been decided to discontinue the daily clinic to visiting physicians at the City Hospital for several reasons. We have quite a number of patients, and it is absolutely necessary that they receive prompt and efficient treatment. We must give them our undivided attention, and it necessarily requires more time to treat patients where there are a large number of doctors present at the clinic.[65]

They added,

It is our belief that there is a liability of so many doctors spreading the infection by being constantly in attendance at these clinics. We dislike to be compelled to discontinue these clinics but feel that it is to the best interest of our patients and the people in general for them to be discontinued. Furthermore, we feel that perhaps most of the physicians who have the time and inclination to visit our hospital have already done so, and that the clinic has already served its purpose in that way.[65]

As the cerebrospinal meningitis epidemic in Dallas pounded on, Dr. Sophian and Dr. Nash worried about the waning protective effect of the subcutaneous antimeningitis serum on which they and many of the City Hospital staff depended for protection. Dr. Sophian felt strongly that contracting cerebrospinal meningitis was a worse fate than developing serum sickness with repeat subcutaneous inoculations of antimeningitis serum. He took a second subcutaneous inoculation of antimeningitis serum and advised the City Hospital staff to follow suit.

Dr. Sophian developed hives, the most common form of serum sickness. While he itched, he realized that eventually the second subcutaneous inoculation of antimeningitis serum would lose *its* efficacy and that he, the staff members of the City Hospital, and others in close contact with victims would require a third inoculation. This scenario was a specter, begging more serious forms of serum sickness. Moreover, antimeningitis serum was becoming scarce because the demand for it was outstripping the horses' ability to produce it.[66]

Dr. Sophian returned to his idea of a meningococcal vaccine that would provide long-lasting protection without producing serum sickness. On Saturday, January 20, 1912, he discussed the feasibility, safety, and efficacy of his idea with Dr. Frank Johnson Hall,[67] a nationally-renowned clinical pathologist and rabies-vaccine virus expert who lived and worked in Kansas City, Jackson County, Missouri. At this time, Dr. Hall was combatting the Kansas City version of the ongoing multi-state cerebrospinal meningitis epidemic.[68] After hearing the details of Dr. Sophian's plan to manufacture a killed meningococcal vaccine, Dr. Hall commended the idea.[69] Dr. Hall's affirmation gave Dr. Sophian the boost he needed to move forward with his plan.

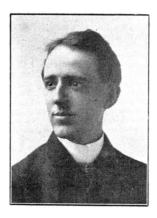

FRANK JOHNSON HALL.
M. D., 1897, (Kansas City Medical College).
*Associate Professor of Clinical Pathology, and
Director of the Pathological Laboratory,* 1905.

Dr. Frank Johnson Hall (1875–1946), *The Jayhawker* (yearbook),
University of Kansas, 1907, p. 16. The image is courtesy of
the Kenneth Spencer Research Library, University of Kanas
Libraries, University of Kansas, Lawrence, Kansas.

At the Dallas Medical Lunch Club on Saturday, January 20,
1912, about seventy-five physicians listened to Dr. Sophian's weekly
cerebrospinal meningitis update.[70] Dr. Sophian surprised them by
saying, "I am both glad and sorry to appear before you today. I am
glad because we have a good report to make. I am sorry, because in
a few days I shall leave Dallas. The so-called epidemic is practically
over in this city. Dallas is not worse, if she is not much better,
than those places which are quarantining."[70] Dr. Sophian added
that most of the City Hospital cases were getting well and that
he expected to discharge twelve to fourteen of them on Monday,
January 22, 1912. By the end of the week, he expected most of
the patients in the City Hospital to be gone. From now on, he
anticipated "sporadic cases—the sort we are dealing with now."[70]
Dr. Sophian continued,

> I started out with very high ideas as to what the
> cities ought to do in such emergencies as you have

had here. I stated to you in the first conference we had, the things I believed you ought to do. In all my experience of ten years, I have never seen them carried out and I did not expect you to do so in Dallas. But I am glad to say to you that in Dallas they have been carried out and carried out well … I am frank to admit that I did not believe that so large a community would, or could, take the thing over and regulate it as Dallas has done. I told you at first of the prophylactic measures, giving some of the most common, the sprays, the gargles, and the habits of cleanliness. They have all been carried out.[70]

Dr. Sophian then expressed remorse for failing to carry forward his idea of a meningococcal vaccine.[70] He declared his high regard for the efficiency and the organizing ability of Dr. Nash and the excellent nursing staff led by the day and night superiors, Miss Nielsen[71] and Mrs. Barnes, respectively. Dr. Nash, who also attended the meeting, said that the mortality at the hospital had been about 24 percent and that most of the fatal cases had arrived moribund to the hospital after driving ten to twenty miles across Texas country roads.[70]

That same Saturday, January 20, 1912, Dr. Rudolph H. von Ezdorf arrived in Austin and spent the entire day in conference with Dr. Steiner and Dr. Key.[72] Dr. von Ezdorf reported the following data, provided to him by Dr. Steiner, to Dr. Rupert Blue,[73] the US Surgeon General[74] of the Federal Public Health Service in Washington: "The principal points of prevalence [of cerebrospinal meningitis in Texas] were Austin (five cases, one death), Dallas (about 200 cases), Waco (100 cases, 39 deaths), Fort Worth (37 cases, 18 deaths), Houston (eight cases)," and 95 cases in 36 towns and counties in various parts of the state.[75] On Sunday, January 21, 1912, Dr. von Ezdorf set out on a tour of these high-prevalence Texas to assess for himself the meningitis situation in each. He started in Dallas.

[The prevalence, mortality, and case fatality rates for the above cities between October 1911 and January 20, 1912, calculated, respectively, to:

- Austin (population in 1910, 30,000[76]): *1.7 cerebrospinal meningitis cases per 10,000 Austin residents, .33 cerebrospinal meningitis deaths per 10,000 Austin residents,* and *20 percent.*
- Dallas (population in 1910, 92,000[76]): *21.7 cerebrospinal meningitis cases per 10,000 Dallas residents.* (Dr. von Ezdorf received incomplete data from Dr. Steiner for Dallas.)
- Waco (population in 1910, 26,000[76]): *38.5 cerebrospinal meningitis cases per 10,000 Waco residents, 15 cerebrospinal meningitis deaths per 10,000 Waco residents,* and *39 percent.*
- Fort Worth (population in 1910, 73,000[76]): *5.1 cerebrospinal meningitis cases per 10,000 Fort Worth residents, 2.4 cerebrospinal deaths per 10,000 Forth Worth residents,* and *49 percent.*
- Houston (population in 1910, 79,000[76]): *1.0 cerebrospinal meningitis cases per 10,000 Houston residents.* (Dr. von Ezdorf received incomplete data from Dr. Steiner for Houston.)]

Also, on Saturday, January 20, 1912, the *Journal of the American Medical Association*, headquartered in Chicago, Illinois, described the Texas cerebrospinal meningitis epidemic:

An epidemic of meningitis has been prevalent for several weeks chiefly in northern and eastern Texas, some cases being reported as far south as Houston and Austin, the disease centering chiefly in the neighborhood of Dallas, where up to January 10, 160 patients with 65 deaths had been reported; Waco also reported at that time 83 cases with 20 deaths. Fort Worth and many other cities and towns in northern Texas also report cases.[77]

The article continued,

> Secretary of the State Board of Health, Dr. Ralph Steiner, called a meeting of the state board at Dallas to discuss the situation and take up such measures as were deemed necessary. The board passed resolutions advising communities in which the disease appeared to close schools, theaters, and other places of amusement and establish quarantine, and the local authorities in the various cities and towns have instituted a cleanup campaign.[77]

The article concluded,

> Dr. Abraham Sophian of the Rockefeller Institute has been in northern Texas delivering addresses and advising with the local authorities in regard to the management of the epidemic. A sufficient quantity of the antimeningitis serum approved by the New York Board of Health has been rushed to Texas and is being employed. The situation while serious is now improving and will not, it is believed, under the energetic measures adopted, spread widely.[77]

On Sunday, January 21, 1912, Dr. von Ezdorf embarked on a tour of Texas cities with a high prevalence of cerebrospinal meningitis, beginning in Dallas. That same day, Mr. Babcock offered his analysis of Texas statewide meningitis mortality data for 1910 and 1911. The numbers of deaths from meningitis in 1910 and 1911 were 349 and 261 persons, respectively. The population of Texas in 1910 and in 1911 was close to four million. Mr. Babcock disparaged people who believed that Dallas was in the throes of a cerebrospinal meningitis epidemic, as follows:

As has been repeatedly stated by the State Board of Health, the City Boards of Health and all health authorities, the meningitis situation is not alarming, and the people are doing themselves and the State a great injustice by thus needlessly exciting themselves ... These figures [the number of deaths: 349 for 1910 and 261 for 1911] speak for themselves and the thinking people of the state will readily see the mistake they make by becoming so easily and unnecessarily excited, receiving and believing all the unsubstantiated rumors, working themselves into an unwarranted ferment of needless excitement, thereby rendering themselves more susceptible to the disease.[78]

CHAPTER 4 NOTES

1 "Expert Visits Cases upon Reaching City; Dr. Sophian Has Begun Study of Local Meningitis Situation; Arrived in Dallas Last Night and Confers with Physicians—State Health Officer Here," *Dallas Morning News*, January 6, 1912, 5.

2 Dr. John Oliver McReynolds (1865–1942) was born in Elkton, Todd County, Kentucky, as one of the seven children of Richard Bell McReynolds (1832–1908), a farmer, and Victoria Campbell (1836–1930). He earned his bachelor's degree from Transylvania University in Lexington, Fayette County, Kentucky, in 1890 and his medical degree from the College of Physicians and Surgeons of Baltimore in 1891. He served an internship at the Baltimore City Hospital (1891–1892) and studied at eye and ear clinics in New York City, Chicago, and various capitals in Europe. He moved to Dallas in 1892 and joined the oculist practice of Dr. Robert Henry Chilton (1844–1901). He and other physicians organized the Texas College of Physicians and Surgeons in 1903; the school closed in 1915. Dr. McReynolds married Katherine Lee Seay (1877–1941); they had one child. He died of stomach cancer at the age of seventy-six years. See "Famed Dallas Eye and Ear Doctor Dies; Dr. J. O. McReynolds' Skill as Physician, Writer, and Teacher Known All Over World," *Dallas Morning News*, July 8, 1942, 1; and Kathryn Pinkney, "John Oliver McReynolds," *Handbook of Texas Online*, accessed October 23, 2017, https://tshaonline.org/handbook/online/articles/fmccj.

3 Dr. William Alexander Boyce (1881–1961) was born in Boyce, Ellis County, Texas, as one of the eleven children (he had ten sisters) of Captain William Alexander Boyce (1842–1913), a Confederate military hero during the American Civil War and a farmer, and Mary Elizabeth Aldredge (1848–1906). William Alexander Boyce earned his medical degree from the Tulane University Medical Department in New Orleans, Louisiana, in 1905. He moved to Dallas to practice ophthalmology. He was a medical director of Southland Life Insurance Company in Dallas before serving in World War I. In 1919, he moved to Los Angeles, California, where he practiced ophthalmology until his retirement in 1950. He married Lillian E. Boyce; they had one child. Their divorce was national news in 1940. At the time of his death, he was married to Estelle Merrill. See "William Alexander Boyce," in "California, Occupational Licenses, Registers, and Directories (1919)," California State Archives,

Sacramento, California, Board of Medical Examiners Registers of Licensed Physicians, 1901–1939; and "Dr. William A. Boyce," *Los Angeles Times*, April 25, 1961, 71.

4   Dr. Manton Marble Carrick (1879–1932) was born in Keatchie, DeSoto Parish, Louisiana, as one of the two children of White L. Carrick (born in 1859) and Cammie Rozina Thompson (1862–1901). He moved with his family to Waxahachie, Ellis County, Texas, as a boy. He graduated from the Dallas Academy in 1897 and earned his medical degree from Fort Worth University Medical Department in 1901. He worked as a house physician at the City Hospital in Dallas and as an assistant house surgeon at the Texas and Pacific Railroad Company Hospital in Marshall, Harrison County, Texas. He also served as assistant quarantine inspector for the port of Galveston in 1908, assistant superintendent of the Texas State Epileptic Colony in Abilene in 1910, and the superintendent of the Texas State Leper Colony in 1912. He taught preventive medicine at Baylor University College of Medicine (1914–1917); served four years in the US Army; received disability retirement in 1921 for contracting diabetes mellitus; and served (1921–1925) as the Texas state health officer under Governor Pat Morris Neff. From 1927 to 1929, he served as the Dallas city health officer. He married Elizabeth Mai Connor Gordon (1880–1961) in 1926. He died from diabetes at the age of fifty-three years. See "Dr. M. M. Carrick Appointed," *Dallas Morning News*, January 4, 1912, 7; "Becomes Quarantine Inspector," *Fort Worth Star-Telegram*, August 7, 1908, 5; and David Minor, "Carrick, Manton Marble," *Handbook of Texas Online*, accessed January 14, 2018, https://tshaonline.org/handbook/online/articles/fca62.

5   "State Health Officer Coming," *Dallas Morning News*, January 5, 1912, 3. A grainy image of Dr. Sophian in his bowler hat and long coat, taken around January 7, 1912, in Dallas, Texas, by the famous photographer, Henry Clogenson (1861–1924), is available at "Visiting Doctors Hear Dr. Sophian," *Dallas Morning News*, January 7, 1912, 8.

6   Thomas William Field (1847–1909) chartered the Oriental Hotel Company in 1889 and announced plans to build a six-story luxury hotel on land he had purchased two years earlier at Akard and Commerce Streets in Dallas. In 1893, he sold his interest in the nearly completed Oriental Hotel to another group of investors headed by St. Louis beer magnate Adolphus Busch (1839–1913). The latter's

group completed the $500,000 hotel and opened it to customers in October 1893. The hotel boasted 150 fully-electrified guest rooms. The ground floor contained a grand dining room, a barbershop, a cigar stand, billiard rooms, and a huge ballroom with one of the first tile floors in the city. The second floor held parlors and a bridal room. For years, the Oriental Hotel was considered the finest hotel in Dallas. It was torn down in 1924 to make way for the Baker Hotel. See Sam Childers, *Historic Dallas Hotels* (Charleston, SC: Arcadia Publishers, 2010), 21–23.

7   Dr. Leake, Dr. McReynolds, and other St. Paul's Sanitarium medical staff members organized the Southwestern University Medical Department in 1903. From 1903 to 1911, it was associated with Southwestern University in Georgetown, Williamson County, Texas (about 170 miles south of Dallas). From 1911 to 1915, Southwestern University Medical Department became the medical department of Southern Methodist University in Dallas. See John S. Fordtran, "Medicine in Dallas 100 Years Ago," *Proceedings of Baylor University Medical Center* 13, no.1 (January 2000): 34–44.

8   "Doctors Confer with Serum Expert; Dr. Abraham Sophian of New York Invited for Meningitis Lecture; Cleanliness Is Urged; Flexner's Assistant Says Disease Is Communicated by Contact—No New Cases," *Fort Worth Star-Telegram*, January 6, 1912, 3.

9   Wade W. Oliver, *The Man Who Lived for Tomorrow: A Biography of William Hallock Park, MD* (New York: E. P. Dutton, 1941), 300.

10   The Dallas Medical Lunch Club was organized in 1909 to promote a better social acquaintance among the members of the Dallas County Medical Society. The popular physician club met every Friday (or Saturday) at one o'clock in the afternoon at the Oriental Hotel. There were no dues, and each physician paid fifty cents for each meal he ate and nothing when he was absent. See "The Dallas Medical Lunch Club," *Texas State Journal of Medicine* 7, no. 3 (July 1911): 99.

11   "Visiting Doctors Hear Dr. Sophian; Many from Other Texas Cities Attend Dinner by Physicians Lunch Club; Treatment of Disease; Advises Administering Meningitis Serum on First Day—Outlines Precautions Advisable," *Dallas Morning News*, January 7, 1912, 8.

12   A ladies' ordinary was a women-only dining space in North American hotels and restaurants beginning in the early nineteenth century. At the time, women required a male escort in restaurants and the public rooms of luxury, mainly urban hotels. See "Ladies' Ordinary,"

Wikipedia, accessed December 20, 2017, https://en.wikipedia.org/wiki/Ladies%27_ordinary.

13 Dr. Clay Cory Johnson (1867–1948) was born in Dawsonville, Dawson, Georgia, as one of the six children of Samuel Caraway Johnson (1831–1870), an attorney at law, and Emily Martha Johnson (1836–1912). Clay C. Johnson earned his medical degree from the College of Physicians and Surgeons of Baltimore, Maryland, in 1891; his preceptor was Dr. Samuel Wister Johnson, his eldest brother. He returned to Georgia to practice medicine before moving to Texas to join another brother, Cone Johnson, in Tyler, Smith County, Texas. Dr. Clay Johnson next practiced medicine at Corsicana, Navarro County, Texas, before moving to Fort Worth in 1905. He owned a sanitarium in Fort Worth and worked at a number of railroads as their company surgeon. He married Alice Jester (1875–1963) in 1898; they had four children. See *Annual Announcement and Catalogue of the College of Physicians and Surgeons, Baltimore, Maryland, 1890–1891* (Philadelphia, PA: College of Physicians and Surgeons, 1891), 21; "Dr. Clay Johnson Dies at Fort Worth," *Amarillo Daily News*, March 8, 1948; and "Dr. Clay Johnson Funeral Services Monday Afternoon," *Corsicana Daily Sun* (Corsicana, TX), March 8, 1948, 1.

14 In 1896, Dallas's only hospital was the City Hospital. Several prominent Dallas physicians and civil leaders appealed to Edward Joseph Dunne (1848–1910), the bishop of Dallas (1893–1910), to encourage the Daughters (Sisters) of Charity of St. Vincent de Paul to open a hospital in Dallas. They sent two sisters by covered wagon the 1,200 miles from Emmitsburg, Frederick County, Maryland, to Dallas to open the hospital in a small cottage on Hall Street in June 1896. In 1898, the sisters moved into the new, spacious building designed by a local architect, Harry A. Overbeck (1861–1942), on Bryan Street. St. Paul's Sanitarium changed its name to St. Paul's Hospital (1927) and to Saint Paul Hospital (1958). The original hospital and all its annexes were demolished in 1968. See John Roppolo, "St Paul Hospital," *Dallas County Chronicle* 14, no. 4 (December 2015): 1–3; "The End of St. Paul Medical Center," University of North Texas Libraries, Discovering the Southwest Metroplex, accessed October 24, 2017, https://blogs.library.unt.edu/southwest-metroplex/2015/12/16/the-end-of-st-paul-medical-center/; and Paula Bosse, "Saint Paul's Sanitarium, 1910," *Flashback*

Dallas, accessed October 24, 2017, https://flashbackdallas. com/2015/08/23/st-pauls-sanitarium-1910/.

15 Alexander Sanger (1847–1925) was born in Obernbreit, Kitzingen, Bavaria, as one of the eight children of Elias Sanger (1800–1877) and Babette Mandelbaum (1813–1886). In 1865, he followed his two older brothers to Cincinnati, Hamilton County, Ohio, to work for Heller Brothers, a wholesale produce company. He later worked for Sanger Brothers, a dry-goods wholesale and retail firm in Corsicana, Navarro County, Texas. He then moved to Dallas in 1872 to open and manage a branch store of Sanger Brothers. Alex Sanger was actively involved in the civic affairs of Dallas. He married Fannie Fechenbach (1848–1898); they had one child. See Natalie Ornish, "Sanger, Alexander," *Handbook of Texas Online*, accessed January 14, 2018, https://tshaonline.org/handbook/online/articles/fsa54; and Diana J. Kleiner, "Sanger Brothers," *Handbook of Texas Online*, accessed January 14, 2018, https://tshaonline.org/handbook/online/articles/ijsqj.

16 Dr. Sophian trumpeted urotropin (hexamethylenamine) at a dose of fifteen to thirty grains daily. He explained that urotropin was "split up into formaldehyde and ammonia, which are excreted for the most part in the urine, but also find their way into the CSF [cerebrospinal fluid] and through the nasal mucous membranes into the nose." He personally used copious amounts of urotropin. See "Epidemic Meningitis: Editorial," *Medical Herald* 32, no. 2 (February 1913): 75–77; and Phebe L. DuBois, "Differential Diagnosis and Treatment of Epidemic Cerebrospinal Meningitis," *Journal of the American Medical Association* 60, no. 11 (March 15, 1912): 822.

17 Dr. Sophian meant by "active community treatment" the use of a typhoid vaccine to prevent typhoid from spreading in a community. The British pathologist Almroth Edward Wright (1861–1947) originated the typhoid vaccine, as well as the idea of using a heat-killed vaccine (1897), while he was a professor of pathology at the Royal Army Medical College in England. Dr. Wright attributed his idea for the typhoid vaccine to reading about the success of the Russian (Ukrainian) bacteriologist Waldemar Mordecai Haffkine (1860–1930), who developed cholera and plague vaccines for use in British India. Dr. Sophian believed that a heat-killed meningococcal vaccine could prevent cerebrospinal meningitis as well as the heat-killed typhoid vaccine prevented typhoid fever. See Leonard Colebrock, "Sir Almroth Wright and Anti-Typhoid Inoculation,"

British Medical Journal 2, no. 4471 (September 14, 1946): 398; Almroth Edward Wright, *Vaccine Therapy: Its Administration, Value, and Limitations* (London: Longmans, Green, and Company, 1910), 98, 191; William Cecil Bosanquet and John William Henry Eyre, S*erum, Vaccines, and Toxines* [sic] *in Treatment and Diagnosis* (New York: Funk and Wagnalls Company, 1910), 52–54; W. Bulloch, "Waldemar Mordecai Wolff Haffkine," *Journal of Pathology and Bacteriology* 34, no. 2 (1931): 125–29; and Barbara J. Hawgood, "Waldemar Mordecai Haffkine, CIE (1860–1930): Prophylactic Vaccination against Cholera and Bubonic Plague in British India," *Journal of Medical Biography* 15, no. 1 (2007): 9–19.

18 "A Communication: Serum Sickness," *Texas State Journal of Medicine* 7, no. 12 (April 1912): 336.

19 "Meningitis Toll Saturday Is Light," *Dallas Morning News*, January 7, 1912, 4.

20 "City Hospital Is Reserved for Cases; Mayor Directs Removal of Other Patients for Handling Meningitis; Gives Free Treatment; City Furnishes Serum, through Health Department, Patients Unable to Pay for It," *Dallas Morning News*, January 7, 1912, 4.

21 See "Physicians Confer; Warning Is Issued; People Are Advised to Avoid Congregating in Public Places; Dr. Leake's Statement; President Board of Health Reviews Situation regarding Meningitis and Gives Advice," *Dallas Morning News*, January 8, 1912, 4.

22 "Addresses Doctors at Night Meeting; Dr. Sophian Speaks at Session of Dallas County Medical Society; Situation Not Serious; Declares Presence of One Hundred Cases; No Cause for Alarm—Suggests Immunitization [sic]," *Dallas Morning News*, January 7, 1912, 4.

23 Typhoid fever often killed more soldiers than did combat during wars. Clara Councell wrote, "[Typhoid fever] was apparently the most fatal disease of the American Civil War and was very common in the Franco-Prussian War when it spread through France, in the Russo-Turkish War of 1877–1878, and in the Boer War of 1899–1902 between the British and the Dutch. During the Spanish American War (1898), the incident rate was 142 per 1,000 per annum. Large numbers of soldiers contracted typhoid, diarrhea, and dysentery in the Russo-Japanese War of 1904." See Clara E. Councell, "War and Infectious Disease," *Public Health Reports* 56, no. 12 (March 21, 1941): 547–73; Harry Morel, "Inoculation and Typhoid Fever," *Public Health Journal* 6, no. 5 (May 1915): 244–46; and R. W. Marsden, "Inoculation with Typhoid Vaccine as a Preventive of

Typhoid Fever," *British Medical Journal* 1, no. 2052 (April 28, 1900): 1017–18.

24 "Back from Winning War on Meningitis; Dr. Sophian Reports Epidemic in Dallas and Other Texas Cities Practically Stamped Out; Treated Over 300 Cases; Brings Back Many Presents from Grateful Citizens and Loving Cup Presented by City," *New York Times*, February 15, 1912, 5.

25 Dr. John Spencer Davis (1881–1947) was born in Blooming Grove, Navarro County, Texas, as the youngest of the nine children of Dr. John Marion Davis (1815–1888) and Sarah Simpson (1840–1918). He earned his medical degree (1908) from Tulane University Medical Department in New Orleans, Louisiana, and attended summer school at Harvard Medical School in 1910. He returned to Dallas to open the Davis Diagnostic Clinic. He married Gertrude Greene (1883–1958); they had child. Dr. Davis died of a coronary occlusion and hypertensive heart disease at the age of sixty-six years. See "Davis Funeral to Be Friday," *Dallas Morning News*, May 2, 1947, 5; *Announcement of the Medical School of Harvard University, 1909–1910* (Cambridge, MA: Harvard University, 1909), 139; and "Dallas Doctor Ends Own Life, Liddell Spencer Davis, Harvard Student, Had Just Got on Staff," *Dallas Morning News*, April 8, 1930, 4.

26 See "Physicians Confer; Warning Is Issued; People Are Advised to Avoid Congregating in Public Places; Dr. Leake's Statement; President Board of Health Reviews Situation regarding Meningitis and Gives Advice," *Dallas Morning News*, January 8, 1912, 4.

27 See Rudolph H. von Ezdorf, "Cerebrospinal Meningitis in Texas," *Public Health Reports* 27, no. 8 (February 23, 1912): 274; and "Meningitis Serious All over Texas; State Health Officer Orders Schools Closed Wherever a Case Develops," *El Paso Herald-Post*, January 8, 1912, 2.

28 "Calls State Board to Meet in Dallas; State Health Officer Steiner Asks for Meeting Here Wednesday; Advice to Physicians; Makes Suggestions to City and County Health Officers regarding Precautions to be Urged," *Dallas Morning News*, January 9, 1912, 3;

29 "Assemble Patients at City Hospital; Dr. Sophian Is Now Treating Fifteen Meningitis Cases at That Place; Expert Is 'Vaccinated'; Takes Injection of Flexner Serum to Immunize Himself—Statement by Dr. Leake," *Dallas Morning News*, January 9, 1912, 3.

30 "One Death Tuesday from Meningitis; Only Three New Cases Reported, Indicate Much Improved Situation; City Orders Clean-Up," *Dallas Morning News*, January 10, 1912, 4.

31 Recall that the City Hospital steward during the Dallas meningitis epidemic in 1912 was Dr. George White Howard. See "Dr. Sophian Lectures to Medical Students; Tells Them of Importance of Laboratory Work; Will Leave Tonight for Other Texas Cities— Two New Cases and One Death Saturday," *Dallas Morning News*, February 4, 1912, 3.

32 The City Hospital interns during the Dallas meningitis epidemic were Dr. C. F. Card, Dr. S. M. Hill, Dr. V. E. Robbins, Dr. Orren Presley Gandy (1890–1949), Dr. Robert August Trumbull (1889–1958), Dr. Emmet Smith, and Dr. J. E. Jones. See "Dr. Sophian Lectures to Medical Students; Tells Them of Importance of Laboratory Work; Will Leave Tonight for Other Texas Cities—Two New Cases and One Death Saturday," *Dallas Morning News*, February 4, 1912, 3.

33 The City Hospital nurses were Rose Emma Nielsen (day-nurse supervisor), Mrs. Jesse Barnes (night-nurse supervisor), Minnie Greer (Grier), Jessie Smith, Miss Menefee, Katherine Chamberlain, Josephine Oster, Mrs. Dearborn, Miss Bonderplas, Ann Corbett, Jane Gordon, Katherine Ott, E. Bierbaum (Brierbaum), Mary Kelly, E. Fitzgerald, Annie Van Arsdale, Margaret Howard, Grace Pierce, Mary Suggs, Mrs. Roberts, L. E. Payne, Miss Payne, Katherine Kortebin, and Miss Rushing. The following seven volunteer nurses, who served without pay and credited their time to their training course, came from the Texas Baptist Memorial Sanitarium (C. I. Smith, A. C. Smith, Miss Calloway, Miss Justice) and from St. Paul's Sanitarium (Miss Kern, Miss Fahey, and Miss Mims). The ambulance drivers were Officers Dick Haney and Charles Collier. Officer Cheek drove the automobile for the diagnosticians. See "Dr. Sophian Lectures to Medical Students; Tells Them of Importance of Laboratory Work; Will Leave Tonight for Other Texas Cities— Two New Cases and One Death Saturday," *Dallas Morning News*, February 4, 1912, 3.

34 "State Board Gives Advice to Public; Suggests Cities Close Theaters When Meningitis Makes Its Appearance; Situation Well in Hand; Compliments Dallas Officials upon Their Method of Handling the Epidemic Here," *Dallas Morning News*, January 11, 1912, 8.

35 Dr. Hugh Love McLaurin (1863–1916) was born in Brandon, Rankin County, Mississippi, as one of the seven children of Dr. Hugh

Calhoun McLaurin (1813–1880) and Harriet Emily Love (1828–1918). Hugh Love McLaurin earned his bachelor's degree from the University of Mississippi and his medical degree from Tulane University Medical Department (1884) in New Orleans, Louisiana. He served for two years as superintendent of the Mississippi State Sanitarium at Vicksburg before moving to Dallas in 1886 to open a medical practice. He served on the Texas State Medical Board through two administrations and was serving in this role at the time of his death. He married Kate Gano (1862–1944) in 1890; they had four children. He died of Bright's disease and cerebral apoplexy at the age of fifty-two years. See *Historical Catalogue of the University of Mississippi (1849–1909)* (Nashville, TN: Marshall and Bruce Company, 1910), 179; "Dr. H. L. M'Laurin Dead, End Came at His Home," *Waxahachie Daily Light*, August 11, 1916, 2; "Deaths," *Texas State Journal of Medicine* 12, no. 6 (October 1916): 278; "Dr. H. L. M'Laurin Dies Suddenly at His Home; Was Practicing Physician in Dallas for 30 Years; Death Comes Quickly after Stroke of Apoplexy—Funeral Service to Be Held Today," *Dallas Morning News*, August 12, 1916, 5.

36 Dr. Benjamin Milton Worsham (1862–1918) was born in Hopkins County, Texas, as the youngest of the eight children of James Albert Worsham (1817–1890), a farmer, and Maria Grimes (1825–1912). He taught school before earning his medical degree from the University of Louisville Medical Department (1886). He practiced medicine at Sulphur Springs, Hopkins County, Texas, and Waxahachie, Ellis County, Texas. He then served as an assistant at the State Lunatic Asylum in Austin, superintendent of the Southwestern Insane Asylum in San Antonio, and superintendent of the State Epileptic Colony in Abilene. In 1909, he retired from the practice of medicine, moved to El Paso, and became the original stockholder of the Two Republics Life Insurance Company, of which he served as director and president. He married Margaret Ozora Boone (1872–1958) in 1892; they had one child. Dr. Worsham died of organic heart disease and acute dilatation of the heart at the age of fifty-two years. See "Death Claims Dr. Worsham, Alienist of Note, President of Life Insurance Company, Dies," *El Paso Herald-Post*, May 3, 1918, 5; and "Benjamin M. Worsham," in "Deaths," *Journal of the American Medical Association* 70, no. 21 (May 25, 1918): 1,555.

37 Dr. Sidney Mainer Lister (1875–1946) was born in Colita, Polk County, Texas, as one of the four children of Walter Charles Sidney

Lister (1850–1918), a stockman and rancher, and Emma Virginia Mainer (1855–1900). He earned his medical degree (1898) from Barnes Medical College (in existence from 1892 to 1918) in St. Louis, Missouri. Dr. Lister served on the Texas Prison Board (1931–1941); as president of the Harris County Medical Society; as president of the Houston Board of Health; as chief of the medical staff at Memorial Hospital in Houston; and as a founder of a city-county hospital that ultimately grew into the Jefferson Davis Hospital of Houston and Harris County. He married Lucille Wilson (1879–1946) in 1903; they had three children. He died of auricular fibrillation, cerebral thrombosis, and hypertensive and arteriosclerotic heart disease. "Former Prison Board Head; Dr. Sidney Lister, Is Dead," *Abilene Reporter-News*, November 17, 1946, 13; and "Prominent Physician of Houston Passes," *Dallas Morning News*, November 16, 1946, 9.

38 Dr. Ashley Wilson Fly (1855–1919) was born in Waters Valley, Yalobusha County, Mississippi, as one of the four children of Anderson Boswell Fly (1825–1895), a Methodist minister, and Margaret Jane Giles (1825–1879). He earned his medical diploma from the University of Louisville Medical Department (1875); moved to Galveston, Texas, the same year; and opened a medical practice. He served as the mayor of Galveston (1893–1899), and as a regent of the University of Texas for eight years. He married Kate Wilson (1857–1905) in 1878 and Frances Brand (1881–1971) in 1915. He and Frances had one child. He died of a cerebral hemorrhage at the age of sixty-three years. See "Galveston Doctor Dies after Illness of Week; Dr. A. W. Fly Was Prominent in Political Circles; Was at One Time Mayor of City and Served as University Regent for Several Years," *Galveston Daily News*, January 25, 1919, 3.

39 In 1912, the Dallas population was about 92,000, of whom about 18,000 (about 20 percent) were African American. In 1912, the *Dallas City Directory* listed the following fourteen African-American physicians and surgeons: Drs. Benjamin Rufus Bluitt, J. W. Anderson, Frank M. Brooks, F. A. Bryan, R. T. Hamilton, M. P. Penn, David W. Shields, J. M. Dodd, W. M. Hames, A. J. Johnson, M. H. Leach, A. L. Runyan, P. M. Sunday, and J. T. Welch. The first African American physicians to practice medicine in Dallas were Dr. George F. Smith, who arrived as early as 1885, and Dr. Majors, according to oral tradition. See "Bluitt Sanitarium," Dallas Landmark Structures and Sites, Dallas Landmark (2001), National Register of Historic Places (2005), accessed January 15, 2018, http://dallascityhall.com/

departments/sustainabledevelopment/historicpreservation/Pages/
Bluitt-Sanitarium.aspx; "Dallas," in Campbell Gibson and Kay Jung,
*Historical Census Statistics on Population Totals by Race, 1790
to 1990, and by Hispanic Origin, 1970 to 1990, for Large Cities
and Other Urban Places in the United States* (Washington, DC:
US Census Bureau, 2005); and *Worley's 1912 Directory of Dallas,
Texas* (Dallas, TX: John F. Worley Directory Company, 1912).

40 Dr. Benjamin Rufus Bluitt (1864–1946) and Dr. David W. Shields
    (1862–1937) were two of the fourteen African-American physicians
    practicing medicine in Dallas during the cerebrospinal meningitis
    epidemic in 1912. Dr. Shields was born in Alabama in 1862 as the
    eldest of the five children of David Shields (born in 1834) and Amelia
    Shields (born in 1845). He grew up in Claiborne County, Mississippi;
    attended Alcorn University (Claiborne County, Mississippi); and
    earned his medical degree (1881) from Flint Medical College,
    the medical department of New Orleans University (a Methodist
    Episcopal Church school). He practiced medicine for forty years,
    part of the time in Denison, Grayson County, Texas, and part of
    the time in Dallas (as early as 1905 to 1930, when he retired). His
    wife was Sadie Shields; she predeceased him; they had no children.
    He died of a cerebrovascular stroke and senility. Dr. Bluitt was
    born in Freestone or Limestone County, Texas, as one of the four
    children of Jarriet Bluitt (1835–1870) and Mariah Bonner (died
    1903); both were former slaves who, like all Texas slaves, received
    news of their freedom two years and an indeterminate number of
    months (depending on their former owners) after President Abraham
    Lincoln issued the Emancipation Proclamation in 1862. Benjamin
    Bluitt attended Wiley College, a white-missionary-run college for
    African Americans established in Marshall, Harrison County, Texas;
    he graduated with the class of 1882. He then attended Meharry
    Medical Department of Central Tennessee College in Nashville,
    Tennessee, graduating in 1885. He moved to Dallas in 1888 and
    opened a medical practice to serve the 5,000 African Americans
    then living in the city. Around 1920, Dr. Bluitt moved to Chicago to
    head the medical staff of Fort Dearborn Hospital. He married three
    times. His first wife was Cornelia J. Ford (1882–1934). His second
    wife was Geneva Bluitt (1899–1940), who died of tuberculosis at
    the age of twenty-eight years. His third wife was twenty-three-year-
    old Violet. Dr. Bluitt died of stomach cancer in Chicago at the age
    of eighty-one years. Jennifer Bridges, "Bluitt, Benjamin Rufus,"

Handbook of Texas Online, accessed January 13, 2018, https://tshaonline.org/handbook/online/articles/fbl69; "The Metropolitan," *Grayson County TX GenWeb*, accessed January 13, 2018, http://txgenwebcounties.org/grayson/Ethnic/AfricanAmerican/TheMetropolitan_newspaper/Metropolitan.html; and Desha P. Rhodes, *A History of Flint Medical College, 1889–1911* (New York: iUniverse, 2007).

41 "Fatal Meningitis Gets Hold in Texas; Cerebrospinal Disease Is Developing Rapidly, 325 Cases Are Reported; These Are in Northern and Eastern Part of State; Experts Put to Work; State Board of Health Meets at Dallas in Effort to Combat the Deadly Disease—Several Cities of the State Have Declared Quarantine against the Afflicted Districts," *Macon Telegraph* (Macon, GA), January 11, 1912, 1; and "Meningitis in Texas," *Arkansas Gazette* (Little Rock, AR), January 13, 1912, 6.

42 See "Fifty Families Are Fleeing from Epidemic Cerebro Spinal Meningitis," *Pensacola Journal* (Pensacola, FL), January 11, 1912, 2; and "Meningitis Epidemic Kills Many Texans," *Philadelphia Inquirer*, January 11, 1912, 2.

43 See "Sophian's Mother Dying; He Will However Remain to Fight Meningitis," *Marshall Messenger* (Marshall, TX), January 12, 1912, 5; "Meetings Abandoned, Account Meningitis," *Omaha World-Herald* (Omaha, NE), January 12, 1912, 2; "Panic Over Meningitis; Public Gatherings Are Being Abandoned in Texas," *Springfield Republican* (Springfield, MA), January 12, 1912, 2; "No Meetings Held; Even Church Services Abandoned in Meningitis District," *Abilene Daily Chronicle*, January 12, 1912, 1; "Situation Serious at Dallas," *Bryan Daily Eagle*, January 10, 1912, 2; and "Health Board Meets," *Fort Worth Star-Telegram*, January 10, 1912, 14.

44 "Physicians Discuss Dallas Situation; Are Charged with Having Gone from Extreme of Indifference to That of Panic; Indorse [sic] Health Officer; Express Confidence in Efficiency of Dr. Nash's Method of Handling Epidemic," *Dallas Morning News*, January 13, 1912, 3.

45 "'Can Now Control Situation Easily,'—Dr. A. Sophian; Meningitis Expert Says City Now Prepared to Cope with Disease; Force Well Organized; Effectiveness of Treatment and Cooperation of Physicians Improve Conditions—Record for Day," *Dallas Morning News*, January 13, 1912, 3.

46 Drs. Clemens Freiherr Von Pirquet (1874–1929) and Béla Schick (1877–1967) first described serum sickness in 1905 as fever, skin eruptions (mainly urticaria, or hives), joint pain, and lymphadenopathy in regions draining the site of injection following injections of horse serum antitoxin. Clemens F. von Pirquet and Béla Schick, *Serum Sickness* (Philadelphia, PA: Williams and Wilkins, 1951).

47 Dr. Thomas J. Crowe (1862–1948) was born on a farm near Rochester, Wayne County, New York. At the age of seventeen years, he began clerking for the Pacific Express Company, which transferred him to Austin in 1883 at the age of twenty-one years. He began to study homeopathic medicine on his own and later took courses at the Homeopathic Medical College of Missouri (in existence from 1857 to 1909) in St. Louis, from which he eventually earned his homeopathic medical degree (1887). He also took courses at the Lying-in College of Philadelphia, the Philadelphia Post-Graduate School of Homeopathy, the Philadelphia Polyclinic, and the Rush Hospital for Consumptives in Philadelphia. He moved to Dallas in 1895, where he served as the chairman of the Dallas Board of Health and the secretary of the Texas State Board of Medical Examiners (1921–1948). He married Mallie (Julia?) Elinor Crowe (1871–1960); they had two children. See "T. J. Crowe Succumbs to Heart Attack; Physician, Surgeon Practiced in Dallas More than 50 Years," *Dallas Morning News*, January 2, 1948, 1; and "Thomas J. Crowe, MD," in Phillip Lindsley and Luther B. Hill, *A History of Greater Dallas and Vicinity* (Chicago, IL: Lewis Publishing Company, 1909), 117–18.

48 Homeopathy "is a therapeutic method using preparations of substances whose effects when administered to healthy subjects correspond to the manifestations of the disorder (symptoms, clinical signs, pathological states) in the individual patient" (Edzard Ernst, "A Systematic Review of Systematic Reviews of Homeopathy," *British Journal of Clinical Pharmacology* 54, no. 6 [December 2002]: 577). Dr. Samuel Hahnemann (1755–1843) originated the homeopathic method. Homeopathy was popular among the upper classes in Europe and the United States during the mid-to-late nineteenth century. John D. Rockefeller, for example, patronized a homeopath. Allopathy, by contrast, is the scientific system of the mainstream medical profession. In the early twentieth century, some homeopathic schools drew closer to the teachings of allopathic schools. See Samuel Hahnemann, *The Homoeopathic Medical Doctrine* (Dublin, Ireland: W. F. Wakeman, 1833); and Woodson

C. Merrell and Edward Shalts, "Homeopathy," *Medical Clinics of North America* 86, no. 1 (2001): 47–62.

49 Dr. Abraham Sophian's Texas medical license was conferred by the Texas State Board of Medical Examiners, which formed in 1907. The board consisted of eleven physician members appointed biennially by the Texas governor and confirmed by the Texas State Senate.

50 "Says No 'Epidemic' in Dallas; Major E. H. Roach Thinks Number of Cases of Meningitis Here Does Not Warrant Use of Term," *Dallas Morning News*, January 12, 1912, 8.

51 Erskine Horton Roach (1873–1940) was born in Memphis, Shelby County, Tennessee, as the eldest of the four children of Andrew Jackson Roach (1830–1884), a commercial traveler, and Ida Tennessee Horton (1853–1918). He was the manager of a wholesale grocery house and a major in the US Army 158th Infantry. He married Pearl Isabel Compton (1875–after 1940) in 1898; they had no children.

52 "Clinics in Dallas Control Meningitis; Dr. Sophian of the Rockefeller Institute Directs Texas Doctors in Use of Serum; Quarantine at 10 Cities; About 500 Cases in All—Schools Closed in Dallas—Disease Spreads through the State," *New York Times*, January 13, 1912, 5.

53 *Texas Almanac: City Population History of Selected Cities, 1850–2000*, accessed December 8, 2017, https://texasalmanac.com/sites/default/files/images/CityPopHist%20web.pdf.

54 Estelle Felix (1882–1972) was born in Warta, Posen, Prussia, as the sixth of the eight children of Arthur A. Felix (1855–1930), a merchant, and Emilie Leitner (1855–1912). The family immigrated in two groups, with Arthur A., Sarah, Pauline, Eva, and Joseph arriving in Buffalo via New York City in December 1890 and Emilie, Flora, Estelle, Louis, and Eugenia joining them in Buffalo via New York City in May 1891. The family subsequently moved back to New York City, where Estelle attended the Normal College of the City of New York for four years, graduating at the age of seventeen years in 1900. For the next decade, she worked as a primary school teacher in New York City's public schools. Her younger sister, Jane Felix (1888–1945), married Harry Sophian (1882–1945), Abraham's older brother, in 1907. Estelle Felix and Dr. Abraham Sophian married on April 26, 1911, in New York City.

55 "Sophian's Mother Not Dead; 'Twas Mother-in-Law of Meningitis Expert Who Died,'" *Houston Post*, January 13, 1912, 5.

56 "Dr. Sophian Collapsed; Overwork and Loss of Sleep Causes Partial Collapse of Specialist—Was Soon Back at Work," *The Times* (Shreveport, LA), January 14, 1912, 8.

57 "March of Disease Checked in Dallas; Only Two Deaths and Four New Cases Are Reported for Saturday; Outlook Is Brighter; Dr. Nash Says Force Organized Now so as to Cope with Any Condition That Might Arise," *Dallas Morning News*, January 14, 1912, 8.

58 Walter E. Flanders (1871–1923) founded the Flanders Automobile Company in Detroit, Michigan, in 1910. The Flanders Model 20 had a four-cylinder, water-cooled engine with twenty horsepower and a hundred-inch wheelbase. At $750, it cost less than Ford's Model Ts in 1911, but as Ford cut its prices, the Flanders remained more expensive than the Model T. The company went out of business in 1913. See "Dr. Sophian Uses a Flanders, Manager C. W. Hartman Places Car at His Disposal," *Dallas Morning News*, January 14, 1912, 5; and "Flanders (automobile company)," *Wikipedia*, accessed December 20, 2017, https://en.wikipedia.org/wiki/Flanders_(automobile_company).

59 "Meningitis Situation Improving; State Health Officer Says County Officials Are Slow in Filing Reports; Commissioner Kone Suspends Lecturing," *Bryan Daily Eagle*, January 15, 1912, 2.

60 Wade W. Oliver, *The Man Who Lived for Tomorrow: A Biography of William Hallock Park, MD* (New York: E. P. Dutton, 1941), 301–2.

61 Dr. Rudolph Hermann von Ezdorf (1873–1916) was born in Philadelphia, Pennsylvania, as the eldest of the five children of Richard von Ezdorf (1848–1926), an architect, and Anna Lutz (1848–1944). Richard von Ezdorf and Anna Lutz were born in Venice, Italy, and Innsbruck, Austria, respectively. Richard von Ezdorf immigrated to the United States around 1873 and became the chief designer of the State, War, and Navy Building in Washington, DC. Rudolph von Ezdorf grew up in Washington, DC, where he earned his medical degree from the George Washington University Medical School (1894). He joined the US Public Health Service as an assistant surgeon (1898), advanced to passed assistant surgeon five years later, and reached the grade of surgeon in 1912. He served as quarantine officer at Santiago de Cuba during the intervention of the United States; worked in the office of the consul general at Havana; and served as the quarantine officer at Matanzas, Cuba. He also worked in the ports of Colon and Cristobal and, in 1907,

assumed charge of the New Orleans Quarantine Station. He had extensive experience in the diagnosis and suppression of yellow fever and contracted the disease in the Mississippi epidemic of 1898. He also saw service in the yellow fever epidemics of Hampton, Virginia; Miami, Florida; and Laredo, Texas. He served in many other capacities and considered malaria his forte among diseases. He married Mary Charlotte Thompson (1872–1965) in 1898; they had one child. Dr. von Ezdorf died suddenly near Lincolnton, Lincoln County, North Carolina, from heart disease. He was only forty-three years old. See "Obituary," *British Medical Journal* 2, no. 2917 (November 25, 1916): 746; and "Obituaries," *Military Medicine* 39 (1916): 453.

62 Assistant surgeons, passed assistant surgeons, and surgeons in the US Public Health and Marine Hospital in 1911 earned $1,600, $2,000, and $2,500 per year, respectively. For more information on the qualifications and performance requirements for each grade, see "Bureau of Public Health and Marine Hospital Service," *Texas State Journal of Medicine* 7, no. 1 (May 1911): 31–32.

63 See "Cerebrospinal Meningitis in Texas," *Public Health Reports* 27, no. 4 (January 26, 1912): 128; and "Says Serum Offsets Usual Bad Effects; Dr. Sophian Declares Sequalae Are Not Noticeable," *Dallas Morning News*, January 22, 1912, 2.

64 "Marine Surgeon Is Coming," *Dallas Morning News*, January 17, 1912, 5; and "US Surgeon May Aid in Meningitis Fight," *Fort Worth Star-Telegram*, January 18, 1912, 7.

65 "Situation Shows Improvement Here," *Dallas Morning News*, January 18, 1912, 2.

66 "So-Called Epidemic Practically Over," *Dallas Morning News*, January 21, 1912, 8.

67 Dr. Frank Johnson Hall (1875–1946) was born on a farm near Liberty, Clay County, Missouri, as the only child of Allan Reed Hall (1851–1889), a cattleman, and Theodora (Dora) Johnson (born in 1858), the daughter of Dr. Francis Marion Johnson (1835–1893). Frank Hall grew up on the family's Liberty farm and on a cattle ranch in Oklahoma before moving to Kansas City after his father's death in 1889. His mother married William E. Wilson (born in 1857), a grocer, in 1898; they had no children. Frank Hall graduated from Garfield Grade School in Kansas City in 1892, from Central High School in Kansas City in 1897, and from the Kansas City Medical College (existed from 1881 to 1905) in 1900. He performed

post-graduate work at the University of Chicago in 1901, 1902, and 1903. He served as a consultant pathologist at the Kansas City General Hospital and founded the American Biologic Company, which held a license to propagate the rabies virus vaccine after the method of Pasteur for use in preventing rabies in exposed humans during the virus's incubation period. Dr. Frank Hall also gained fame nationally during the murder trial of Dr. Bennett Clark Hyde, the alleged murderer of Thomas H. Swope (1827–1909), the Kansas City notable and philanthropist who donated the land for the new Kansas City General Hospital in 1905. Dr. Hall also served as the Kansas City-based pathology department editor for the newly-reorganized *Medical Herald*, beginning in November 1911. Dr. Hall married Mary Eleanor Whitney (1881–1952) in 1898; they had eight children. He retired in 1943 and died three years later at the age of seventy-one years. See Dr. Frank Hall Dies; Pathologist Here 46 Years Was 71; Retirement in 1913 Follows Active Career in Medical Profession—A Member of Many Groups," *Kansas City Star*, February 25, 1946, 12; "More Victories over Death; A Serum Reduces the Proportion of Fatal Meningitis," *Kansas City Star*, May 4, 1911, 3; and "Meningitis Serum Used Here; Dr. Frank Hall Says the Flexner Treatment is Not New Here," *Kansas City Star*, October 30, 1911, 5. For more information on Dr. Hall's involvement in the Swope trial, see Giles Fowler, *Deaths on Pleasant Street* (Kirksville, MO: Truman State University Press, 2009), 79–81, 102, 135–136; "How Did Swope Die; A Medical Examination Made of the Body of the Millionaire," *Kansas City Star*, January 14, 1910, 1; "'Give the Barber Glasses'; How a Kansas City Physician Used Sherlock Holmes Methods," *Kansas City Star*, January 17, 1910, 2; "One Grain! Dr. Hektoen Says 1/6th Grain of Strychnine Was Found in Col. Swope's Liver; Strychnine Injected: Nurse Testifies Dr. Hyde Ordered Hypodermics After Convulsions Began; Dr. Hektoen Is Called; The Chicago Chemist Tells of the Analysis Which Showed the Presence of Strychnine," *Kansas City Star*, February 8, 1910, 1; "Dr. Frank Hall Testifies: The Tonic Could Not Have Caused the Death, the Physician Says," *Kansas City Star*, February 9, 1910, 12; "At the Hypothetical Stage; Lawyer in the Hyde Trial Begun Practice for Scientists Yesterday, *Kansas City Star*, April 30, 1910, 2; and "Dr. Hyde Arrested as Swope's Slayer; Accused of First Degree Murder, He Has Hearing and Is Released on Bail, *New York Times*, February 11, 1910, 1.

68 See Margaret R. O'Leary and Dennis S. O'Leary, *The Kansas City Meningitis Epidemic, 1911–1913: Violent and Not Imagined* (Bloomington, IN: iUniverse, 2018).

69 On Saturday, January 20, 1912, Dr. Sophian said, "One more thing I would like to have seen more largely done and *I have only today* [January 20, 1912] *received from Dr. [Frank Johnson] Hall*[69] [emphasis added] an eminent authority, commendation of the suggestion for the vaccination or use of the [antimeningitis] serum as a preventive, a serum prophylaxis. "So-Called Epidemic Practically Over," *Dallas Morning News*, January 21, 1912, 8.

70 "So-Called Epidemic Practically Over," *Dallas Morning News*, January 21, 1912, 8.

71 Rose Emma Nielsen (1891–1934) was born in Galveston, Galveston County, Texas, as one of the five children of Jens Peter Nielsen (1861–1916) and Mary Schirmer (1861–1910). She married Dr. Albert Ware Nash in 1913; they had three children. She died of a streptococcal throat infection and throat hemorrhage at the age of forty-two years. Her husband died hours later of a heart attack. They had a double funeral. "Dallas Doctor and Wife Die within Two Hours Each Other," *Corsicana Semi-Weekly Light* (Corsicana, TX), February 13, 1934, 7; "Double Funeral Services Held," *Galveston Daily News*, March 15, 1934, 17.

72 "Dr. von Ezdorf in Austin; Representative of United States Marine Hospital to Assist in Meningitis Infection in Texas," *Dallas Morning News*, January 20, 1912, 11; "Dr. von Ezdorf To Be in Dallas: Representative of Marine Hospital Service Will Be in City This Morning," *Dallas Morning News*, January 21, 1912, 8; and "No Need of Local Quarantine," *Bryan Daily Eagle*, January 22, 1912, 3.

73 Dr. Rupert Blue (1867–1948) was born in Richmond County, North Carolina, as one of the eight children of John Gilchrist Blue (1829–1889), a lawyer, and Annie Marie Evans (1830–1911). He was raised in Marion, Marion County, South Carolina. He attended the University of Virginia in Charlottesville, Virginia (1889–1890) and the University of Maryland School of Medicine, where he earned his medical degree in 1892. He spent his entire medical career in the US Public Health Service, entering in 1893. He worked as an intern at the Cincinnati Marine Hospital; studied in Galveston; and, in 1899, went to Italy to inspect passengers and freight en route to the United States for plague. He next went to Milwaukee, Wisconsin, and then to California, where the plague had broken out. He aided

in the discovery that bubonic plague was carried by fleas on rats and was not transmitted by humans, as was believed. He then had charge of the Marine Hospital in Norfolk, Virginia, and then went to New Orleans, which was besieged by a yellow fever epidemic. He continued in this peripatetic manner until he became US Surgeon General (1912 to 1920). He was the president of the American Medical Association in 1915. He married Juliette Downs (1874–1895) in 1895. She died the same year at the age of twenty-one years. He never remarried. He died of heart disease at Roper Hospital, Charleston, South Carolina, at the age of eighty years. See Thomas F. Logan, "What I Am Trying to Do; An Authorized Interview with Dr. Rupert Blue, Surgeon General of the United States Public Health and Marine Hospital Service," in Walter Hines Page and Arthur Wilson Page, *The World's Work: A History of Our Time, November 1911 to April 1912* (Garden City, NY: Doubleday, Page, and Company, 1912), 23:653–57; "Ex-PHS Director, Dr. Blue, Is Dead; Famed Medic Noted for Plague Campaigns, *Times-Picayune*, April 14, 1948, 25; and "Dr. Rupert Blue Dies at 80; Former Surgeon General, AMA Head," *Evening Star* (Washington, DC), April 13, 1948, 12.

74 The Federal Public Health Service was a bureau of the US Treasury Department. Through successive acts of Congress, it underwent a process of evolution so that all its duties became essentially of a public health character. The US Surgeon General presided over the central bureau in Washington. The bureau in January 1913 consisted of seven divisions: personnel and accounts, foreign and insular quarantine and immigration, domestic (interstate) quarantine and sanitation, sanitary reports and statistics, scientific research, marine hospitals and relief, and miscellaneous. An assistant surgeon general oversaw each of the first mentioned six divisions. J. W. Kere, "Organization of the Federal Public Health Service," *Public Health Reports* 28, no. 3 (January 17, 1913): 117–19.

75 "Cerebrospinal Meningitis in Texas," *Public Health Reports* 27, no. 4 (January 26, 1912): 128.

76 *Texas Almanac: City Population History of Selected Cities, 1850–2000*, accessed December 8, 2017, https://texasalmanac.com/sites/default/files/images/CityPopHist%20web.pdf.

77 "Texas," *Journal of the American Medical Association* 58, no. 3 (January 20, 1912): 206.

78 "Former Meningitis Statistics," *Dallas Morning News*, January 21, 1912, 6.

CHAPTER 5

A MENINGOCOCCAL VACCINE AND A TEXAS FAREWELL, FEBRUARY 1912

O n Monday, January 22, 1912, two days after Dr. Abraham Sophian announced at the Dallas Medical Lunch Club that he planned to return to New York City, Dr. Ralph Steiner submitted his first known report on the Texas meningitis epidemic to Texas Governor Colquitt.[1] Dr. Steiner wrote,

> Dear Sir: In view of the prevalence of epidemic cerebrospinal meningitis in the state, I have felt it advisable to submit a short report upon this disease. By invitation of the city of Dallas and upon request of the state board of health, Dr. A. Sophian of the Rockefeller Scientific Research Institute [sic] at New York was sent to Dallas with the view of investigating the disease and assisting the local health authorities in its management and control.

Dr. Steiner added, "I wish to make public acknowledgement of the valuable service rendered by this talented gentleman and to assure him the state of Texas will always remember him with gratitude."[1] Dr. Steiner continued,

At my request, the surgeon general of the United States detailed Passed Assistant Surgeon R. H. von Ezdorf to service in Texas. Dr. von Ezdorf is a man of large experience in public health work and of recognized ability ... He is now in this state and, in connection with the health department, is investigating the epidemic of meningitis. I trust and believe, with his assistance, I may be able to submit in the near future a report which will prove of inestimable value.[1]

Dr. Steiner next argued against quarantines as a method to control the Texas meningitis epidemic, saying,

[I] assure your excellency that general quarantine in the present instance is unscientific and unnecessary. Our larger cities have avoided this error, but a number of our smaller towns have quarantined against infected points and some even against the world. The result has been extreme annoyance to the traveling public, heavy losses, inconvenience to railroads and the commercial interests of the state.

He noted that the Texas State Health Board supported the isolation and quarantine of individual cases and contacts as the only precaution in the nature of quarantine[1] and concluded,

I have also the pleasure of informing your excellency [*sic*] that general conditions throughout the state are rapidly improving. Epidemic meningitis is a cold weather disease. I look for a marked decrease in cases on return of seasonable condition.

Signed, Ralph Steiner, State Health Officer.[1]

On Wednesday, January 24, 1912, Dr. Steiner and Dr. Key signed a circular sent to all Texas physicians to announce the availability of Dr. Key's diagnostic services in interpreting nose and throat specimens sent to him by physicians from their convalescing meningitis patients and contacts. The circular said,

> Dear Doctor: It is doubtful whether a definite quarantine period is sufficient to control the spread of meningitis, as it is known that carriers may carry the meningococcus in their nasal and throat secretions for a period of several weeks. To prevent the spread of the disease in this manner, a bacteriological examination of these secretions from all convalescent meningitis patients or persons directly exposed to the disease must be made ten days after the subsidence of the disease. We have arrangements for such examinations and request you to assist us. Whether you will continue quarantine will depend in each case upon our findings.[2]

Also, on Wednesday, January 24, 1912, Mayor Holland, Dr. Nash, and Dr. Sophian agreed to shutter the cerebrospinal meningitis headquarters in the Oriental Hotel, as the City Hospital staff now could perform the screening work previously performed by Dr. Turner, Dr. Carrick, and Dr. Neel. At the same meeting, Dr. Sophian agreed to remain in Dallas for an additional week and to spend an additional week speaking on cerebrospinal meningitis to physicians in Texas cities with a high disease prevalence.[3]

On Wednesday, January 24, 1912, Dr. von Ezdorf, who had been touring the cerebrospinal meningitis high-prevalence cities of Dallas and Fort Worth since Sunday, January 21, 1924, rolled into Waco. There he shared that Dallas health officials had counted 249 cerebrospinal meningitis cases and 110 cerebrospinal meningitis deaths (October 1, 1911, to January 22, 1912) and that Fort Worth health officials had counted sixty-one cerebrospinal meningitis cases and twenty-seven cerebrospinal meningitis deaths. Waco health officials reported to Dr. von Ezdorf 114 cerebrospinal meningitis cases and forty-two cerebrospinal meningitis deaths.[4]

[Based on these case and death counts, the prevalence, mortality, and case fatality rates for the above three cities between October 1911 and January 24, 1912, calculated to:

- Dallas (population in 1910, 92,000[5]): *27.1 cerebrospinal meningitis cases per 10,000 Dallas residents, 12.0 cerebrospinal deaths per 10,000 Dallas residents, and 44 percent.*
- Fort Worth (population in 1910, 73,000[5]): *6.6 cerebrospinal meningitis cases per 10,000 Fort Worth residents, 2.9 cerebrospinal deaths per 10,000 Forth Worth residents, and 44 percent.*
- Waco (population in 1910, 26,000[5]): *43.9 cerebrospinal meningitis cases per 10,000 Waco residents, 16.2 cerebrospinal meningitis deaths per 10,000 Waco residents, and 37 percent.*]

On Friday, January 26, 1912, Dr. Leake convened a meeting of the Dallas Board of Health to discuss reopening the Dallas schools on Monday, January 29, 1912. Even though the cerebrospinal meningitis situation appeared to be improving, Dr. Nash advised against reopening schools on Monday, February 5, 1912, because of lingering public anxiety. Dr. Leake and the board agreed.[6]

Sometime between Saturday, January 20, 1912, and Saturday, January 27, 1912, Dr. Sophian asked Dr. Thayer about manufacturing a meningococcal vaccine. Dr. Thayer agreed to starting the project. At the Dallas Medical Lunch Club on Saturday, January 27, 1912, Dr. Sophian announced to the audience that Dr. Thayer was working on a meningococcal vaccine. Dr. Sophian added that a meningococcal vaccine would not cause serum sickness or anaphylaxis and could be used more generally and more freely than could antimeningitis serum as a preventive agent.[7–8]

Also, on Saturday, January 27, 1912, the *Journal of the American Medical Association* updated its readers on the Texas cerebrospinal meningitis situation: "It is reported by the health authorities of Dallas that the poliomyelitis [*sic*] situation is distinctly more favorable and that the epidemic is well in hand. Up to January 20 [1912], there had been 225 cases reported; of these 202 are said to have been actual cases of meningitis, and of these, 99 patients died." The article added, "Of the patients, 128 were white, of whom 68 died, and 74 were colored [sic], of whom 33 died. There are at present under quarantine in Dallas 64 houses, in some of which there are cases of meningitis and from others cases have been removed to the city hospital. Disinfection of the premises and discharge from quarantine has already commenced."[9]

The article continued,

> The City Hospital, Dallas, was cleared of all other patients and placed in charge of Dr. A. Sophian from the Rockefeller Institute for Medical Research, as a meningitis hospital. He is said to be making from 40 to 45 injections of serum a day and is toiling almost incessantly. In proportion to the population, Waco had a more severe epidemic than Dallas. At Waco, up to the evening of January 9, there had been 105 cases, with 42 deaths.[9]

The article next described the lumbar puncture procedure technique advanced by Dr. Sophian: "The patient undergoes the usual cleansing preparation, then, while a careful watch is kept of the blood pressure and pulse, from 15 to 45 cubic centimeters of cerebrospinal fluid is withdrawn, or fluid is withdrawn until the blood pressure drops from five to ten millimeters, depending on the condition of the patient. Many patients are unconscious at the time the operation is made."[8] After the withdrawal of the cerebrospinal fluid, the "serum is injected in varying quantities, but almost always in smaller amounts than that of the fluid removed."

The journal article concluded, "Some cases are of very rapid progress: One girl is reported to have had the first symptoms at seven in the morning and had died four hours later. The disease is said to have a larger mortality in white people than in Negroes [sic]. It is a matter of surprise also that the majority of patients are adults. It is said that all the available serum of Rockefeller Institute has been sent to Dallas."[9]

The time for Dr. Sophian's Dallas departure was fast approaching. On Sunday, January 28, 1912, Dallas leaders announced their intention to hold a banquet to honor Dr. Sophian, Dr. Nash, and other physicians on the Thursday evening, February 1, 1912, at the Oriental Hotel. Approximately 250 people received invitations.[10]

On Monday, January 29, 1912, Dr. Sophian traveled to Austin to meet with Governor Colquitt and Dr. Steiner in the Texas State Capitol building. Dr. Sophian assured the governor that conditions in Dallas generally were improving, as measured by a decline in disease lethality since the introduction of intraspinal antimeningitis serum. Between October 1, 1911, and January 8, 1912, 44 percent of cerebrospinal meningitis patients had succumbed; since the opening of the City Hospital on January 8, 1912, 10 percent of children and 10 to 15 percent of adults had succumbed.[11]

During the meeting with Governor Colquitt, Dr. Steiner expressed concern about the scarcity of antimeningitis serum. He had ordered six hundred liters from the Research Laboratory in New York City, hoping to receive the product to meet demand. Governor Colquitt proclaimed that the Texas State Board of Health should manufacture its own sera for all contagious diseases, as was being done in other states, notably New York.[11] The Texas State Board of Health laboratory could produce the sera for less money and avoid the problem of chronic shortages. The poor people of Texas would benefit, he said. Dr. Steiner duly noted the governor's orders. Dr. Sophian returned to Dallas, arriving by noon.

A *Dallas Morning News* editorial on Wednesday, January 31, 1912, deemed "sensible" Governor Colquitt's call for the Texas State Board of Health to manufacture sera for use in Texas but noted, presciently, "There is apt to be some complaint on behalf of the druggists, if this suggestion shall reach the stage of legislative consideration, that this would be an interference with their business." Furthermore, said the editor, "*It is at least questionable if the service could not be better performed at the*

University's school of medicine than by the State Health Board" [emphasis added].[12]

Also, on Wednesday, January 31, 1912, Dr. von Ezdorf left Houston for Washington to write and publish his final report on the Texas meningitis epidemic (October 1, 1911, to January 22, 1912). He tabulated a total of 550 Texas cases, with 210 deaths since the beginning of the epidemic in October 1911. Of the 550 cases and 210 deaths in Texas, 249 and 110, respectively, had occurred in Dallas, as earlier noted.[13] The prevalence, mortality, and case fatality rates for Texas between October 1, 1911, and January 22, 1912, calculated to *1.4 cerebrospinal cases per 10,000 Texans, .5 cerebrospinal deaths per 10,000 Texans*; and 38 percent, respectively. These figures understandably did not raise alarm in Washington. However, the statewide figures did not accurately reflect the meningitis experience of high-prevalence Texas cities, where the disease prevalence was high.

Furthermore, on Wednesday, January 31, 1912, the Dallas city commissioners met to discuss remuneration for Dr. Sophian's services. Finance Commissioner Walter Tillou Henderson[14] said that the action to pay Dr. Sophian was taken without consulting Dr. Sophian and without any request from him. The city commissioners felt that some compensation should be offered; the question was whether Dr. Sophian would accept it.[15]

Finally, at a meeting of the Dallas Chamber of Commerce on Wednesday, January 31, 1912, Herbert Marcellus Hughes,[15] an owner of the Wiley Blair Wholesale Grocery Company, told his fellow businessmen that during his recent mercantile trips to both New York City and Chicago, the northern people were remarkably conversant with the current affairs and the meningitis situation in Dallas. In addition, they had a favorable idea of the city because of its efficient and open way of handling the epidemic, considering the calling in of outside expert advice one of the best features.[15] He commented, "New York people [were] especially well acquainted with the work of Dr. Abraham Sophian and [held] a very high opinion of his scientific abilities." Mr. Hughes declared that even though the meningitis epidemic had harmed business, the good impression of the handling of the epidemic would be "of lasting benefit such as offset the other."[16]

On Thursday evening, February 1, 1912, the business and professional elite of Dallas met in the main dining room of the Oriental Hotel to honor Dr. Sophian, Dr. Nash, Dr. Thayer, Dr. Walter Henrik Moursund,[17] Dr. Neel, Dr. Turner, Dr. Carrick, and Dr. Davis. The latter four were the diagnosticians who ran the meningitis headquarters in the Oriental Hotel. The elaborately decorated hall held sixty tables placed so that attendees faced the speakers.[18] Dr. Frank Johnson Hall of Kansas City, Missouri, was among the fifty-four physicians present at the banquet.[19]

Dr. Cary, in the role of toastmaster, introduced "General" Martin McNulty Crane,[20] who boomed,

> We have seen the ravages of this disease change laughter to sorrow. When at the worst, Dr. Abraham Sophian has come to our help, and he has put this monster at our feet. For us to be grateful to this man, who has come without hope of reward, is saying little. We are not trying to compensate him, but we want to show him that we are grateful. And now, Dr. Sophian, all I can do for you is to present this memento. It has no intrinsic value but take it and keep it in memory of this time.[21-22]

"Loving Cup Presented to Dr. Sophian," *Dallas Morning News*,
February 2, 1912, p. 2. The photographer is unknown.

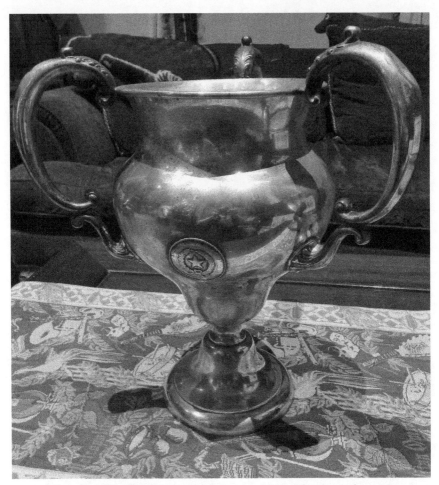

The actual Dallas, Texas, loving cup, 2018. Photographer: M.
R. O'Leary, 2018. The Dr. Abraham Sophian Dallas, Texas,
Loving Cup is part of the Dr. Abraham Sophian Archive.

The sterling-silver loving cup, according to a *Dallas Morning News* article on February 2, 1912, was twenty inches tall, held eighteen pints, and carried a four-inch-diameter 14-karat-gold relief of the seal of the United States[22] on one of its three rounded sides. The following words were engraved on one side of cup, "To Doctor Abraham Sophian in recognition of his unselfish devotion to the cause of science and in appreciation of his masterly leadership in preventing the spread of disease and in saving lives among us.

This token is given by grateful citizens, Dallas, Texas, February First, Nineteen Hundred Twelve."[22]

Dr. Sophian took the beautiful loving cup in his hands and said with much feeling,

> With my heart is the only way I can talk tonight. I wish to express my appreciation, and I have remarked on your hospitality. My stay here has been a busy one, but pleasant. The plans I formulated on my way have nearly all been carried out. I think there would have many times as many cases without the cooperation I have had. We have had 170 [cerebrospinal meningitis] cases and a mortality of less than 20 per cent. One of my plans I have not quite carried out—that is, of preparing a vaccine. But it is ready and I took a dose of it last night [Wednesday, January 31, 1912]. I advise it for all who have been exposed.[20]

Dr. Sophian continued, "I desire to say a word for those who have worked with me, and especially for Dr. Nash. He deserves more than I. I think the work is highly organized now, and *if it is kept up* [emphasis added] and all the people help, I think Dallas has little need for fear. The mortality has been lower than for typhoid." He added,

> I wish to express my admiration for your mayor and commissioners. If they had not turned over everything we could not have done anything. Your body of physicians have done nobly, and I never knew any physicians could do so much. Of the particular [City Hospital] doctors, Dr. Henry Smith, Dr. S. M. Hill, Dr. [Robert August] Trumbull, Dr. V. E. Robbins, and others are to be thanked. Of the nurses, Miss Nielsen, Mrs. Barnes, Miss Jessie Smith[23] and others deserve great praise.

He concluded, "I thank you very much for your courtesy. In years to come this will always be my happiest memory."[20]

A resolution, typed on Dallas City Chamber of Commerce stationery and adopted by the Dallas Chamber of Commerce at an earlier special session, thanked Dr. Sophian, saying,

> Realizing the great service rendered the citizenship of Dallas; recognizing the personal devotion and self-sacrifice of Dr. Abraham Sophian in coming to this city and serving it so wisely and so well, therefore be it resolved by the Dallas Chamber of Commerce, representing the commercial interest of the city, that we the Board of Directors of this organization publicly express our appreciation and that of our membership for the invaluable aid which Dr. Sophian has rendered this city during the past weeks.

The resolution continued,

> In our opinion, the presence of Dr. Sophian has done much to educate our people, enabling them to deal with the meningitis situation wisely and in cooperation with the medical profession of Dallas. Dr. Sophian has rendered a great service, not only to this city but to the state of Texas as a whole. We therefore publicly express our thanks for his work and on behalf of the 1,110 businessmen of the organization acknowledge our gratitude for his devotion and self-sacrifice.[24]

John Robert Babcock (secretary, Dallas Chamber of Commerce),[25] Rhodes Semmes Baker,[26] Herbert Marcus [Sr.],[27] Joseph Sutton Kendall,[28] George Bannerman Dealey (publisher, *Dallas Morning News*),[29] Thomas Elbert Jackson,[30] Joseph Loose

Brown,[31] Louis Lipsitz,[32] Harold Sutherland Keating,[33] and Charles Harry Platter[34] signed the resolution.

The Dallas City Chamber of Commerce letter, 1912. Photographer, M. R. O'Leary, 2018. The letter is part of the Dr. Abraham Sophian Archive.

Mayor Holland next said,

> I had desired to pay a tribute to Dr. Sophian, but
> General Crane has done that. But we all know in
> such warfare as we have had against disease, no
> general can win without able lieutenants, and I
> desire to present a token to Dr. Nash and his helpers.
> I indorse [sic] Dr. Sophian's sentiments about our
> doctors. It is unusual in any city for physicians to
> work as ours have without pay. Dr. A. E. Thayer,
> the nurses, the interns, the students of the two
> medical colleges should not be forgotten. The four
> diagnosticians deserve thanks, as do our Board of
> Health and all their helpers, including the boys who
> drove the doctors' cars and the ambulance.[20]

Mayor Holland then presented Dr. Nash with a gold watch in a 14-karat solid-gold case, with nineteen jewels of modern size. The outer case had an elaborate monogram: "A. W. N." On the cover of the inside lid was the following inscription: "In appreciation of the untiring devotion of Dr. Albert W. Nash to his duties as Health Officer in a grave emergency, this token is given by grateful citizens. Dallas, Texas, February First, Nineteen Hundred Twelve."[20]

Dr. Nash accepted the gift and said,

> I have lived with you nearly always, and I cannot
> speak my gratitude for this gift. Before the hospital
> opened [for the exclusive care of cerebrospinal
> meningitis patients], the mortality was 62.5 per
> cent. Counting everything since, it has been 25 per
> cent. Leaving out the country patients, it has been
> 8.8 per cent. But it has not been entirely our skill.
> The doctors' cooperation has done wonders. With
> this kept up, we have little more to fear. Of course,
> our mayor and commissioners have been back of
> all. Our other doctors have been of great help—the

able privates in the ranks. Diagnosticians, nurses, interns, drivers, and all have done their part. I have only done my duty and I expect to continue doing my duty.[20]

Reverend James Frank Smith,[35-36] pastor of the Dallas Cumberland Presbyterian Church, next lauded the skill of Dr. Thayer and presented him with a diamond locket on a 14-karat solid-gold fob with a safety attachment. It was inscribed, "From grateful citizens to Dr. Alfred E. Thayer. Dallas, Texas, February 1, 1912."[20] Dr. Thayer responded, "I appreciate this gift and I wish to remember my helper at the laboratory, Dr. Moursund. The [cerebrospinal meningitis] vaccine is still experimental, but we have tried it without bad results. It may be of great value also as a substitute for the serum."[20]

George Bannerman Dealey[29] next announced,

> Mr. Toastmaster, Honored Members of the Medical Profession and Common Citizens: Dallas is one of the most remarkable places on earth and it does some of the biggest things. State Fair, hotels, musicians and all show this. In planning for a great city, we send for one of the best men at city planning. In a crisis, a scare, not an epidemic, we send and get the best to be had anywhere, and we got him.

Mr. Dealey continued, "If Dallas becomes what I think it will—the prettiest and cleanest city in the Southwest—we will look on this as a warning that we are not doing what we should. In the Dallas situation it is gratifying to know how the doctors have gotten together, and also to hear them speak of the nurses and interns." He then presented gold-headed silk umbrellas to Drs. Neel, Turner, Davis, and Carrick.[20]

Dr. Turner responded for the group, saying,

We feel we have only done what we should have done. This occasion ought to have been made to give proper recognition to Dr. Sophian. He has left his family, even remained in a time of calamity in his home, the loss of his mother [*sic*]. He has been the cohesive force for the public and the profession. He has given the confidence and the power to fight the disease. We of the "Big Four" ... deserve no praise. He who is not willing to do all he can is not worthy of the name of "doctor." The true doctor knows no sense of personal danger, particularly in the presence of disease. And here I want to say a word for the drivers of our cars—ever at our beck and call. Health is wealth. For this good city to have wealth, she must have health. What was this city's wealth worth when its health was gone? I think it's well to look to the future for the things to promote the city's health as well as its wealth.[20]

Dr. Leake next said, "I wanted to be here tonight for two reasons. First, because I have felt uncertain about the use of Flexner's serum. I felt I should await the figures to make up my mind. These showings have been marvelous. Dr. Sophian should be known as Hypocrates [*sic*] IV, if he has done all we have seen here. He is the fourth father of medicine."[20]

Dr. Samuel Palmer Brooks,[37] president of Baylor University in Waco, next remarked,

It happens that I come from a neighboring city that has shared with you the perplexity of the recent situation. I have watched with a great deal of interest every report from Dallas and of the work you have been doing. It is a blessed time that brings all men together to appreciate the work of the man who lives in his laboratory looking through pieces of window glass and discovering facts that will benefit mankind. As a citizen of Waco and of Texas, I wish to express our appreciation of the efforts of the men who have come to us from New York to aid us and for men who make possible institutions like the Rockefeller Institute.[20]

Following a brief benediction by Dr. William M. Anderson Sr,[38] the elderly pastor of the First Presbyterian Church of Dallas, the attendees filed out of the Oriental Hotel. A list of the banquet contributors (e.g., Studebaker Bros. Co. of Texas, Huey and Philip Hardware Company, and Dallas Cotton Exchange) and a list of the physicians in the audience were printed in the newspaper.[20] The flowers on the sixty tables were sent to the nurses at the City Hospital as an "attestation of esteem for their heroic work."[20]

On Friday, February 2, 1912, Dr. Steiner in Austin, who had not attended the Dallas banquet the previous night, acknowledged the death from cerebrospinal meningitis of Miss Frankie Bettis, a University of Texas coed.[39] She had become ill twenty-four hours before her death in the Chi Omega sorority house in Austin. She had been visiting her family in Beaumont two weeks earlier; had spent Monday, January 29, 1912, in Houston; and had returned by train to Austin on Tuesday, January 30, 1912. Miss Bettis did not feel well on Wednesday, January 30, 1912, according to Dr. Margaret Roberta Holliday,[40] the University of Texas Health Services physician for women, who was among the physicians caring for her. On Thursday morning, Miss Betts had stayed in bed but was able to get up to use the bathroom. That same afternoon, she experienced alarming symptoms. The next morning (Friday, February 2, 1912), she had died.

Dr. Steiner announced, "The case of Miss Bettis is similar to other cases of cerebrospinal meningitis that have occurred in Austin in that it did not originate here. No case that has developed in Austin has been a source of infection. The people of Austin, and especially university students, are safer here than on trains or in other places more favorable to infection and the spread of the disease." He advised university students to stay in Austin, confining themselves as closely as possible to their classrooms and boardinghouses. He noted that the house in which Miss Bettis's death occurred was in strict quarantine and that the health officers and university authorities were taking all necessary precautionary measures.[39]

Also, on Friday, February 2, 1912, Dr. Thayer regaled the members of the Tarrant County Medical Society with information on manufacturing a meningococcal vaccine.[41] His experimentation had not proceeded so far that he could quantify the vaccine's efficacy and safety. However, he was happy the vaccine had ended his own chronic nasal colonization with meningococci.[42]

At the same meeting, Dr. Thayer expressed his disapproval of the use of subcutaneous antimeningitis serum as a preventive because of its propensity to cause serum sickness. He mentioned the case of a physician who had developed a severe case of serum sickness following the subcutaneous injection of antimeningitis serum at the cerebrospinal meningitis clinic held by Dr. Sophian in the basement of St. Paul's Sanitarium on January 6, 1912.[43] The same anonymous physician praised Dr. Thayer's meningococcal vaccine, which he had received without ill effect.[44] Dr. Thayer disparaged the overuse of urotropin, which he said could cause kidney problems. Much of the rest of his speech described the work of the "swabbers"—the medical students who obtained smears of the mucus in the noses and throats of suspected meningococcal carriers, as described earlier.

On the evening of Friday, February 2, 1912, the Dallas County Medical Society separately honored Dr. Sophian and Dr. Nash. Fifty-five members and eleven visitors were present. Dr. William R. Blailock[45] presented a five-piece silver tea service to Dr. Sophian to signify the society's esteem for him. Dr. Blailock had a long-standing interest in cerebrospinal meningitis dating to 1899, when he managed two patients with the disease, surveyed Texas physicians on cerebrospinal meningitis, and published his survey results.[46] Dr. Blailock said the physicians in the audience looked forward to hearing Dr. Sophian's final report that evening on what he had learned in Dallas.[47]

Dr. Sophian did not disappoint his audience, presenting a wide-ranging speech available elsewhere, entitled "Observations during the Present Epidemic."[47] Dr. Sophian thanked the medical society for the tea service, saying, "I feel more honored by the good will which has inspired it than by the generosity of this gift. I have enjoyed my stay here and I leave with much good will and friendship for Dallas people. I leave here many friends with whom I hope to keep in touch in the future."[47]

Dr. Sophian said the following about the meningococcal vaccine:

> On the first night I was here, as you remember, we outlined a plan for our campaign, including prophylactic measures against spread of the disease, including sprays with peroxide of hydrogen, use of antiseptic throat and nose sprays and gargles, and taking of urotropin. Also, we planned use of [antimeningitis serum] as preventive of a negative nature and we planned to work out an active vaccine which shall serve for more permanent immunity against the disease than we may hope for from serum immunity, and isolation of all patients and exposed cases to prevent spread of disease through carriers and patients.[47]

Dr. Sophian added,

> Of those plans, we have succeeded well in all except that we have not quite completed our vaccine plan … I have suggested my plans for the vaccine to Dr. A. E. Thayer and he has worked them out. We now have a quantity of vaccine ready for distribution and use and I myself as well as some others have taken it without harmful or even inconvenient after-effects. Offhand, we cannot yet accept the vaccine

as beyond the experimental stage, but we think it will prove itself.[47]

Dr. Sophian continued,

> As I said, the vaccine is still experimental, but knowing what we do, it ought to work out all right. To immunize patients for a period of a year or more we are using 500,000,000 of the bacteria in the first dose and following that up with two doses of 1,000,000,000 of the bacteria at intervals of a week to ten days ... The local reaction has been slight in each case where the vaccine has been used and the danger is very much smaller than with the serum injection as preventive. There is not the serum sickness to so great extent and almost no danger, I think. The use of this vaccine is like that of typhoid vaccine, and I see no reason why it should not prove itself as readily when there has been time for a trial.[47]

Dr. Howard, the City Hospital steward, next presented Dr. Nash with a pair of diamond-studded cuff buttons on behalf of the Dallas County Medical Society. Dr. Nash said that he did not deserve such a gift, having done only what he had promised to do when he took his office. He added,

> I wish to say that I feel we have done a great deal here, but the major part of it, at least, is due to Dr. Sophian. In this emergency, a great part of our success has come from the cooperation of the physicians of Dallas and Dallas County. Now that Dr. Sophian is leaving, *it depends almost entirely upon you physicians to keep up that cooperation and to finish what has been begun* [emphasis added]. I wish to fully to thank all of my associates. Of the

interns and nurses, none have failed, and I think all of you know how they have worked. I thank you.[47]

On Saturday, February 3, 1912, the Dallas city commissioners presented Dr. Sophian with a check for $2,500 to recognize his service to the city during the cerebrospinal meningitis epidemic and to defray Dr. Sophian's traveling expenses.[48] The city commissioners arrived at the dollar amount after conferring with the leading physicians of the city. The commissioners also presented Dr. Sophian with a hand-inked parchment containing the following resolutions adopted by the board of commissioners of Dallas City:

> Whereas, Doctor Abraham Sophian, in his service to the people of Dallas and the State of Texas, has exemplified the highest attributes of a true physician in ministering to the sick and staying the spread of a dread disease; Whereas, by his conservative and modest conduct, has maintained the cordial cooperation not only of the medical profession but our citizenship in general; Therefore, be it resolved by the Board of Commissioners of the City of Dallas that we take this opportunity in behalf of the Citizens of Dallas, of expressing our sincere appreciation of the services rendered by Dr. Sophian, and wish for him a continuation of that success which he so richly deserves ... Adopted by the Board of Commissioners of the City of Dallas, February 2nd AD 1912. Signed, Mayor Holland, Water Works and Sewage Commissioner, Police and Fire Commissioner, Commissioner of Streets and Public Property, and Commissioner of Finance and Revenue.[48–49]

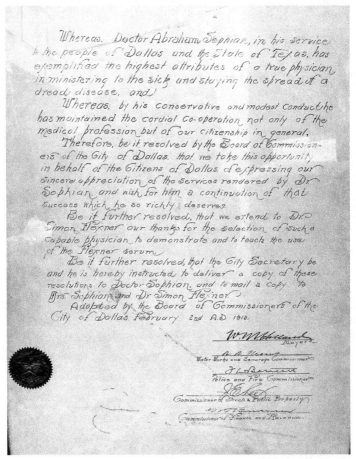

The parchment given by the Dallas City Board of Commissioners to Dr. Abraham Sophian on February 2, 1912. Photographer: M. R. O'Leary, 2018. The document is in the Dr. Abraham Sophian Archive.

Later in the afternoon of Saturday, February 3, 1912, Dr. Sophian formally addressed the students of the Southwestern University Medical Department[50] about the importance of pathology as a promising new branch of medicine. He said,

> I want to speak to you in a general way of the significance of some branches of medicine which are not yet in general use. To talk of my own experience in college [Cornell University Medical College, New

York City], I was much impressed with internal medicine, and soon after I entered one of the large hospitals [Mount Sinai Hospital] of New York City, I found out how much I had to learn.[51]

Dr. Sophian continued,

Fortunately, I had had both laboratory and clinical training, and I spent three and a half years in this hospital, gaining actual experience at the bedside of patients. It was not until I had left the hospital that I realized the importance of laboratory training. Until I took a fellowship in laboratory work there, I had thought of laboratory work applied to internal medicine as of value but not very useful. It gave me an insight into a branch which is not generally made use of, and I want to urge each of you in entering the profession to consider laboratory work and, if possible, arrange to give it a fair trial.[51]

He added,

In the last analysis, diagnosis of disease is far more important than treatment. If a physician can recognize a disease, it is not hard to treat it. The chief question with every physician should be not so much what to give the patient as what is the trouble with him. Good diagnostic work is the most important thing in treatment. After that, judgment counts. I can never tell, in meningitis, for instance, what a dose will be. There is no state of treatment, but when the dose will be given and how much must depend altogether on the judgment of the physician. Judgment simply means diagnosis of the case. And that is where the laboratory comes in.[51]

For example, said Dr. Sophian,

> A physician cannot really diagnose typhoid fever by symptoms alone, for he must know what bacteria are present. There are other diseases so much like typhoid in their appearance that the difference cannot be detected without bacteriological examination. It is the same with all septicemia. While training in college is mostly clinical, there is some laboratory work which does not usually appeal much to students. It seems less practical, but the student who pays more attention to such work will make a far better diagnostician.[51]

Dr. Sophian next said,

> Medicine is now drifting rapidly into a field of prevention, which is certainly more important than active medicine. In treatment of meningitis cases here, I have been quite as much interested in prevention as I have been in treatment and trying to cure patients. Far more good may be done by preventive medicine. For instance, take the work done in preventive medicine for typhoid where the statistics of vaccination in the army show how much more important is preventive medicine than treatment. In that work, all results must originate in the laboratory, and they consist principally of vaccine and serum therapy, which are made in laboratories. It is only a short time, I am sure, until all medicines will be placed on such a high scientific basis as to require laboratory work of every doctor.[51]

Dr. Sophian concluded, "In treatment of any disease, we must have scientific knowledge ... I wanted simply to impress the great importance of the laboratory in modern medicine and to convince you that at least a fair knowledge should be had of such work."[51]

After the lecture, Dr. James Harvey Black,[52] a professor of bacteriology and pathology at Southwestern University Medical Department, led Dr. Sophian on a tour through the new 250-bed Texas Baptist Memorial Sanitarium.[53] Dr. Sophian remarked that the Texas Baptist Memorial Sanitarium was as nice in its appointments as any to be found in New York City.[51]

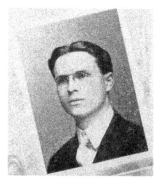

Dr. James Harvey Black (1884–1958) in his senior class photo from Southwestern Medical Department, 1906–1907. The photographer is unknown. The image was scanned from *The Sou'Wester* (Georgetown, TX: Southwestern University, 1907), 160–161.

At six thirty in the evening on Saturday, February 3, 1912, Dr. Sophian and Dr. Nash took a train to Fort Worth to speak to members of the Tarrant County Medical Society in the auditorium of the Fort Worth University Medical Department.[54-55] In his speech, Dr. Sophian predicted that the cerebrospinal meningitis epidemic in Texas had reached its peak and would soon wane. He based his prediction on the "history of all meningitis epidemics of this kind, [which] flourish for about three months and then very abruptly disappear." He added, *"The epidemic [in Texas] has run its course and I expect to see it disappear very abruptly"*[56] [emphasis added].

The same night (Saturday, February 3, 1912), Dr. Nash announced that 8.8 percent of infected individuals treated with antimeningitis serum at the City Hospital had died of their cerebrospinal meningitis. About 25 percent of infected individuals in Dallas had died from cerebrospinal meningitis between the inception of the epidemic in Dallas in October 1911 and February 3, 1912. Dr. Nash seconded Dr. Sophian's opinion that the disease epidemic was waning.[56]

On Monday, February 5, 1912, Dr. Sophian visited San Antonio and Fort Sam Houston,[57] about 275 miles southwest of Dallas. He declared San Antonio practically immune to the meningitis epidemic because of its warmer climate and told the surgeon general at Fort Sam Houston that the soldiers faced little danger from the ongoing cerebrospinal meningitis epidemic in other parts of Texas.[58-59] The next day, in Galveston,[60] a delegation of physicians met Dr. Sophian at the train station and escorted him to Hotel Galvez. He gave two speeches that Tuesday, February 6, 1912. The first speech was at four o'clock in the afternoon in the large auditorium of the University of Texas Medical Branch, and the second was in the Galveston County Courthouse before the combined medical societies of Galveston and Harris Counties.[61]

In his two addresses, Dr. Sophian noted that cerebrospinal meningitis epidemics appeared periodically in history. The question as to why the disease made a periodic appearance was difficult to answer. The immediate causes of the disease were predisposing factors, especially the climate. The months of the year that affected the secretions of the nose and throat were associated with cerebrospinal meningitis epidemics. The direct infection of cerebrospinal meningitis was almost always from a group of organisms finding lodgment in the nose and throat. Infection by inoculation was possible but rare.[61]

Dr. Sophian said the troubles of cerebrospinal meningitis epidemics rested least in people afflicted with the disease and most in the healthy carriers of the meningococci in the nose and throat. For every 100 people ill with cerebrospinal meningitis during an epidemic, there were 500 to 1,000 healthy carriers—no one knew exactly how many. As was true in the case of other diseases, perfectly healthy people could become disastrously effective permanent carriers of the meningococcal bacteria.[61]

Dr. Sophian urged disinfection of the nose and throat with a one-half-of-1-percent solution of hydrogen peroxide. He described the symptoms experienced by someone becoming ill with cerebrospinal meningitis. As a rule, the insidious symptoms developed within twelve to thirty-six hours, ending in a sudden explosion of violent symptoms. At times, however, the explosion of symptoms was the first observed. So easily distinguishable were the symptoms, however, that the disease could be strongly suspected by clinical observation in most instances. Dr. Sophian said he had never seen a second attack of cerebrospinal meningitis in a person who had survived a first attack.[61]

Dr. Sophian exhaustively covered the method of preparation and the means of introducing the antimeningitis serum into the spinal canal. He advised against the use of anesthetics during the procedure, except in extreme cases. After his speech, the combined Galveston and Harris County Medical Society members feted Dr. Sophian at a Galveston Island oyster roast.[61]

On Wednesday, February 7, 1912, Dr. Sophian spoke in Houston to a large audience of physicians and others assembled in the Houston Chamber of Commerce building.[62] In his address, Dr. Sophian noted that meningococci entered the system by establishing colonies in the upper air passages of the nose and throat. During the months of October, November, December, January, and February, these meningococci commonly were found in the noses and throats of most people wherever the epidemic prevailed. The meningococci passed from the air passages directly into the blood to lodge in the spinal column. The infection rarely entered the system through the skin. In the early stage of the disease, before the septicemic condition was reached, spraying the nose and throat with a good antiseptic solution prevented the disease from progressing further.[62]

Dr. Sophian then stated, "Healthy people are the only carriers of the disease, for the very simple reason that the sick are not able to be about. One disease carrier, while he may not contract the disease in any except its first stage, can easily infect thousands with whom he comes in contact. For this reason, people who are disposed to the disease should be quarantined to prevent the spread of the epidemic." He added, "A strict quarantine should be maintained, cultures of the nose and throat should be made at short intervals, and the persons quarantined should not be released until every vestige of the disease is gone."[62]

Dr. Sophian recommended the use of urotropin for cases that had advanced beyond the first stage. The drug was secreted into the spinal fluid soon after administration and, when used promptly enough, was effective.[63] The usual early symptoms of cerebrospinal meningitis were slight fever, headache, occasional vomiting, dilated pupils, a rigid neck, and marked tenderness at the angle of the jaw. Dr. Sophian emphasized many times during his lecture the importance of "taking the case in hand as soon as possible." He emphasized that people who exhibited any of the symptoms of the disease should consult a physician at once, thereby avoiding all the worst stages of the disease. Complications other than pneumonia were not frequent, although a few afflicted patients in Dallas had developed blindness, deafness, and paralysis as a result of their infection.[62]

On Wednesday, February 7, 1912, Dr. Sophian boarded a train for New York City. He held his Texas loving cup, carefully wrapped, on his lap.[62] He had been gone from his home for one month. Even after arriving home, Dr. Sophian remained in the national public eye because of his work in Dallas.[64-70]

CHAPTER 5 NOTES

1   "Health Officer Steiner's Report on Meningitis," *Bryan Daily Eagle*, January 23, 1912, 3; and "Dr. Steiner Makes Report; Shows Quarantine against Meningitis Unscientific; Authority Is Cited; Medical Works Quoted in Support of View of Health Board— Situation Is Improved," *Cleburne Morning Review*, January 23, 1912, 8.

2   "Fair Prospect; Quarantine against Meningitis May Be Raised Soon Says Steiner; Are Not Scientific; State Health Officer Says No Definite Term of Isolation May Be Fixed as All Cases Differ," *Houston Post*, January 24, 1912, 9.

3   "Close Headquarters; Pleased at Outlook; Improvement Such No Special Diagnosticians Required; Meningitis Situation Causing Officials to Grow Optimistic—Dr. Sophian Plans Trip to the South," *Dallas Morning News*, January 24, 1912, 4.

4   See "Dr. von Ezdorf's Meningitis Report; Says Texas Cities and Physicians Are Working Together to Eradicate the Disease—Deaths About Forty Per Cent," *Bryan Daily Eagle*, January 26, 1912, 2; and "Cerebrospinal Meningitis in Texas," *Public Health Reports* 27, no. 4 (January 26, 1912): 128.

5   *Texas Almanac: City Population History of Selected Cities, 1850– 2000*, accessed December 8, 2017, https://texasalmanac.com/sites/ default/files/images/CityPopHist%20web.pdf.

6   "Public Schools Will Resume Work Feb. 5; Health Board Decides upon That Date, after Conference; Dr. Nash Says There Is No Actual Danger Now—Nine New Cases Friday," *Dallas Morning News*, January 27, 1912, 3; and "Advises Medical Inspection; Dr. R. H. Von Ezdorf Reports on Health Conditions to Governor," *Dallas Morning News*, January 28, 1912, 6.

7   Dr. Sophian's exact words were, "The serum administered as a prophylactic remedy against meningitis confers a certain degree of protection against the disease for about two weeks, perhaps longer. The average dose is about ten cubic centimeters. When it is administered in this way, in a large percentage of cases, a condition occurs called serum sickness, consisting principally of hives or nettlerash." He continued, "This, while a temporary annoyance, has not further results, except in very rare cases. Exceedingly rare among thousands upon thousands of cases where the serum has been administered, a condition of shock or antiphylaxis [*sic*] may occur."

He added, "We have advised this prophylactic immunization only for those who are intimately exposed to the disease, always describing the foregoing conditions. I personally have taken it, realizing the conditions, but feeling that the temporary annoyance of the hives and the very small risk of antiphylaxis [sic] was as nothing compared with the risk and danger of meningitis." He concluded, "We are now preparing a vaccine which, we hope, will produce an active and long immunity. The after-effects of using such a vaccine will be unimportant. This may be used more generally and freely than the serum." "Preparing a Banquet for Sophian and Nash; Dallas to Compliment Doctors for Faithful Services; Dr. Sophian Issues Statement Concerning Antiphylactic Effect of Serum; Physicians' Lunch Club Meets," *Dallas Morning News*, January 28, 1912, 6.

8   "Dr. Sophian Gives History of Fight," *Dallas Morning News*, February 3, 1912, 13.

9   "Texas: The Meningitis Situation," *Journal of the American Medical Association* 58, no. 4 (January 27, 1912): 287.

10 "Preparing a Banquet for Sophian and Nash; Dallas to Compliment Doctors for Faithful Services; Dr. Sophian Issues Statement Concerning Antiphylactic Effect of Serum; Physicians' Lunch Club Meets," *Dallas Morning News*, January 28, 1912, 6.

11 "Dr. Sophian Visits Governor," *Dallas Morning News*, January 30, 1912, 3.

12 "Editorial," *Dallas Morning News, January* 31, 1912, 6.

13 "Surgeon Von Ezdorf to Deliver Meningitis Lectures in Louisiana Centers," *Times-Picayune*, January 31, 1912, 7; and "Dr. von Ezdorf Here from Texas Fight; Gives Local Physicians the Benefit of His Studies in Connection with Cerebrospinal Meningitis Visit; Holds There Is No Need for State [Louisiana] Quarantines; Has Delivered Several Addresses in Louisiana, and Will Speak at Forum Today," *Times-Picayune*, February 4, 1912, 7.

14 Walter Tillou Henderson (1869–1936) was born in La Grange, Troup County, Georgia, as one of the three children of James Claude Henderson (1838–1913) and Cornelia Forbes (1845–1922). He moved with his family to Sherman, Grayson County, Texas, and thence to Honey Grove, Fannin County, Texas, where he graduated from Honey Grove High School. He then attended Eastman Business College (in operation from 1859 to 1931, one of the largest commercial schools in the United States) in Poughkeepsie, Dutchess County, New York. In 1894, he married Lillian Alice Ware (1871–1966) in Honey

Grove, and they moved to Dallas the next year. He did mercantile bookkeeping and bank work until 1908, when he became the Dallas auditor. In 1911, he became the Dallas commissioner of finance and revenue. In 1915, he completed his second term in office and began practicing law. He became the corporation court judge in Highland Park in 1934. He and Lillian had two children. He died at the age of sixty-seven years. See "Highland Park Official Passes Away Late Monday Night at His Home," *Dallas Morning News*, May 26, 1936, 12.

15 "Plans Are Announced for Sophian Banquet," *Dallas Morning News*, January 31, 1912, 3.

16 Herbert Marcellus Hughes (1883–1918) was born in Oakton, Hickman County, Kentucky, as one of the six children of Thomas Davis Hughes (1853–1902), a farm laborer, and Josephine Tolley (1854–1922). His father died when he was young. As the eldest son, he supported his mother and the younger children. He moved to Texas in 1898, when he was eighteen years old. In 1901, he became connected with Wiley Blair in the wholesale grocery business at Wichita Falls, Wichita County, Texas. He later became a partner and then one of the principal stockholders of the company, which was one of the largest wholesale grocery concerns in the Southwest. He was a member of the Chamber of Commerce and Manufacturers' Association of Dallas. He married Josephine Blair, the daughter of Wiley Blair, in 1906; they had two children. He was vice president of the Dallas Railways Company. He died of Spanish influenza pneumonia at the age of thirty-five years. See "About People," *Electric Traction* 14 (November 1918): 754; "Herbert M. Hughes Is Called by Death; Well-Known Business Man and Civic Worker Victim of Pneumonia," *Dallas Morning News*, October 10, 1918, 6; and "Resolutions Adopted on Death of Herbert Hughes," *Dallas Morning News*, October 17, 1918, 6.

17 Dr. Walter Henrik Moursund (1884–1959) was Dr. Alfred E. Thayer's assistant pathologist in the Ramseur Science Building at Baylor University College of Medicine during the meningitis epidemic in Dallas in 1912. He was born in Fredericksburg, Gillespie County, Texas, as one of the eight children of Albert Waddell Hansen Moursund (1845–1927), a lawyer and judge in Fredericksburg, and Henrikke Mowkinckel (1854–1942); both of his parents were natives of Norway. Walter Henrik Moursund graduated from the Fredericksburg High School and earned his medical degree from

the University of Texas Medical Branch at Galveston (1906). He practiced medicine in several Texas towns before joining the pathology faculty at Baylor University College of Medicine in Dallas (1911). He remained at Baylor University College of Medicine for his entire medical career, serving as a professor of physiology, pathology, clinical pathology, bacteriology, and hygiene; secretary and registrar; acting dean; and dean (1923–1953). He wrote *A History of Baylor University College of Medicine, 1900–1953* (Houston, TX: Gulf Printing Company, 1956). He married Freda Adelide Plate (1884–1979); they had five children. He died of acute myelomonocytic leukemia at the age of seventy-four years. See "Dr. Walter H. Moursund, Medical Educator, Dies," *Dallas Morning News*, April 3, 1959, 3; and "Dr. Moursund, Ex-Dean of Medical School, Dies," *Dallas Morning News*, April 6, 1959, 6.

18 "Dallas Will Honor Meningitis Expert; Citizens Plan Banquet Tonight for Drs. A. Sophian and A. W. Nash; To Express Gratitude; Desire to Acknowledge Faithful Services of Men Who Have Labored to Stamp Out Disease," *Dallas Morning News*, February 1, 1912, 4.

19 "Gifts Presented to Foes of Meningitis; At Banquet to Drs. Sophian and Nash Citizens Express Appreciation; Win Battle for Dallas; Fight against Disease Has Reduced Death Rate from 62.5 to Less than 25 Per Cent," *Dallas Morning News*, February 2, 1912, 2.

20 Martin McNulty Crane (1853–1943) was born in Grafton, Taylor County, West Virginia, as the youngest of the three sons of Martin Crane (1812–1860) and Mary McNulty (died in 1857). When Martin McNulty Crane was four, his mother died, and his father took him to Stewart County, Tennessee, where his father died. Family members raised Martin M. Crane. At the age of seventeen years, he left Tennessee for Johnson County, Texas, where he taught himself law. He entered the Texas Bar in 1877 at the age of twenty-four years and opened a law practice. He soon entered Democratic politics, serving as Johnson County attorney, state representative of the Nineteenth Texas State Legislature, state senator of the Twenty-Second Texas State Legislature, Texas lieutenant governor, and Texas attorney general (1894–1898). He declined to run for governor. He had a successful law practice for forty years. He married Eula Olatia Taylor (1854–1940) in 1879; they had ten children. He died in Dallas at the age of eighty-nine years. See "M. M. Crane, Attorney General," in E. H. Loughery, *Texas State Government: A Volume of Biographical*

Sketches and Passing Comment (Austin, TX: McLeod and Jackson, 1897), 10.

21 The actual loving cup received by Dr. Sophian is fourteen inches high and holds thirteen pints. In addition, the relief is trimmed in 14-karat gold, the seal is two inches in diameter, and the seal is of the state of Texas. The engraved words are exactly as noted in the text.

22 "Loving Cup Is Presented to Dr. Sophian," *Dallas Morning News*, February 2, 1912, 2.

23 Miss Jessie Smith (1888–1971) was born in Odessa, Russia, as one of three children. Her parents and two brothers died during one of the anti-Jewish pogroms in Odessa in 1905. Stabbed and cut, she dragged herself to the Odessa Hospital, recovered from her wounds over the winter, escaped across the Russian border, and sailed from a German port to New York City. In 1911, she graduated from the nurse training program at the Har Moriah Hospital on Second Street and Avenue A in New York City. See "Left for Dead Now Becomes Nurse," *Jewish Herald* (Houston, TX), November 17, 1911, 2.

24 The Chamber of Commerce resolution document is part of the Dr. Abraham Sophian Archive.

25 John Robert Babcock (1874–1938) was born in Leonardsville, Madison County, New York, as one of the five children of Henry Dwight Babcock (1845–1924), a machinist, and Nancy Brown (1846–1908). He moved to Dallas in 1909 to improve his health. In Dallas, he worked as the secretary and assistant to the president of the Dallas Chamber of Commerce from 1909 to 1918. He moved back to New York (1919) to become associated with the National Bank of Commerce. He soon became its district representative for New England (1920), business development department director, and western representative on the Pacific Coast, 1926–1931. He continued his services in the West for the Guaranty Trust Company, with which the Bank of Commerce had merged, and eventually returned to the main office in New York to serve as the second vice president of the Guaranty Trust Company. He married Jennie Maude Dakin (1875) in 1904; they had four children. He died unexpectedly at the age of sixty-four years. See "Former Chamber Aid Buried in New Jersey," *Dallas Morning News*, July 3, 1938, 4; "Industrialist Dies," *Corpus Christi Caller-Times*, July 1, 1938, 6; "J. R. Babcock Rites Conducted," *Courier-News* (Bridgewater, NJ), July 1, 1938, 11; and "J. R. Babcock, Bank Official, Buried Here," *Courier-News* (Bridgewater, NJ), July 2, 1938, 16.

26 Rhodes Semmes Baker (1874–1940) was born in Duck Hill, Montgomery County, Mississippi, as one of the children of Andrew Jackson Baker (1842–1912), a planter, and Billie "Bettie' Newsome Kearney (1854–1909). The family migrated from Mississippi to Texas (1884), where Rhodes graduated from the law department of the University of Texas at Austin (1896). He opened a law practice, Spence and Baker, and became prominent in civil law adjudication. He also became active in public affairs, at one time holding the office of land commissioner of the state of Texas and the vice presidency of the Dallas Chamber of Commerce. In 1908, his fellow workers in the 150,000 Club honored him by electing him their president. He married Edna M. "Pansy" Rembert (1878–1955) in 1899; they had three children. He died of renal failure and pneumonia at the age of sixty-five years. See "Rhodes S. Baker," *Dallas Morning News*, February 8, 1940, 2; "Rhodes Baker Paid Tribute at Funeral," *Dallas Morning News*, February 8, 1940, 7; and "Flag at Half-Mast for Denning, Baker," *Dallas Morning News*, February 8, 1940, 16.

27 Herbert Marcus Sr. (1878–1950) was born in Louisville, Jefferson County, Kentucky, as one of the five children of Jacob Marcus (1846–1929), a cotton buyer and dry-goods merchant, and Delia Bloomfield (1848–1919). He left public high school in Louisville for financial reasons at the age of fifteen years; moved to Hillsboro, Hill County, Texas, in 1893; and took successive jobs as a janitor at a general store owned by a brother-in-law and as a salesman at Sanger Brothers. He and his brother-in-law, Abraham Lincoln Neiman (1875–1970), worked at the Coca-Cola Company in Atlanta, Georgia; sold their rights to sales territories for $25,000; and used their money to open Neiman Marcus, a women's shop stocked with ready-made clothing imported to Texas from New York City and elsewhere, in 1907. He bought out his brother-in-law in 1928. He married Minnie Lichtenstein (1882–1979) in 1902; they had four children. He died of a cerebral hemorrhage at the age of seventy-two years. See "Herbert Marcus Critically Ill Following Stroke at His Home," *Dallas Morning News*, December 11, 1950, 1; and "Herbert Marcus Dies at Dallas Home Early Today," *Waxahachie Daily Light*, December 11, 1950, 6.

28 Joseph Sutton Kendall (1884–1919) was born in Honey Grove, Fannin County, Texas, as one of the two children of Joel Sutton Kendall (1849–1906), an educator and superintendent of public instruction in Texas, and Lorena "Lunie" Ellen Woodson (1852–1940). He

left Honey Grove for Dallas to work as a clerk in a real estate firm. Within a year, he went into business for himself and, in one year, became one of the most powerful businessmen in Dallas. He financed and sold properties in Munger Place and Highland Park and represented the Busch interests in Texas, which included financing the purchase of the land for erection of the Adolphus Hotel. During the Liberty Loan campaign (World War I), he raised an enormous amount of money and had a mental breakdown. He declined a position in the US Treasury by Secretary William Gibbs McAdoo. He managed the financial coup by which the Great Southern Life Insurance Company obtained control of a big block of the controlling stock of the Missouri State Life Insurance Company, which resulted in his accession to the latter's presidency. He married Bess Walcott (1885–1970) in 1904; they had three children. He died of pandemic influenza at Bellevue Hospital, New York City; he was thirty-four years old. He had been in New York City to confer with financiers regarding business expansion plans. See "J. S. Kendall Dies in New York; Sold $10,000,000 in Liberty Loan Bonds in Day," *Fort Worth Star-Telegram*, February 13, 1919, 1; "Head of State Life Co. Dies in New York; J. S. Kendall Succumbs to Influenza in Bellevue Hospital after Brief Illness—Wife with Him When End Came; Came to St. Louis Last October from Dallas; Health Had Been Undermined by His Efforts as Chairman of Dallas Liberty Loan Organization Last Fall," *St. Louis Star and Times*, February 13, 1919, 1; and "J. S. Kendall Dies in Hospital in New York City; Was President of the Missouri State Life Insurance Co. and Went to Metropolis on Business; He Was Giving Away $10 Tips in Hotel; One Estimate Stated that He Had Disposed of $2000 in a Few Hours—Taken to Psychopathic Ward," *St. Louis Post-Dispatch*, February 13, 1919, 1.

29 George Bannerman Dealey (1859–1946) was born in Manchester, England, as the fourth of the nine children of George Dealey (1828–1894), a bookmaker, and Mary Ann Nellins (1829–1913). The family moved from Manchester to Liverpool before immigrating to Galveston, Texas, in 1870, when he was eleven years old. He took evening classes at the Island City Business College while working at the *Galveston News*, beginning in 1874. He became business manager of the *Dallas Morning News* at its incipiency in 1885. He rose through the ranks of the *Dallas Morning News*, finally buying it and two other publications from the heirs of Alfred Horatio Belo (1839–1901) in 1926. He had other business interests in addition

to the newspaper and pursued civic activities during the next two decades. He married Olivia Allen (1863–1960) in 1884; they had five children. Dealey Plaza in Dallas was named in honor of George Bannerman Dealey. He died of a coronary occlusion at the age of eighty-six years. See Judith Garrett Segura, *Belo: From Newspapers to New Media* (Austin, TX: University of Texas Press, 2008); and "Journalism Dean Loved His Job All 71 Years," *Dallas Morning News*, February 27, 1946, 13.

30 Thomas Elbert Jackson (1881–1972) was born in Jo Daviess County, Illinois, as one of the six children of Milton W. Jackson (1851–1915), a blacksmith, and Susan E Mankey (1858–1930). He moved to Dallas around 1907 and, three years later, became the southwestern manager of the Pittsburgh Plate Glass Company, a position he held for the next sixty-two years. He served as a director of the Dallas Chamber of Commerce (1911–1936). During World War II, he chaired the Dallas County Rationing Board. He held many civic positions throughout his adult life. He married Virginia Elizabeth Fall in 1903; they had one child. Thomas E. Jackson died of a stroke at the age of ninety years. See "Business Leader, T. E. Jackson Dies," *Dallas Morning News*, August 31, 1972, 6; and "T. E. Jackson," *Dallas Morning News*, September 1, 1971, 2.

31 Joseph Loose Brown (1867–1935) was born in Mercersburg, Franklin County, Pennsylvania, as one of the seven children of Reverend Isaac Getz Brown (1828–1885) and Elizabeth Matilda Loose (1835–1920). Fourteen-year-old Joseph L. Brown moved to Wichita, Sedgwick County, Kansas, to farm and sell books at a bookstore. He then moved to Kansas City to work for his uncles, Jacob Leander Loose (1850–1923) and J. Schull Loose (1845–1922), owners of the Loose-Wiles Biscuit Company. Several years later, he managed a biscuit factory in Fort Worth. Finally, he owned and operated the Brown Cracker and Candy Company in Dallas (1907–1935). The company was the largest manufacturer of biscuits and candy in the Southwest United States. He also remained a director of the Loose-Wiles concern. He was a lifelong bachelor and lived for many years at the Adolphus Hotel in Dallas. He died of a stroke at the age of sixty-eight years. See "Death Claims J. L. Brown, Cracker, Candy Firm President Dies at Dallas; Rites at Wichita," *Amarillo Globe-Times*, July 9, 1935, 1.

32 Louis Lipsitz (1872–1927) was born in Detroit, Wayne County, Michigan, as one the five children of Joseph Lipsitz (1842–1910), a

merchant, and Rebecca Soraski (1837–1899). The family moved to Tyler, Smith County, Texas, in 1877. Louis Lipsitz attended public schools and the Eastman Business College in Poughkeepsie, Dutchess County, New York, before returning to Tyler, Smith County, Texas, to work as a clerk in the dry-goods firm of A. Harris and Company, which was owned by his father and an uncle. By 1900, Louis had become a partner in the company, which had expanded into lumber sales. In 1907, he moved to Dallas to run the Harris-Lipsitz Company, a wholesale dry-goods firm, and the Harris Lumber Company, a wholesale lumber establishment. He was president of the Dallas Chamber of Commerce in 1915. He was a lifelong bachelor. He died at the age of fifty-four years after dancing on the roof garden of the Crazy Hotel at Mineral Wells, Texas. See "An Outstanding Figure," *Dallas Morning News*, April 4, 1927, 10; and "Louis Lipsitz Laid to Rest; Dallas Civic and Business Leader Buried in Emanu-El Cemetery," *Dallas Morning News*, April 5, 1927, 15.

33 Harold Sutherland Keating (1859–1921) was born in Halifax, Nova Scotia, Canada, as one of the children of William H. Keating and Eliza W. Forbes (1840–1907). At the age of eighteen years, Harold moved to Kansas City, Jackson County, Missouri, to work in the Smith and Keating Implement Company. He moved to Dallas in 1888 to enter the Keating Implement and Machinery Company, the firm owned by his brother, A. C. Keating. When his brother retired, Harold became president of the company. He married Mary Victoria Leake (1865 1944) in 1878; their two children died as infants. He died after a long illness at the age of sixty-two years. See "Retired Dallas Business Man Who Died Thursday," *Dallas Morning News*, January 22, 1921, 10.

34 Charles Harry Platter (1869–1941) was born in Chillicothe, Livingston County, Missouri, as one of the two sons of Thomas McCague Platter (1839–1873), a hotel keeper, and Elizabeth A. Harry (1845–1933). He left Chillicothe at the age of sixteen years for Denison, Grayson County, Texas, to work for the Waples-Platter Wholesale Grocer Company, of which his uncle, A. F. Platter, was an official. He moved to Dallas in 1901 to establish the Platter Tobacco Company and later became associated with the Boren-Steward Grocery Company. He married Mary Hanna (1867–1940); they had two children. He died after a long illness at the age of seventy-two years. See "Death Calls C. H. Platter, Food Broker;

Was Civic Worker, Helped in Early-Day Planning of City," *Dallas Morning News*, October 31, 1941, 18.

35 Reverend James Frank Smith (1868–1920) was born on a farm in Greenfield, Weakley County, Tennessee, as one of the ten children of John Wesley Smith (1846–1915) and Emily Ellen Combs (1846–1922). He earned degrees from Bethel College in McKenzie, Tennessee, and Cumberland University in Lebanon, Tennessee. In 1896, he received his bachelor of divinity degree from the Union Theological Seminary and his master of arts degree from Columbia University, both in New York City. In the fall of the same year, he was called to the pastorate of the Cumberland Presbyterian Church in Dallas, where he remained until his death two decades later from Banti's disease. He married Lillian Duff Neal (1876–1970) in 1903; they had two children. See "Prominent Dallas Preacher Is Dead; Was Church Leader," *Fort Worth Star-Telegram*, July 17, 1920, 3.

36 Reverend James Frank Smith had Banti's disease, which Dr. Thayer apparently diagnosed. Reverend Smith died of his disease eight years after the banquet for Dr. Sophian, Dr. Nash, and others. Banti's disease was first described in 1883 by the Italian pathologist Dr. Guido Banti (1852–1925) as "a group of cases characterized by primary enlargement of the spleen, a more or less characteristic secondary hypochromic anemia, leukopenia, thrombocytopenia, gastrointestinal bleeding, and a chronic course leading to terminal ascites and liver cirrhosis." See "Banti's Disease or Syndrome," *Journal of the American Medical Association* 115, no. 17 (October 26, 1940): 1,456–57.

37 Dr. Samuel Palmer Brooks (1863–1931) was born in Milledgeville, Baldwin County, Georgia, as one of the five children of Samuel Erkine Brooks (1831–1906), a farmer and clergyman, and Aurelia Elizabeth Palmer (1836–1880). In 1868, the family moved to Texas, where Samuel Palmer Brooks worked as a laborer for the Santa Fe Railroad, began study at the Baylor University Preparatory School at the age of twenty-four years, graduated from Baylor University at the age of thirty years, earned another bachelor's degree at Yale College (New Haven, Connecticut), taught at Baylor University for four years, and earned a master's degree from Yale University. In 1902, the trustees of Baylor University recruited him as president of the university; he was thirty-nine years old. He served in this capacity from 1902 until his death in 1931. He married Martha "Mattie" Sims (1868–1940) in 1895; they had two children. He died

of cancer at the age of sixty-seven years. See "Dr. S. P. Brooks, Head of Baylor, Dies of Cancer; Death Takes Beloved College President after Long Illness; Injured in Europe; Strength Never Fully Returned after His Trip Abroad," *Dallas Morning News*, May 14, 1931, 1, 3; and "Brooks Burial Is Set for 3:30 This Afternoon, Follows 30 Years to Day Funeral of Former Head of Baylor," *Dallas Morning News*, May 15, 1931, 1.

38 Dr. William Madison Anderson Sr. (1862–1924), known as the "marrying parson," was born in Gibson County, Tennessee, as the only son of William J. Anderson (1839–1900) and Martha Krenn Holmes (1839–1913). He married Sarah "Sadie" Knott Anderson (1862–1945); they had seven children (all sons). Their eldest son, William Madison Anderson Jr. (1889–1935), became a Presbyterian minister in Austin, Texas, in 1914; assisted his father at the First Presbyterian Church of Dallas, which the senior Reverend Anderson had helped to build; and assumed his father's pastorate upon his father's death in 1924. Dr. William Madison Anderson Sr. died at the age of sixty-two years after a lingering illness that began in 1916. See "Dr. Anderson, Well Known Pastor, Dies," *Marshall News Messenger*, April 6, 1924, 1; and "Body of Minister Is Held in State; Funeral for Presbyterian Pastor at Dallas to Be Held Today," *Galveston Daily News*, April 7, 1924, 5.

39 Frankie Bettis (1892–1912) was born in Beaumont, Jefferson County, Texas, as the eldest of the three children of Frank Jewell Bettis (1867–1913), a manufacturer, and Sarah "Sadie" Letitia Baldwin (1871–1952). See "Another Meningitis Case; Miss Frankie Bettis Dies at Sorority House after a Brief Illness—Contracted Disease Elsewhere," *Austin American-Statesman*, February 2, 1912, 2; "Death of University Student; Young Lady Dies in Sorority House after Brief Illness—President Mezes Issues Statement to Patrons," *Dallas Morning News*, February 3, 1912, 13; "Austin, Tex.," *Dallas Morning News*, February 10, 1912, 3; and "Frankie Bettis," Texas Death Certificate No. 1312/5687, Texas State Board of Health Standard Certificate of Death, February 2, 1912.

40 Dr. Margaret Roberta Holliday (c. 1882–1923) was born in Goliad, Goliad County, Texas, as one of the seven children of William Burroughs Holliday (1853–1895), a stock raiser, and Nancy L. Cromwell (1859–1957). She earned her bachelor's and master's degrees from the University of Texas at Austin in 1901 and 1902, respectively, and her medical degree from the University of Texas

Medical Branch at Galveston in 1906. She moved to Austin, where she served as assistant physician at the State Lunatic Asylum and, beginning in 1909, as University of Texas Health Services physician for women students. She married Dr. Simon John Clark (1878–1960) in 1918. She died five years later of tuberculosis; she was about forty-one years old. Arthur Wayne Hafner, *Directory of Deceased American Physicians, 1804–1929* (Chicago, IL: American Medical Association, c. 1993); "Dr. Margaret Holliday Clark," *Austin American-Statesman*, December 30, 1912, 3; and "Margaret Holliday Clark," Texas Death Certificate No. 35118/ 33, Bureau of Vital Statistics, Texas State Board of Health, December 31, 1929.

41 "Hear Address by Dr. Thayer, Dallas Pathologist Tells Tarrant County Medical Society Good Results of Meningitis," *Dallas Morning News*, February 3, 1912, 13; and "Use of Serum for Immunigation [*sic*] Opposed, Dr. Thayer Tells of Experiences of Dallas Physicians in Fighting Meningitis in Dallas," *Fort Worth Star-Telegram*, February 2, 1912, 13.

42 "A Communication: Serum Sickness," *Texas State Journal of Medicine* 7, no. 12 (April 1912): 336.

43 The anonymous physician who had developed severe serum sickness in January 1912 took three subcutaneous doses (five hundred million dead meningococci in sterile saline solution) of Dr. Thayer's heat-killed meningococcal vaccine at one-week intervals in February 1912. He said he developed no systemic reaction and believed but could not prove that he had longer-lasting immunity. "A Communication: Serum Sickness," *Texas State Journal of Medicine* 7, no. 12 (April 1912): 335–36.

44 "Northern District, Society News," *Texas State Journal of Medicine* 7, no. 11 (March 1912): 313–14.

45 Dr. William Russell Blailock (1849–1919) was born in Leake County, Mississippi, as the youngest of the eight children of Henry Eldridge Blailock (1797–1895) and Evaline Elizabeth "Lena" Currie (1811–1900). He earned his medical degree from the Tulane University Medical Department in 1875; practiced medicine at Carthage, Mississippi; and moved to Texas in 1883, first working in Waco and McGregor before moving to Dallas in 1904. He was vice president of the Texas Medical Association. He married Zelda Madaline Datson (1851–1937); they had three children. See "Deaths in Dallas," *Dallas Morning News*, Mary 23, 1919, 8.

46 William R. Blailock, "Meningitis in Texas and Indian Territory during First Three Months of 1899," *Transactions of the Texas State Medical Association, Thirty-First Annual Session Held at San Antonio, Texas* (Austin, TX: Von Boeckmann, Schutze, and Company, 1899), 121–38.

47 "Dr. Sophian Gives History of Fight," *Dallas Morning News*, February 3, 1912, 13.

48 Alex Sanger, president of the Dallas Chamber of Commerce, praised the $2,500 gift to Dr. Sophian. On hearing some unfavorable comments upon the action of the Dallas commissioners, Mr. Sanger asked some of the best physicians in Dallas whether Dr. Sophian had taught them and other physicians throughout the state anything about meningitis. They replied that Dr. Sophian had reduced the mortality of the disease from 90 percent to less than 10 percent; had remained in Dallas, risking his own life, even while there was sickness in his own home in New York; and had taught knowledge of inestimable value to Texas physicians. It was appropriate that he receive the gift. Mr. Harry L. Seay added that if there had been any criticism, it should have been that the commissioners did not pay Dr. Sophian $5,000. See "Dallas Will Pay Dr. Sophian $2,500; City Officials Decide to Make Him Present of Check for That Sum; Services Appreciated; Commissioners Adopt Resolution Lauding Efforts of Physician to Control Meningitis Situation," *Dallas Morning News*, February 3, 1912, 18; and "Chamber Commerce Meeting Is Lively; Much Debate Accompanies Election of Directors and Report on Constitution," *Dallas Morning News*, February 18, 1912, 1.

49 The parchment containing the resolutions and signatures of the Dallas mayor and the Dallas Board of Commissioners is part of the Dr. Abraham Sophian Archive.

50 Southwestern University Medical Department (in existence from 1903 to 1911, also called Southwestern Medical College) was located in a four-story gray brick building at 1420 Hall Street, Dallas. Southwestern University, the parent organization of the Southwestern University Medical Department, was located in Georgetown, Williamson County, Texas, about 170 miles south of Dallas. Dr. Leake, Dr. McReynolds, and other physicians on the medical staff of St. Paul's Sanitarium in Dallas organized the Southwestern University Medical Department in 1903. On April 14, 1911, Southwestern University Medical Department became the

Medical and Pharmaceutical Departments of Southern Methodist University, following the recommendation of a commission of clergy and laity appointed by the Methodist Episcopal Church South. On May 31, 1913, fourteen medical school graduates received their Southern Methodist University medical degrees as the second graduating class of Southern Methodist University. In the summer of 1915, the board of trustees of Southern Methodist University disbanded the medical faculty, citing as reasons financial concerns and the need for increasingly stringent admissions requirements. The suspension of the Medical and Pharmaceutical Departments of Southern Methodist University was temporary, lasting only a year, but the programs never resumed operation. The medical building was sold to the Texas State Dental College, and much of its medical equipment was purchased by the Baylor University College of Medicine. See "Medical Colleges of the United States, Dallas," *Journal of the American Medical Association 59*, no. 8 (August 24, 1912): 632; "Historical Note," Southern Methodist University Medical and Pharmacy School Records: A Guide to the Collection, *Texas Archival Resources Online*, accessed November 1, 2017, http://www.lib.utexas.edu/taro/smu/00088/smu-00088. html; and John S. Fordtran, "Medicine in Dallas 100 Years Ago," *Proceedings of Baylor University Medical Center* 13, no. 1 (January 2000): 34–44.

51 "Dr. Sophian Lectures to Medical Students; Tells Them of Importance of Laboratory Work; Will Leave Tonight for Other Texas Cities— Two New Cases and One Death Saturday," *Dallas Morning News*, February 4, 1912, 3.

52 Dr. James Harvey Black (1884–1958) was born in Huntington, Cabell County, West Virginia, as one of the six children of Reverend James Adam Black (1854–1902) and Mary Nancy Murphy (1856–1942). James Harvey Black moved with his family to Fannin, Goliad County, Texas, in 1900; his father died two years later. James Harvey Black graduated from the Paris (Texas) High School in 1900 and spent two years preparing for medical college at the Academic Department of Southwestern University in Georgetown, Williamson County, Texas. He then moved to Dallas, where he earned his medical degree from the Southwestern University Medical Department (1907). Dr. Black served an internship at nearby St. Paul's Sanitarium (1906–1907) and returned to Southwestern University Medical Department at 1420 Hall Street to work as a bacteriology professor (1907–1911). In 1911,

Southwestern University Medical Department became Southern Methodist University Medical Department, and Dr. Black became professor of bacteriology and pathology at Southern Methodist University Medical Department. He was also dean of Southern Methodist University Medical Department (1914–1915), when the trustees of Southern Methodist University closed the medical department and merged the school's assets with Baylor University College of Medicine. From 1915 to 1942, Dr. Black was professor of bacteriology and pathology, preventive medicine, and clinical medicine at Baylor University College of Medicine in Dallas. In 1942, he became a professor of clinical medicine at Southwestern Medical School, a new medical school. Dr. Black maintained a private practice in clinical pathology in the Wilson Building in the Main Street district of downtown Dallas (1907–1932); he subsequently limited his practice to allergies. He married Allena Marie Patton (1886–1978) in 1913; they had two children. He died of a coronary occlusion at the age of seventy-four years. See *Sou'wester Yearbook 1907*, Southwestern University (Georgetown, TX: Athletic Association of Southwestern University, 1907), 160–61; "Dr. J. H. Black Dies, SMS [*sic*] Allergy Specialist," *Dallas Morning News*, December 1, 1958, 5; "In Memoriam, James Harvey Black, 1884–1958," *American Journal of Clinical Pathology* 32, no. 2 (August 1959): 172–73; "On Trail of Hay Fever; Allergy Causes Are Elusive, Physician Concludes," *Kansas City Times*, September 21, 1950, 3; "SMU's Forgotten Medical School," *SMU Magazine*, accessed January 3, 2018, http://blog.smu.edu/smumagazine/2011/12/smus-forgotten-medical-school/; and "Banquet to Dr. J. H. Black; Southwestern Medical Dean Going to Kentucky to Wed," *Dallas Morning News*, August 20, 1913, 6.

53 The Texas Baptist Memorial Sanitarium originated as the two-story, fourteen-room, brick Good Samaritan Hospital of Dallas (1903). In 1904, the Baptist General Convention of Texas renamed Good Samaritan Hospital as the Texas Baptist Memorial Sanitarium. In 1909, the Texas Baptist Memorial Sanitarium moved out of the brick building into a new 250-bed facility. In 1921, the Texas Baptist Memorial Sanitarium became Baylor University Hospital in Dallas to reflect its relationship with Baylor University in Waco, Texas. See "Our History," Baylor Scott and White Health, accessed November 1, 2017, http://news.bswhealth.com/pages/history.

54 The Fort Worth Medical College was established as the Medical Department of Fort Worth University in 1894 by a group of Fort Worth physicians. In 1918, the school closed after merging with Baylor University College of Medicine in Dallas. During its twenty-four years in Fort Worth, the Medical College graduated approximately 400 medical students. See "Fort Worth Medical College, accessed November 1, 2017, http://www.waymarking.com/waymarks/WM5V45_Fort_Worth_Medical_College_Fort_Worth_Texas; and John S. Fordtran, "Medicine in Dallas 100 Years Ago," *Proceedings of Baylor University Medical Center* 13, no. 1 (January 2000): 34–44.

55 "Dr. Sophian, Expert on Meningitis, to Speak Tonight," *Fort Worth Star-Telegram*, February 3, 1912, 7.

56 "Meningitis Epidemic to End Abruptly Now, Says Sophian; Dr. Flexner's Assistant Speaks to Tarrant County Medical Society—Two New Cases Here," *Fort Worth Star-Telegram*, February 4, 1912, 8.

57 Fort Sam Houston is a US Army base in San Antonio, Texas. Founded in 1845, it was named after Sam Houston (1793–1863), the first president of the Republic of Texas. In 1912, Fort Sam Houston was the largest US Army post. It contained the headquarters of the Southern Department, the San Antonio Quartermaster Depot, and a garrison of an infantry regiment, a regiment of cavalry, a field artillery battalion, and signal and engineer troops. See John Manguso, *Fort Sam Houston* (Charleston, SC: Arcadia Publishing, 2012); and John Manguso, "Fort Sam Houston," *Handbook of Texas Online*, accessed November 1, 2017, https://tshaonline.org/handbook/online/articles/qbf43.

58 "Reports from Affected Points," *Dallas Morning News*, February 6, 1912, 2.

59 "Eminent Specialist Coming, Dr. A. Sophian, Meningitis Expert, Due in Galveston Today—San Antonio Almost Immune, He Says," *Galveston Daily News*, February 6, 1912, 8.

60 "Expert on Meningitis Spends Strenuous Day; Dr. A. Sophian Addresses Medical College Students; Galveston and Harris County Physicians Join as Hosts in Oyster Roast Down on the Island," *Galveston Daily News*, February 7, 1912, 12.

61 "Sophian Lectured, Meningitis Expert Made Address at Galveston; Spoke before Medical Students and County Medical Society—Will Visit Houston Today," *Houston Post*, February 7, 1912, 5.

62 "Heard Dr. Sophian; Meningitis Specialist Was Here Yesterday; Houston Medical Men Entertained and Then Listened to Expert on Present Epidemic Situation," *Houston Post*, February 8, 1912, 9; and "The Fight on Meningitis; Work Accomplished by City Pathologist through the Laboratory during the Epidemic," *Houston Post*, March 3, 1912, 8.

63 "State," *Galveston Daily News*, February 8, 1912, 1.

64 On February 8, 1912, the editors of the *Waco Morning News* wrote, "While we are sleeping, others are toiling in laboratories and in workshops, endeavoring to discover something to lessen human misery or make life more endurable. In every epidemic that carries off the human race, sympathetic hands minister to suffering bodies and tender hearts endeavor to make the agony less awful, and if possible bring back to the pale and sunken cheeks the radiant glow of health ... There never was such a time in the history of the world when there was so much genuine human interest in the general welfare ... We cannot all be Maude Ballington Booths, nor Dr. Sophians, nor yet Miss McMasters, but we can in our own way do a little good as we go along." "Editorial by Murphy and Tupper, Editors and Owners," *Waco Morning News*, February 8, 1912, 8.

65 On February 15, 1912, the *New York Times* published Dr. Sophian's analysis of the Texas meningitis situation. Excerpts follow. Dr. Sophian said, "One great question, of course, is the reason for the appearance of spinal meningitis, and why some may carry the germs of the disease for months in nose and throat and give the germs to others, or finally be stricken themselves. It is necessary for something to predispose to the development of the disease, and in the case of meningitis it is most likely climatic changes. It is not necessary for the weather or climate to be bad, for I consider Texas weather superior to our weather in winter, at least. But there are sudden and unexpected changes, and in Texas there have been many of these recently ... In all, there have been about 300 cases of meningitis in Dallas since October [1911]. During the month I was there, we had in the special hospital about 185 cases, of which only about 45 per cent were children. This is unusual, for usually 83 per cent are children. Later in the epidemic, the relative proportion of children was larger. The rich and poor were sent to the hospital, and that was probably one of the reasons we had such good results not only in the treatment, but in the control of the epidemic. The disease spread all over the Southwest but was more centralized in Texas ...

The recoveries obtained resulted usually for three reasons: First, the cooperation of the physicians, by which we were able to get cases early, and, second, to the fact that we were able to control the cases and watch them carefully in the hospital. The third reason was the serum treatment, in the use of which I employed a new method of controlling the doses and administering it. The results exceeded our expectations. Excluding the cases which were hopeless when brought in, our mortality was ten per cent, which is extremely good, considering the many cases past middle life, some over 60, and others where the disease was unusually severe. Our mortality among children was only from five to six per cent ... The serum used was prepared in the Research Laboratory of the [New York City] Health Department under the direction of Dr. William H. Park. I took down 110 liters, making approximately 3,500 doses. The City of Dallas paid for this serum. I used that city as a center of distribution for the rest of the state. I established a special meningitis hospital and appointed a staff of four volunteer physicians." Dr. Sophian continued, "As soon as a case of meningitis was discovered, it was taken to the hospital and the home fumigated and those within quarantined. The average period was ten days ... Meningitis appears periodically. That cannot be prevented, but when it does appear, it can be checked and reduced to a minimum. I cannot say too much in praise of the mayor, the commissioners, and the physicians of Dallas for the hard work and good work done by them in meeting the situation and the cooperation of all." See "Back from Winning War on Meningitis; Dr. Sophian Reports Epidemic in Dallas and Other Texas Cities Practically Stamped Out; Treated Over 300 Cases; Brings Back Many Presents from Grateful Citizens and Loving Cup Presented by City," *New York Times*, February 15, 1912, 5.

66 On February 17, 1912, the *Journal of the American Medical Association* published the following update: "Dr. Abraham Sophian of the Rockefeller Institute for Medical Research left Texas, where he went to assist in combating the epidemic of spinal meningitis, on February 3. In appreciation of his services, the city of Dallas gave him $2,500 and Waco and a number of smaller towns presented him with $5,000, besides which he received a number of gifts in jewelry from local health departments and private individuals." See "Personal," *Journal of the American Medical Association* 58, no. 7 (February 17, 1912): 492.

67 Editors of the February 1912 issue of the *Texas Journal of Medicine* praised Dr. Abraham Sophian, who, "more than any other agency, saved the day, not only for Dallas, but for the entire state. He came to [Texas] gladly and freely, and to him [Texas] undoubtedly owes a debt of gratitude beyond our ability to pay." See "The Meningitis Situation," *Texas State Journal of Medicine* 7, no. 10 (February 1912): 265.

68 On March 2, 1912, the editors of the *Journal of the American Medical Association* published "Faithful Work" about Dr. Sophian: "When the meningitis epidemic broke out in Texas, it was necessary that the serum to combat the disease be administered by one familiar with its use. When Dr. Sophian—the physician chosen—was sent to the field, he may not have realized the hard work that lay before him, but we find no record of his flinching from his task." The article continued, "At any rate, a few days later he was in the midst of the epidemic, working 20 or more hours a day, bending all his energies to the humanitarian work he was sent to perform. When medical men work like this and fall a prey to disease, exposure or strain, we honor them as martyrs." The article concluded, "It is not unfitting that we occasionally chronicle a fine piece of self-sacrificing devotion to duty, even though the recipient of the praise has returned to his routine work and will doubtless deplore the publicity thrust upon him." "Faithful Work," *Journal of the American Medical Association* 58, no. 9 (March 2, 1912): 641; and "Faithful Work," *Evening News* (Ada, OK), March 6, 1912, 2.

69 In the March 2, 1912, issue of the *Journal of the American Medical Association*, Jerome Davis Greene, the general manager of the Rockefeller Institute for Medical Research, wrote the following letter to the editor to clarify that Dr. Sophian, mentioned in the "Medical News" columns (*Journal*, Jan. 27, 1912, 287), was not sent to Texas by the Rockefeller Institute for Medical Research. Instead, the latter, after receiving an application for relief by physicians and health department officials in Texas, "merely took the responsibility of seeing that a physician familiar with the serum treatment of meningitis was sent to Texas with the necessary supplies, and that his traveling expenses were paid." Mr. Greene added, "It appeared at once that a very competent physician to undertake this mission was Dr. A. Sophian of the Research Laboratories of the New York Department of Health, to whose immediate charge, under an arrangement with the department, the institute had recently given over the routine

manufacturing and dispensing of the meningitis serum." Mr. Greene concluded, "Although the institute very gladly made itself responsible for the mission, it is only fitting that the generous cooperation of the department of health in immediately giving Dr. Sophian leave of absence and in supplying a large quantity of serum at cost should be recognized. Signed, Jerome D. Greene, New York, General Manager, Rockefeller Institute for Medical Research." "The Texas Meningitis Epidemic," *Journal of the American Medical Association* 58, no. 9 (March 2, 1912): 649.

70 Jerome Davis Greene (1874–1959) was born in Yokohama, Kanagawa, Japan, as one of the nine children of Reverend Daniel Crosby Greene (1843–1913) and Mary Jane Forbes (1845–1910), both missionaries. He earned his bachelor's degree from Harvard College (1897); served as secretary to Harvard University president Charles William Eliot (1901–1905); served as secretary to the Harvard Corporation under Eliot and to President A. Lawrence Lowell (1905–1910); and served as secretary under Harvard University President James B. Conant (1934–1943). From 1910 to 1912, he served as the general manager of the Rockefeller Institute for Medical Research. He worked at a Boston investment banking firm (1917–1932), selling millions of dollars of the fraudulent securities of the Swedish Match king Ivar Kreuger. After losing most of his fortune, Mr. Greene recovered and spent many years serving on various boards and promoting the causes associated with Thomas Woodrow Wilson. He married May Tevis (1875–1941) in 1901 and Dorothea R. "Thea" Dusser de Barenne (1913–2000) in 1942. He and May Tevis had one child. He died at the age of eighty-four years. See "Jerome Greene Funeral Tomorrow at Harvard," *Boston Traveler*, March 30, 1959, 14.

CHAPTER 6

THE TEXAS MENINGITIS EPIDEMIC GRINDS ON, FEBRUARY-MAY 1912

The Texas cerebrospinal meningitis epidemic did not let up in February 1912 as predicted by Dr. Sophian and Dr. Nash.[1] The publication of cerebrospinal meningitis data dried up after Dr. Sophian left.[2] Nevertheless, there were ways to learn about meningitis activity. For example, there were about 116 new cases of the disease reported to Dr. Nash in Dallas during February 1912,[2] and the City Hospital in Dallas contained seventy-six cerebrospinal meningitis on Thursday, February 15, 1912.[3]

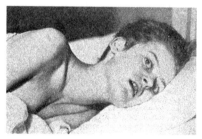

A young girl stricken with cerebrospinal meningitis, 1912. The original caption accompanying this image is: "Patient actively ill six days with epidemic meningitis. She was apathetic but otherwise clear and responded to questions. Note the anxious expression; the retraction of the head; the dilated pupils; the right facial paralysis; right external strabismus, and the sordes on the teeth." The photographer is unknown. The image was scanned from Abraham Sophian, *Epidemic Cerebrospinal Meningitis* (St. Louis, MO: C. V. Mosby, 1913), 72.

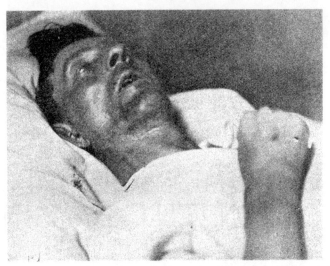

A male patient with cerebrospinal meningitis, 1912. The original caption accompanying this image is: "An alcoholic patient, ill thirty-six hours with epidemic meningitis. Violently delirious and deeply stuporous at intervals. Note the blank expression and the rigidity of the neck." The photographer is unknown. The image was scanned from Abraham Sophian, *Epidemic Cerebrospinal Meningitis* (St. Louis, MO: C. V. Mosby, 1913), 74.

Two major meningitis-related initiatives were underway in February 1912 in Austin and Dallas. The first initiative, announced on Thursday, February 8, 1912, by Governor Colquitt and Dr. Steiner, was to establish in Austin a state-run biologics laboratory to manufacture antimeningitis serum and other biologics. Poor Texans needed cheap biologics and all Texans needed a dependable supply of antimeningitis serum. Dr. Steiner claimed that the Texas State Board of Health biologics laboratory would be able to manufacture antimeningitis serum for thirty-five or forty cents per dose, as compared to the five dollars per dose charged by the Research Laboratory in New York City and other biologics establishments.[4]

On Friday, February 9, 1912, Dr. Steiner enthusiastically promoted his state-run biologics laboratory while displaying a batch of Dr. Key's heat-killed meningococcal vaccine before members of the Travis County Medical Society. Dr. Key had manufactured the meningococcal vaccine in the state food department laboratory in a room in the Texas State Capitol building. Dr. Key used meningococcal cultures that he had obtained from the cerebrospinal fluid of Rains County cerebrospinal meningitis patients.[5] The reactions of the Travis County Medical Society members to the meningococcal vaccine display are unknown.

Dr. Steiner lacked the funds and expertise to install and operate a biologics laboratory in Austin. He turned to his sister's husband, US Representative (Texas) Albert Sidney Burleson,[6] for help in identifying an expert. Representative Burleson approached US Surgeon General Blue in Washington about dispatching a public health service research pathologist from Washington, free of charge, to assist Dr. Steiner in the installation and operation of the proposed biologics laboratory in Austin.[7-9] US Surgeon General Blue agreed to the request and began the process of identifying a person to send to Austin. The Texas state attorney, prodded by Governor Colquitt, released state funds to establish the laboratory, promising Dr. Steiner that "everything possible was being done to expedite the matter."[7]

While Dr. Steiner awaited the name of the person US Surgeon General Blue planned to send to Austin, he secured new rooms for the Texas State Board of Health biologics, diagnostic, and state pure food department laboratories on the third floor of the west wing[10] of the Texas State Capitol building in Austin. The rooms were located adjacent to the committee conference rooms of the Texas House of Representatives, the third-floor halls, and the stairways linking the third floor to the floors below, which were in constant use while the House was in session.[10] In addition, the rooms designated for the laboratories opened via tall doors onto a broad balcony on the west side of the House gallery, which overlooked the spacious House Hall below. The representatives, when in session, sat at their wooden desks facing both the House speaker and the tall doors at the west end of the hall. By coincidence, the Texas House of Representatives did not meet at all in 1912.[11] Of note, the heating, plumbing, and ventilation systems of the Texas State Capitol building were antiquated and functioned poorly.[12]

The second meningitis-related initiative during February 1912 was Dr. Thayer's meningococcal vaccine enterprise operation in the laboratories on the second floor of the Ramseur Science Hall of the Baylor University College of Medicine in Dallas. Recall that Dr. Thayer had been working on the meningococcal vaccine since shortly after Saturday, January 20, 1912, when Dr. Sophian spoke with Dr. Hall in Kansas City and soon after asked Dr. Thayer to manufacture the vaccine.

To manufacture his meningococcal vaccine, Dr. Thayer combined live meningococcal cultures grown from the cerebrospinal fluid of several different cerebrospinal meningitis patients in Dallas. He placed a sample of the polyvalent culture in a test tube partially filled with a jelly made of agar (a kind of seaweed), veal broth, and about one-third diluted sheep serum. He incubated the test tube for about forty-eight hours at a temperature slightly less than that of the human body. He then tested the culture for purity.[13-14]

From a demonstrably pure culture, Dr. Thayer propagated secondary massive cultures over a large surface of the same jelly. Forty-eight hours later, he swept off the secondary cultures with sterile salt solution, retested the cultures for purity, and used a Zeiss counting chamber and Gentian violet as the diluting fluid to count the number of meningococci in a cubic millimeter (about fifteen drops). He then diluted the total with sterile salt solution (0.75 percent) to bring the number down to five hundred million meningococci per cubic centimeter.[13-14]

Dr. Thayer next sterilized the suspension of meningococci at 55 degrees Centigrade (131 degrees Fahrenheit)[15] for two hours, retested it for purity, and added one-tenth of 1 percent of carbolic acid as a preservative. He placed one cubic centimeter of the vaccine into a small glass ampoule, which he sealed in the flame of a Bunsen burner. One ampoule contained one cubic centimeter of 500 million heat-killed meningococci, suitable for one inoculation.[13-14]

With a meningococcal vaccine now available, Dr. Thayer proceeded to inject the vaccine. He prepared his own arm with alcohol and iodine, scratched the glass ampoule at its neck with a diamond so as to make it break with a smooth edge, and sucked up the contents into hypodermic syringe. He then slowly injected the serum through the needle attached to the syringe and into the brown spot left by the iodine. He washed off the stain of the iodine so that evidences of local reaction would not be obscured.[13]

Dr. Thayer continued, "Of this I took by hypodermic one cubic centimeter (of 500 million) at intervals of a week for three doses and have vaccinated in the same way about 20 others," including Dr. Sophian around February 2, 1912, as noted above.[16] The local reaction consisted of "only a slight soreness, such as would come from any hypodermic injection." Systemic reactions included "slight nausea, a little headache, fever of one degree, pains in some of the joints and dryness of the throat and nose." He contrasted these symptoms with the use of subcutaneous antimeningitis serum as an immunizing dose, which made some people "seriously ill for a week or ten days" with serum sickness. He added, "[Horse] [s]erum, too, is said to be more dangerous on subsequent doses than on the first. Its immunity is also considered temporary, measured in hours or days, while vaccine immunity may last months longer ... than an epidemic of spinal meningitis would prevail."[13] He concluded, "The reactions have so far been mild, even when the subject had had a prophylactic injection of [antimeningitis] serum two weeks before."[13]

As February 1912 sped by, Dr. Thayer vaccinated "quite a number of persons ..., several for the second time." He stated that the reactions were mild and that the vaccination reduced the number of meningococci in the nose and throat of healthy carriers.[13] In addition to vaccinating volunteers during the first two weeks of February 1912, Dr. Thayer worked on several "crude and preliminary" (his words) vaccine efficacy experiments on young rats. These experiments determined whether doses of vaccine given before inoculation of the rate with live meningococci would prevent its injurious effects. The experiments tended to show that the vaccine protected against an equal quantity of fresh living culture if given either before injecting the live meningococci, or with them, or within a period of three hours. Dr. Thayer said, "Further work of this kind will be done to establish what quantity of vaccine is needed to protect against given quantities of meningococci and within what limits of time."[14]

Unexpectedly, on Saturday, February 18, 1912, Dr. Thayer closed down his meningococcal vaccine operation and research at Baylor University College of Medicine to accept a new job as the medical supervisor of Texas Baptist Memorial Hospital, which was merging with the Baylor University College of Medicine, both in Dallas.[17] He expressed deep satisfaction in having had the opportunity to manufacture and test an autogenous vaccine[18-19] (his words) for cerebrospinal meningitis. He added, "If [the vaccine] proves a success, it ought to be useful both in conferring immunity for a period of months—longer than any epidemic would last, and also for cases which are passing from the acute into the chronic state, when serum is less helpful, to shorten convalescence and prevent complications and sequelae."[19]

Dr. Thayer's exit from his cerebrospinal meningitis research and vaccination operation distressed Dr. Sophian when he learned of it. The manufacture of a meningococcal vaccine was not particularly difficult, but Dr. Thayer was the only pathologist known to Dr. Sophian who was trying to prove that the vaccine actually prevented cerebrospinal meningitis.[20] Dr. Sophian was aware that Dr. Steiner was establishing a Texas State Board of Health biologics laboratory in Austin, but neither Dr. Steiner nor Dr. Key were trained research pathologists. Indeed, an editorial in the *Texas State Journal of Medicine* (February 1912) expressed disappointment with both the Texas State Board of Health and Dr. Steiner, noting that members of the Texas State Health Board were capable but busy and powerless and that Dr. Steiner was actively practicing medicine while overseeing the bureau.[21]

On Friday, February 23, 1912, Dr. von Ezdorf's paper on the Texas cerebrospinal meningitis epidemic appeared in *Public Health Reports*.[3] It was an informative paper in terms of the data and detail[22] it contained but covered the Texas cerebrospinal meningitis epidemic only up to January 24, 1912, the day that Dr. von Ezdorf left Texas for Washington.

On Saturday, March 2, 1912, Dr. Steiner learned that US Surgeon General Blue was sending Passed Assistant Surgeon Arthur Marston Stimson[23] to install the Texas State Board of Health biologics laboratory in the newly-designated rooms overlooking the House Hall in the Texas State Capitol building in Austin. Dr. Stimson possessed expertise in rabies virus vaccine propagation[24] and worked at the Hygienic Laboratory[25] in Washington. On Sunday, March 3, 1912, Dr. Steiner predicted to an Austin newspaper that the new serum laboratory would be in full operation within two to three weeks. Dr. Key would continue using the old pure food and drug department laboratory to manufacture meningococcal vaccine while awaiting the fitting of the new laboratory.[26]

Dr. Stimson arrived in Austin on Wednesday, March 6, 1912,[27] to "advise Texas health authorities in the installation of laboratory facilities for the production of antimeningococcic, antidiphtheritic, and other serums."[9] When newspaper reporters descended upon him, asking for details about the biologics laboratory, Dr. Stimson curtly replied that his review of the situation would take several days and that he did not care to discuss his plans in the meantime.[28]

After only one day of observation, Dr. Stimson saw the impossibility of installing a biologics laboratory in the Texas State Capitol building any time before the fall of 1912.[28] Furthermore, after viewing Dr. Key's meningococcal vaccine manufacturing activities in the state pure food department laboratory, Dr. Stimson told him to stop all further work until the completion of the proposed new laboratory facilities.[9]

Several more days passed. After Dr. Stimson completed his assessment of the local conditions in Austin, he advised Dr. Steiner against carrying out "the project [biologics laboratory] on the scale originally planned ..., as the available funds and accommodations would make its successful realization improbable." Dr. Stimson cited as problematic the proposed laboratory's location inside of the Texas State Capitol building, with its insufficient lighting, its inadequate water supply, and its lack of stable facilities for the horses and other animals needed to produce antimeningitis serum and other biologics. The facilities, declared Dr. Stimson, were simply "inadequate for the work contemplated." [9]

Dr. Stimson instead recommended that Dr. Steiner limit his operation to the installation of a simple diagnostics laboratory, which the Texas State Health Board still lacked, and a biologics laboratory for the production of typhoid vaccine only. [29] He reasoned that even if Dr. Steiner started his antimeningitis serum manufacturing right away, the serum would not be ready for distribution for five or six months. By the time the antimeningitis serum might be ready, the cerebrospinal meningitis epidemic would be over to such an extent as to not justify the manufacture of the antimeningitis serum by the state of Texas. Dr. Stimson also advised Dr. Steiner to postpone the manufacture of antidiphtheritic serum and smallpox vaccine until he could obtain a liberal appropriation from the Texas State Legislature. When Dr. Steiner complained to Dr. Stimson about the cost of obtaining biologics from existing biologics establishments, the latter counseled the former on ways to obtain biologics at a reduced cost. [9]

Dr. Steiner accepted Dr. Stimson's recommendations. [9] On Friday, March 15, 1912, Dr. Stimson handed Dr. Steiner a list of specialized equipment and materials needed to prepare typhoid vaccine [30] and to perform diagnostic examinations on throat swabs, cerebrospinal fluid, stools, blood, water, postmortem tissues, and commercial disinfectants. [31-32] After spending ten days in Austin, Dr. Stimson returned to Washington on Saturday, March 16, 1912. He intended to return to Austin that year but never did. [33]

Eleven days passed. On Wednesday, March 27, 1912, Dr. Key resigned as state bacteriologist to pursue advanced medical studies in the eye, ear, nose, and throat in New York City. [34] Dr. Steiner recruited Dr. Henry Charles Hartman [35-37] to replace Dr. Key.

Meanwhile, the cerebrospinal meningitis epidemic in Texas wore on throughout March 1912, killing 371 Texans—thirty-four more than in February 1912—and, for the second month in a row, surpassing both pneumonia and tuberculosis as the leading cause of death in Texas. [37] Dr. Sophian, still in New York City, followed reports of the cerebrospinal meningitis situation in Texas, including news that some nurses at the City Hospital in Dallas had developed nonfatal cerebrospinal meningitis.[38] Since his return to New York City in February 1912, Dr. Sophian had written and published a paper on the use of blood pressure monitoring to improve the safety of antimeningitis serum administration.[39]

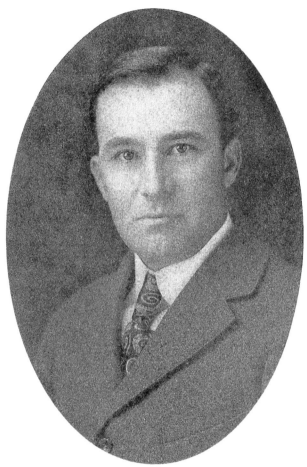

Dr. Henry Charles Hartman (1881–1963), 1917. The image was scanned from the *Cactus Yearbook*, (Austin, TX: University of Texas Student Body, 1917), 341. The photographer is unknown.

After Dr. Thayer abandoned his meningitis research, Dr. Sophian decided to return to Dallas to conduct research on the safety, efficacy, and appropriate dosing pattern of the meningococcal vaccine. He planned to return to Dallas on Monday, April 22, 1912, with Estelle, his wife.[40] Around Tuesday, April 9, 1912, Dr. Sophian was surprised to receive an urgent request from William Perry Motley,[41] the president of the Hospital and Health Board of Kansas City, Jackson County, Missouri, to travel to Kansas City to assist the city in stemming its out-of-control cerebrospinal meningitis epidemic.[42]

Dr. Sophian spoke with Estelle about stopping in Kansas City on their way to Dallas. She agreed and they made plans to leave New York City a week earlier.[42] Dr. and Mrs. Sophian boarded a train in New York City on Saturday, April 13, 1912, and arrived at the Union Depot in Kansas City on Monday, April 15, 1912.[43] He and Mrs. Sophian remained in Kansas City for five days before heading to Dallas. A description of Dr. Sophian's weeklong work in Kansas City, Missouri, in April 1912 is beyond the scope of this book but is available elsewhere.[42]

CHAPTER 6 NOTES

1   "Meningitis Epidemic to End Abruptly Now, Says Sophian; Dr. Flexner's Assistant Speaks to Tarrant County Medical Society—Two New Cases Here," *Fort Worth Star-Telegram*, February 4, 1912, 8.

2   After Dr. Sophian left Dallas, local newspaper reports and data about the cerebrospinal meningitis epidemic in Dallas became scarce. Furthermore, the Dallas health officials did not report their municipal cerebrospinal meningitis data to the US Public Health Service municipal cerebrospinal meningitis database begun on February 17, 1912, because of the epidemic in the Southwestern United States [see "Cerebrospinal Meningitis, Cities of the United States: Table of Cases and Deaths for Weeks Ending February 17–March 9, 1912 ... June 8, 1912," *Public Health Reports* 27, Part 1 (January to June, Inclusive, 1912): 467, 497, 525, 556, 619, 651, 709, 767, 811, 871, 916, 970, 1005, 1004]. The figure of 116 cerebrospinal meningitis cases cited here was derived from data released by to the press by Dr. Nash at the end of May 1912, at which time he reported a grand total of 765 cases of cerebrospinal meningitis in Dallas (October 1, 1911, to May 31, 1912). Of the 765 cases, one, nine, and seventy-three cases occurred in October 1911, November, 1911, and December 1911, respectively, and 156 cases occurred January 1–22, 1912. Using a proportion, the 156 cases for January 1–22, 1912, become approximately 220 cases for January 1–31, 1912. Subtracting 1 + 9 + 73 + 220 (303) from 765 yields the occurrence of 462 cerebrospinal cases to be spread in some way across February, March, April, and May (1912), when the epidemic in Dallas ended. An equal division of 462 cases yields 116 cases per month for February, March, April, and May (1912). It is likely that the number of cases was higher than 116 in February, March, and April 1912 than in May 1912. "Says Meningitis Is Wholly Stamped Out; Last Patient Soon to Be Discharged from Hospital; Total of 450 Treated at Hospital, with Death Rate of 27 Per Cent; Grand Total, 765 Cases," *Dallas Morning News*, May 31, 1912, 16.

3   "Winning Fight on Meningitis; Flexner's Serum is Doing Fine Work in Conquering Epidemic; Death Rate Lower," *Fort Wayne Sentinel* (Fort Wayne, IN), February 12, 1912, 13.

4   Dr. Steiner also envisioned production of diphtheria antitoxin, typhoid vaccine, and smallpox vaccine by the Texas State Health Board biologics laboratory. "To Make Serum, State Will Manufacture

Preventives to Be Sold at Cost, Laboratory Is Planned; Fluid for Cure of Meningitis Which Has Been Selling at $5 Retail Be Provided for Public at Expense of Forty Cents," *Houston Post*, February 10, 1912, 5.

5 "The Travis County Medical Society," *Texas State Journal of Medicine* 7, no. 12 (February 9, 1912): 340.

6 Albert Sidney Burleson (1863–1937) was born in San Marcos, Hays County, Texas, as one of the nine children of Edward Burleson Jr. (1826–1877), a farmer, and Emma Lucy Kyle (1832–1877). He attended public schools and the Coronal Institute in San Marcos; the Agricultural and Mechanical College in College Station, Brazos County, Texas; and Baylor University in Waco, McLennan County, Texas, from which he earned his bachelor's degree (1881). He earned his law degree from the University of Texas at Austin (1884). He was admitted to the Texas bar the same year. He opened a law practice in Austin (1885) and served as assistant city attorney of Austin (1885–1890) and as district attorney of the twenty-sixth judicial district (1891–1898). He was elected as a Democrat to the Fifty-Sixth and the seven succeeding United States Congresses (March 4, 1899, to March 6, 1913). He resigned to become postmaster general for eight years in the cabinet of US President Woodrow Wilson. He then retired from public life and engaged in banking, livestock raising, and other pursuits. He was known as the father of the airmail service and as a fierce federal segregationist who reversed the integration of federal workplaces enacted during the Reconstruction Period (1865–1877) following the end of the American Civil War. He married Adele Lubbock Steiner (1863–1948), the younger sister of Dr. Ralph Steiner, in 1889; they had five children. Albert Burleson died of heart failure at the age of seventy-four years. See "Burleson, Albert Sidney," *Biographical Directory of the United States Congress*, accessed January 16, 2018, http://bioguide.congress.gov/scripts/biodisplay.pl?index=B001110; Adrian H. Anderson, "Albert Sidney Burleson: A Southern Politician in the Progressive Era" (doctoral dissertation, Texas Tech University, 1967); "President Wilson's Politician: Albert Sidney Burleson of Texas," *Southwestern Historical Quarterly* 77 (January 1974): 339–54; "Albert S. Burleson," *News and Observer* (Raleigh, NC), November 25, 1937, 8; and Seymour V. Connor, "Burleson, Albert Sidney," *Handbook of Texas Online*, accessed January 16, 2018, https://tshaonline.org/handbook/online/articles/fbu38.

7 "To Fight Disease; State Laboratory to Make Anti Toxins Planned; During Past Thirteen Months 516 Deaths from Meningitis Occurred in Texas," *Houston Post*, February 14, 1912, 5.

8 "State Preparing to Make Serums and Anti-Toxins; Product of Laboratory Will Be Sold Citizens at Cost; Health Department Actively Pushing Work—Federal Co-operation Is Secured—Meningitis Improvement," *Galveston Daily News*, February 14, 1912, p. 9.

9 "Aid to Texas Authorities in the Installation of a Laboratory," *Annual Report of the Surgeon General of the Public Health Service of the United States for the Fiscal Year 1912* (Washington: Government Printing Office, 1913), 40.

10 "Scattered Are the Legislators; Third Case of Meningitis Has Frightened Them from Capital [*sic*]; No Session until March 3; Speaker Excuses All Members of the House and Lieutenant Governor Agrees to Plan—Hunt Is Ill," *Waco Morning News*, February 16, 1913, 6.

11 "Texas Legislative Sessions and Years," *Legislative Reference Library of Texas*, accessed January 17, 2018, http://www.lrl.state. tx.us/sessions/sessionYears.cfm. Scroll down the list to the Thirty-Second and Thirty-Third regular sessions: no regular session or called session by the governor occurred in 1912. Regular sessions in Texas are held every other year.

12 Dr. A. B. Conley, superintendent of public buildings and grounds of the Texas State Capitol in 1913, wrote the following about the heating and plumbing systems in the Texas State Capitol building: "The present system of heating should be entirely done away with. As the Senate chamber and the hall of the House of Representatives are now heated, the radiators are frequently used as cuspidors. Those who expectorate often deposit disease germs on the radiators. There is not enough heat coming from the radiators to kill the germs, but there is enough heat to vitalize them and to dry the sputum. After the sputum is dried the hot air becomes a menace to all who breathe it, laden as it is with disease-conveying germs. No other public place in Texas would be permitted by the State Department of Health to exist with such an unsanitary system of plumbing as is to be found in the State Capitol." "State Capitol Conditions; Recommendation Made for Improvement as to Heating and Sanitary Systems," *Dallas Morning News*, February 18, 1913, 5; "Judge Duncan Gave Warning; When in Texas House Called Attention to

Unhealthful Condition and Insanitary Practices," *Dallas Morning News*, February 26, 1913, 15; and Tom Finty Jr., "House with Quorum Refuses to Adjourn; Resolution to Suspend Activity until May 2 Is Voted Down; Mexican Question Up; Senate Adopts Long Resolution, but Other Matters Prevent Definite Action in House," *Dallas Morning News*, February 25, 1913, 3.

13 "Dr. Thayer Discovers Meningitis Vaccine; Dallas Pathologist Announces Results of Experiments; Believes Preventive Method for Successfully Fighting Disease Has Been Found," *Dallas Morning News*, February 23, 1912, 6.

14 Alfred E. Thayer, "The Dallas Epidemic of Meningitis; Preliminary Note on the Laboratory Work," *Texas State Journal of Medicine* 7, no. 11 (March 1912): 305–7.

15 Dr. Thayer later revised the temperature at which he killed the meningococci used in his vaccine. He wrote, "In my opinion, it is important to sterilize the vaccine at as low a temperature as possible, and probably 45 degrees Centigrade [113 degrees Fahrenheit] will prove better than 55 degrees Centigrade [131 degrees Fahrenheit], yielding a more potent vaccine. It seems as if its value for prophylaxis were lessened the higher the temperature used. Further work of this kind will be done." Alfred E. Thayer, "The Dallas Epidemic of Meningitis; Preliminary Note on the Laboratory Work," *Texas State Journal of Medicine* 7, no. 11 (March 1912): 305–7.

16 "Dr. Sophian Gives History of Fight," *Dallas Morning News*, February 3, 1912, 13.

17 The merger between the Baylor University College of Medicine and the Texas Baptist Memorial Sanitarium, as the former was located on the campus of the latter. The merger required medical supervision and academic teachers to instruct the medical students and house staff rotating through the hospital to meet the requirements of the Texas State Medical Examining Board. Dr. Thayer was appointed to that person. The two institutions merged to give "Dallas and the surrounding country a medical center equal in its standard to the centers in other parts of the county, North and East." "To Improve Baptist Hospital: Plans Now Being Made for Closer Affiliation with Medical College; Supervisor Is Named," *Dallas Morning News*, February 18, 1912, 7; "Baylor University College of Medicine" (advertisement), *Dallas Morning News*, August 4, 1912, 13; and Walter Henrik Moursund, *A History of Baylor University, College*

of Medicine, 1900–1953 (Houston, TX: Gulf Printing Company, 1956), 37–50, 55–56.

18 The term autogenous vaccine is an old one reflecting an earlier approach to treatment of disease. "An autogenous vaccine is one in which the organism used in making the vaccine is taken from the patient to be treated. This same vaccine would be considered a stock vaccine for any other patient having the same kind of infection. That the use of an autogenous vaccine is scientifically correct must be admitted, since it gives us a vaccine of the exact organism causing the infection, but in practical application it is not an easy matter and is often surrounded with many difficulties. Many infections are of such a nature that it is practically impossible to procure the organism for the production of an autogenous vaccine, and in acute infections where the organism can be procured the necessary delay in making the autogenous vaccine before treatment is started, is often of decided disadvantage. To make an autogenous vaccine, the culture must be procured and incubated 18 hours to obtain a growth. Very often it will be found that the growth shows several kinds of organisms, there being a mixed infection present. Then subcultures to separate the various kinds of germs must be made and again incubated 18 hours, then the vaccine must be made including the count of the organisms, and the sterilizing process. After this sterility tests should be made by incubating at least 24 hours before the vaccine should be used. Imagine an average practitioner hunting around for a culture tube, especially in a small town, then sending it to some place where bacteriological laboratory work is done and waiting until the autogenous vaccine is returned, in a case of puerperal sepsis, infected wound, erysipelas, pneumonia, or any other acute infectious disease. Meantime, the infection will have progressed in many instances to a point where the vaccine will be no longer of any avail, no matter how well made or whether autogenous or not. Such foolish delay is not advocated even by those who urge the use of autogenous vaccines under favorable circumstances where facilities for making them are close at hand. All advocate the use of stock vaccines in such cases to check the progress of the infection while the autogenous vaccine is being prepared." George Henry Sherman, *Vaccine Therapy in General Practice* (Detroit, MI: printed by the author, 1911), 50–51.

19 For examples of the earliest use of an autogenous meningococcal vaccine in two human patients in the United States, see David J.

Davis, "Studies in Meningococcus Infections," *Journal of Infectious Diseases* 4, no. 4 (November 15, 1907): 576–77.

20 On the lack of efficacy and safety studies for bacterial vaccines, including the meningococcal vaccine, the H. K. Mulford Company wrote in March and April 1912 advertisements, "Bacterin therapy is long past the experimental stage, and the immunizing effect of typho-bacterin, for instance, is thoroughly established, the result from its use being sufficient evidence of the worth of this method of controlling the spread of typhoid fever. Remarkable results likewise have followed the use of cholera-bacterin and it is hoped that equally good results will follow the use of meningo-bacterin in controlling epidemics of cerebrospinal meningitis. *While immunization with Meningo-Bacterin has thus far been used in relatively few cases, it is entirely reasonable to believe that it will prove a most valuable aid in the suppression of epidemics of cerebrospinal meningitis*" [emphasis added]. See "An Interesting Announcement Is Made in This Issue by the H. K. Mulford Company Concerning Meningo-Bacterin (Meningococcus Vaccine)," *American Journal of Dermatology* 16, no. 4 (April 1912): 222; and "Vaccine Therapy," *Texas State Journal of Medicine* 8, no. 11 (March 1913): 311.

21 The complete editorial is available at "The Epidemic and the Board of Health," *Texas State Journal of Medicine* 7, no. 10 (February 1912): 267–68.

22 As of January 24, 1912 (when Dr. von Ezdorf stopped counting), there were 550 cases of cerebrospinal meningitis in 49 different Texas localities, with the disease's prevalence greatest in Dallas (249 cases, 110 deaths), Fort Worth (61 cases, 27 deaths), Waco (118 cases, 43 deaths), and Houston (8 cases, 0 deaths). San Antonio, the largest city in Texas (its population in 1910 was about 97,000), had no cases at all as of January 24, 1912. The epidemic began in Dallas in October 1911; struck Waco and Fort Worth on December 20, 1911; and hit Houston on January 1, 1912. Dr. von Ezdorf reported that the weather for the months of December 1911 and January 1912 was unusual because of continuous rain and severe cold. Rudolph H. von Ezdorf, "Cerebrospinal Meningitis in Texas," *Public Health Reports* 27, no. 8 (February 23, 1912): 271–76.

23 Dr. Arthur Marston Stimson (1876–1953) was born in Rome, Oneida County, New York, as one of the four children of William Hamilton Stimson (1842–1903) and Anna Braddock Gallup (1849–1884). He attended the Boys High School in Brooklyn, New York, and earned his

medical degree from Long Island College Hospital (1898). He served on the house staff of Long Island College Hospital before becoming a Louisiana-commissioned medical officer in the US Public Health Service (1902). He became an assistant US surgeon general (1922) and served as chief of the division of scientific research (1922–1930). He retired from the US Public Health Service in 1941. He wrote *A Brief History of Bacteriological Investigations of the United States Public Health Service* (Washington, DC: US Government Printing Office, 1938). During World War II, he served as a sanitation officer in the Navy Department. He married Sarah Boyd Stimson (1880–1978) in 1903; they had four children. See "Arthur Marston Stimson, MD, 1876–1953" in "Notable Contributions to Medical Research by Public Health Service Scientists," National Library of Medicine Reference Division (Washington, DC: US Department of Health, Education, and Welfare, 1960); and *History of the Long Island College Hospital and Its Graduates* (Brooklyn, NY: Association of the Alumni, 1899), 420–21.

24 For more information on Dr. Stimson's rabies virus research, see "Notable Contributions to Medical Research by Public Health Service Scientists," National Library of Medicine Reference Division (Washington, DC: US Department of Health, Education, and Welfare, 1960), 56–57.

25 The Hygienic Laboratory was established in 1887 as a pathology and bacteriology laboratory for the United States Marine Hospital of the Port of New York (Stapleton, Staten Island). For several years, one officer ran the Hygienic Laboratory when he had time away from his hospital duties. In 1891, the laboratory moved with the Marine Hospital Service to Washington, DC. In 1904, it moved into its own separate buildings to house its pathology and bacteriology, chemistry, medical zoology, and pharmacology services. In 1912, the Hygienic Laboratory was located on the grounds of the Old Naval Observatory at Twenty-Fifth and E Streets, NW, Washington, DC. The Hygienic Laboratory is considered the direct ancestor of the National Institutes of Health. See H. D. Geddings, "Research Work in the Hygienic Laboratory of the Public Health and Marine-Hospital Service," *Journal of the American Medical Association* 62, no. 26 (June 25, 1904): 1,686–87; "The Hygienic Laboratory," in James H. Cassedy, *The New Age of Health Laboratories, 1885–1915: An Exhibit, May–October 1987 Marking the Centennial of the Founding of the Pasteur Institute of Paris and the National*

Institutes of Health (Bethesda, MD: National Library of Medicine, 1987), 17–21; Frank G. Carpenter, "Uncle Sam, Doctor," *Los Angeles Times*, November 19, 1911; and David M. Morens and Anthony S. Fauci, "The Forgotten Forefather: Joseph James Kinyoun and the Founding of the National Institutes of Health," *mBio* 3, no. 4 (July–August 2012): e00139-12.

26 "Texas to Have Laboratory for the Manufacture of Disease Preventives," *El Paso Herald*, March 2, 1912, 4.

27 "Toxin Factory to Be in Operation Soon; Expert Due to Arrive at Capitol Wednesday; Laboratory Is Fitted Out; Necessary Apparatus and Instruments Have Been Ordered—Gas and Water Connection Furnished," *Austin Daily Statesman*, March 3, 1912, 4; "Government Expert at Austin; Dr. Stimson to Aid in Manufacture of Serums and Antitoxins at State Capital," *Dallas Morning News*, March 7, 1912, 14; "Dr. Stimson at Austin; United States Employee Will Assist in Manufacture of Serums, Anti-Toxins, Etc., for Combatting Disease," *Galveston Daily News*, March 7, 1912, 9; and "Dr. Stimson on Ground; Is Man Who Will Inaugurate Serum Antitoxin Factory," *Houston Post*, March 7, 1912, 5.

28 "State Serum Factory Plans; Plan Can Not Be Put in Operation before Next Fall—Dr. Stimson, Supervisor of Plant, Here," *Austin American-Statesman*, March 7, 1912, 4.

29 The manufacture of typhoid and meningococcal vaccines was similar. See Almroth Edward Wright, *Vaccine Therapy: Its Administration, Value, and Limitations* (London: Longmans, Green, and Company, 1910), 98, 191; and William Cecil Bosanquet and John William Henry Eyre, *Serum, Vaccines, and Toxines* [*sic*] *in Treatment and Diagnosis* (New York: Funk and Wagnalls Company, 1910), 52–54.

30 The laboratory equipment in 1912 required to produce typhoid vaccine included a sterilizer, culture vessels and media, an incubator, instruments to sow cultures (e.g., Pasteur pipette, platinum wire, or glass needle), pipettes, a darkened cabinet for storing live cultures, a microscope, microscope slides and slide cover glasses, and staining solutions. See R. W. Marsden, "Inoculation with Typhoid Vaccine as Preventive of Typhoid Fever," *British Medical Journal* 1, no. 2052 (April 28, 1900): 1,017–18; A. Besson, *Practical Bacteriology, Microbiology, and Serum Therapy: A Textbook for Laboratory Use* (London: Longmans, Green, and Company, 1913); and "State Laboratory Equipment," *Galveston Daily News*, March 17, 1912, 15.

31 "A Diagnostic Laboratory for the Health Department," *Texas State Journal of Medicine* 8, no. 3 (July 1912): 97.

32 "Equipment for Serum Work; List for State Laboratory Has Been Completed," *Dallas Morning News*, March 16, 1912, 13.

33 "Stimson Returns to Washington," *Dallas Morning News*, March 17, 1912, 14; and "Dr. Stimson to Washington; Will Return to Austin after Laboratory Is Completed," *Galveston Daily News*, March 17, 1912, 15.

34 "State Bacteriologist Resigns; Dr. Sam N. Key Will Leave Service on June 1—Dr. Hartman of Temple Appointed to Fill Vacancy," *Galveston Daily News*, March 28, 1912, 7; "State Bacteriologist Resigns; Dr. Sam Key Succeeded by Dr. Hartman of Temple," *Dallas Morning News*, March 28, 1912, 7; "No title," *Houston Post*, May 2, 1912, 3; and "Dr. Hartman to Accept," *Houston Post*, March 30, 1912, 3.

35 Dr. Henry Charles Hartman (1881–1963) was born in Meyersville, DeWitt County, Texas, as one of the six children of August Christian Hartman (1848–1917), a farmer, and Josephine Hans (1857–1930). He earned his medical degree from the University of Texas Medical Branch at Galveston (1907); worked as demonstrator in the department of pathology at the same medical college for about a year; and moved to Temple, Bell County, Texas, to become the resident pathologist at Smith and White Hospital (see note #36 below). He accepted the state bacteriologist appointment from Dr. Steiner on March 30, 1912, and started work there on Wednesday, May 1, 1912. Eighteen months later (October 1913), he returned to Galveston as chairman of the department of pathology at the University of Texas Medical Branch at Galveston (1913–1926). From 1926 to 1928, he served as dean of the University of Texas Medical Branch at Galveston. He suddenly resigned his deanship and professorship in 1928 to "give attention to private affairs." He subsequently moved to San Antonio, where he worked for many years as a pathologist for the Medical and Surgical Memorial Hospital at 215 Camden Street. He married Nina Duty (1879–1970) in 1906; they had no children. Dr. Hartman died of heart disease, Parkinson's disease, and chronic brain syndrome at the age of eighty-four years. See "Hartman Resigns as Medical Dean; Severs Connection with State College on Sept. 1," *Galveston Daily News*, February 24, 1928, 1; Donald Duncan, *The University of Texas Medical Branch at Galveston: A Seventy-Five Year History* (Austin, TX: University of Texas Press, 1967), 137; "Growth and

Mergers Change Hospital's Name and Ownership," *San Antonio Express-News*, December 12, 2015; and "Dr. Hartman to Accept," *Houston Post*, March 30, 1912, 3.

36 Dr. Arthur Carroll Scott (1865–1916), a native of Gainesville, Cooke County, Texas, and Dr. Raleigh Richardson White Jr. (1872–1917), a native of Tippah County, Mississippi, founded the Scott and White Sanitarium in Temple, a rough railroad town in Bell County, Texas, in 1904. Drs. Scott and White earned their medical degrees at Bellevue Hospital Medical College (1886) and at Tulane University Medical Department (1883), respectively. They first served as the two chief surgeons of Temple's Santa Fe Hospital in the 1890s before working in private medical practice and first opening their sanitarium in a small frame house. Dayton Kelley, *With Scalpel and Scope: A History of Scott and White* (Waco, TX: Library Binding Company, 1970), 33–34; and "Baylor Scott and White Health—Our History—YouTube," accessed November 9, 2017, https://www.youtube.com/watch?v=ebo7lrW97no.

37 "Meningitis Heads State's Death List; Registrar R. P. Paddock's [*sic*] Vital Statistics for March; Total Number of Deaths Was 2,804, with Births Totaling 4,382, Decrease under February," *Dallas Morning News*, April 27, 1912, 16.

38 The following nurses developed cerebrospinal meningitis while working at the City Hospital: M. E. Grier (ten days ill); E. Fitzgerald (ten days), E. Bierbaum (Brierbaum) (ten days) Jessie Smith (twenty-six days), A. C. Kimball (eleven days), A. M. Sankey (twenty days), Blanche Merrill (twenty-three days), G. H. Topping (fifteen days), Katherine Ott (sixteen days), Margaret Howard (nineteen days), and Rose Emma Nielsen (twenty-two days). "Half Pay for Nurses Stricken at Hospital: Eleven Meningitis Victims Are Paid by City," *Dallas Morning News*, June 11, 1912, 16.

39 Dr. Sophian's paper was titled, "A New Method for Controlling the Administration of Serum in Epidemic Meningitis: A Preliminary Note." It described Dr. Sophian's use of blood pressure monitoring in 200 cerebrospinal meningitis patients during 600 lumbar puncture procedures at the City Hospital (Dallas) during January 1912. He noted the error of the assumption that many severe symptoms occurring either during or a few hours after an intraspinal injection of antimeningitis serum were due to the disease, when, in fact, some were the direct result of the injection technique, especially when the symptoms occurred immediately during or after the lumbar

puncture procedure. Dr. Sophian offered four conclusions at the end of his paper. First, the old method of administering serum (without blood pressure monitoring) was inaccurate and sometimes dangerous. Second, blood pressure change was an accurate guide to the quantity of serum that could be safely injected, frequently also indicating the quantity of cerebrospinal fluid that could be withdrawn. Third, the average dose of serum as controlled by blood pressure was smaller than by the old method. Fourth, following an injection of serum controlled by blood pressure, the after-effects were usually much less severe. At the conclusion of his paper, Dr. Sophian acknowledged Dr. Nash for his courtesy in allowing Dr. Sophian to use the hospital records and for his "very valuable cooperation" in the studies. See Abraham Sophian, "A New Method of Controlling the Administration of Serum in Epidemic Meningitis: Preliminary Note," *Journal of the American Medical Association* 58, no. 12 (March 23, 1912): 843–45

40 "Dr. Sophien's [sic] Wife Finds Much Charm in Kansas City; Eminent Specialist's 'Better Half' Call Trip Second Honeymoon; Faith in Mate Great; Expresses Pleasure with Bustle and Window Displays Here on First Visit West," *Kansas City Post*, April 17, 1912, p. 2.

41 William Perry Motley (1858–1938) was born in Tuskegee, Macon County, Alabama, as one of the six children of John Glenn Motley (1823–1908), a minister, and Louisa Perry (1830–1908). He married Sallie Willis Carpenter (1862–1939) in 1887 in Kansas City, Missouri; they had no children. He worked as an agent for the Pacific Mutual Insurance Company and served as head of the Kansas City Hospital and Health Board for many years. "W. Perry Motley Dies; Former Hospital and Health Board Head Ill Since June; About Ten Years Ago He Had Retired from the Life Insurance Business-Known Widely as a Fisherman," *Kansas City Star*, February 6, 1938, p. 11.

42 Margaret R. O'Leary and Dennis S. O'Leary, *The Kansas City Meningitis Epidemic, 1911–1913: Violent and Not Imagined* (Bloomington, IN: iUniverse, 2018).

43 "Meningitis Expert Arrives in K. C. To Combat Disease; Dr. A. Sophien [sic], World Famous Specialist, Surprised at Extent of its Ravages; Consults Local Men; Says He Will Remain Here as Long as Is Necessary to Check Spread," *Kansas City Post*, April 15, 1912, p. 1; and "Sophian Going to Kansas City; Spinal Meningitis Expert Will Aid in Stamping Out Disease in That City," *Dallas Morning News*," April 1, 1912, 7.

CHAPTER 7

MENINGOCOCCAL VACCINE TRIALS AS HOT WEATHER RETURNS, APRIL–AUGUST 1912

D r. and Mrs. Sophian arrived in Dallas, Texas, by train on Friday night, April 19, 1912. As Dr. Sophian registered at the Park Hotel, he told reporters, "My visit to Dallas has no connection with existing conditions."[1] Dr. Sophian was referring to the thriving Texas cerebrospinal meningitis epidemic, which health officials had ranked as the leading cause of death in Texas in both February and March 1912 and that was on track to kill about 270 Texans in April 1912.[2] Rather, Dr. Sophian told reporters that he had returned to Dallas to conduct research studies to measure the efficacy and safety of the meningococcal vaccine in preventing cerebrospinal meningitis. Recall that Dr. Thayer had ended his meningococcal vaccine research in late February 1912, as discussed in Chapter 6.

The next day, Saturday, April 20, 1912, Dr. Sophian met with Dr. James Harvey Black, the professor of bacteriology and pathology at the Southwestern University Medical Department, whom Dr. Sophian first had met during a tour of the Texas Baptist Memorial Sanitarium on February 3, 1912, as noted in chapter 5. The two pathologists were roughly the same age—about twenty-eight years old.

Dr. Black and Dr. Sophian discussed the challenging cerebrospinal meningitis epidemic situation in Texas. Dr. Sophian asked how the epidemic had escaped control in Dallas, as the disease had been "practically stamped out" there when he had departed the city two months earlier.[1] Dr. Black responded that about a hundred people in Dallas had received one or two inoculations of Dr. Thayer's meningococcal vaccine, but very few if any had received the three prescribed injections. Even Dr. Nash had received only two doses of the vaccine because he was unsure that the vaccination was preventive.[3] Two nurses who developed cerebrospinal meningitis while working at the City Hospital received only two injections of the vaccine. Much to Dr. Sophian's additional dismay, Dr. Thayer and others had kept "irregular records" of the vaccinations they had administered.[4] Analyzing the situation, Dr. Sophian attributed vaccine failures to incomplete vaccinations and the unequal development of immunity in those who received the vaccine.[3] These problems, he noted, also existed for typhoid and smallpox vaccines.[3]

Drs. Sophian and Black forged ahead with their plans to study the efficacy and safety of the meningococcal vaccine by quantifying the levels of serum immune bodies induced by various inoculation dosages and regimens in ten healthy medical-student volunteers recruited by Dr. Black.[5] This type of immunology work was new. In 1912, only one documented laboratory and clinical testing of a meningococcal vaccine in the United States existed—that is, Dr. David John Davis[6] of Chicago, who injected himself with the vaccine in 1906.[7] He developed a profound toxemia with headache, vomiting, delirium, and temperature elevation to 103 degrees Fahrenheit. His white blood cell count soared to 44,050 per cubic milliliter (elevated eightfold from his baseline) on the third day, and his opsonic index[8] rose to 2.3 (more than doubled) on the second day before returning to normal day five after the injection.[7]

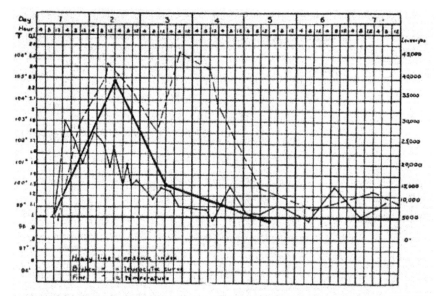

CHART 1.—Opsonic, Leucocytic, and Temperature Curves Following the Injection into a Normal Person of Heated Meningococci.

A graph showing the temperature (fine line), leucocyte (broken line), and opsonin curves (heavy line) following the injection of a heat-killed meningococcal vaccine in a healthy human (Dr. David John Davis) in 1906. Source: David J. Davis, "Studies in Meningococcus Infections," *Journal of Infectious Diseases* 4, no. 4 (November 15, 1907), 578.

Drs. Sophian and Black prepared their meningococcal vaccine from a live meningococcal organism about five generations old, which Dr. Black had obtained from the cerebrospinal fluid of a Dallas meningitis patient. They incubated the live meningococci for eighteen hours on 2 percent glucose agar in slants (test tubes), washed the slants with distilled water, centrifuged the wash for twenty minutes, retained the supernatant and threw away the sediment, heated the supernatant in an incubator for one hour at 50 degrees Centigrade (122 degrees Fahrenheit) to kill the meningococci, tested the killed meningococci for sterility, counted the killed meningococci by the Wright method, and diluted the killed meningococci in normal saline to yield three vaccine strengths for inoculation. The three vaccine strengths were five hundred million, one billion, and two billion bacteria per cubic centimeter vaccine dose.[9]

Drs. Sophian and Black monitored the ten healthy volunteers with blood analyses, agglutination studies, and complement-fixation tests using a polyvalent meningococcus antigen prepared by Dr. Archibald McNeil.[10] After inoculation with the meningococcal vaccine, the volunteers' white blood cell counts rose slightly and returned to normal within days. Using a readily available agglutinin, Dr. Sophian and Dr. Black measured the agglutinin titers of the sera of their vaccinated subjects. The titers ranged from 1:200 to 1:1,500. Complement was fixed in serum dilutions of up to 1:250.[11] All the volunteers demonstrated the presence of serum immune bodies against the meningococcus beginning on the fourth day after their first injection. Three sequential injections appeared to result in the best level of immunity.[12] The volunteers developed local inflammation at the site of injection and generalized aches and fever similar to those occurring with typhoid vaccinations.[13]

Dr. Sophian and Dr. Black concluded from their meningococcal vaccine studies in April 1912,

> All evidence, especially the experimental, points to the efficacy of the injection of dead meningococci for prophylactic vaccination, as a measure which would confer considerable immunity in most cases, probably partial in all, against the infection of epidemic meningitis … It is very likely that only a moderate degree of immunity will give very considerable or complete protection against epidemic meningitis, which is caused by an organism of low virulence, infecting only a very small percentage of those who are exposed, and [who] harbor the organism temporarily in their noses and throats."[14]

Furthermore, Drs. Sophian and Black declared, "It is very likely that if the disease subsequently develops in those vaccinated it will be considerably modified and run a much milder course with a much better outlook for recovery, as is seen in those who develop smallpox after vaccination." The most efficacious vaccination protocol (providing the highest degree of protection) was three injections repeated at intervals of a week in doses of 100 million, 500 million, and 1,000 million.[14]

Dr. Sophian and Dr. Black announced their plans to retest the ten volunteers in one and two years (1913 and 1914) to determine the level of immunity, if any, still present in the volunteers' sera from the original vaccination in April 1912. The excellent results of those retestings in 1913 and 1914 are available elsewhere.[15–16]

On Sunday, April 28, 1912, Governor Colquitt gave a reelection speech in Sherman, Grayson County, Texas, in which he updated the status of the Texas State Board of Health biologics laboratory. He crowed about the performance of Dr. Steiner in enforcing the health laws, extending assistance during the ongoing Texas cerebrospinal meningitis epidemic, and establishing a biologics laboratory in the Texas State Health Board offices in the Texas State Capitol building to manufacture "antitoxin for diphtheria, typhoid fever, and vaccine for smallpox." He was bullish on manufacturing antimeningitis serum, too, announcing,

> We will install necessary apparatus for the manufacture of the [antimeningitis] serum used in the treatment of meningitis, so that when the legislature meets next winter [January through March, 1913], all that will be necessary to put this [antimeningitis] serum within reach of all the people at a very low cost will be a small appropriation to buy a few horses and build a stable where they can be conditioned, so as to extract the blood from which the serum is made ... In times of epidemic like that of this year, the costly meningitis serum, which proved so helpful, is beyond the reach of the poor. As it was, the health department ordered the serum in large quantities from New York and sold it to physicians at a nominal price and to the very poor furnished it free. I shall continue to use the perfection of our laws and bring every means of

prevention of relief from disease within the reach of all the people.[17]

Dr. Sophian remained in Texas until Thursday, May 9, 1912, when he spoke at the Texas State Medical Association convention in Waco (May 7–9, 1912).[18-19] Following his talk, Dr. William Spencer Carter,[20] clinical physiologist and the dean of the University of Texas Medical Branch at Galveston, presented a paper titled, "The Effect of Injecting Ringer's Solution into the Spinal Canal in Varying Amounts and Under Varying Pressures."[23] Dr. Carter commended Dr. Sophian's advocacy of blood pressure monitoring during the administration of antimeningitis serum and presented the results of his own physiological experiments, which showed that fluids injected into the spinal canal extended along its entire length, reached the base of the brain, and covered its entire surface.[21]

Dr. Carter disagreed with Dr. Flexner's original method of injecting large volumes of antimeningitis serum into the spinal canal, as no reliable way existed to determine what amounts and what pressure could be used in making injections into the spinal canal. Dr. Carter demonstrated that hypotension, respiratory distress, and cardiac arrest sometimes occurred during serum injection because of the pressure of the injected fluid upon the lower brain stem, where lie the vital centers controlling the heart and respiration. Dr. Sophian complimented Dr. Carter's experiments and stressed their practical value.[21] After the convention, Dr. Sophian returned with Estelle to New York City.

Dr. Steiner and Dr. Key also attended the Waco conference, presenting talks on diphtheria[22-23] and the nervous diseases as illustrated by moving pictures,[24] respectively. Dr. Key was no longer with the Texas State Board of Health, as Dr. Hartman had become state bacteriologist in Austin on Wednesday, May 1, 1912.[25]

On Monday, May 20, 1912, Mayor Holland released his annual report, which briefly acknowledged the cerebrospinal meningitis epidemic of the previous eight months. He wrote that the cerebrospinal meningitis epidemic "produced considerable scare among our people, owing to the fact that it was an unusual disease for this climate" and that "our health department and city government took hold of the situation with zeal and vigor and successfully coped with the disease."[26]

On Friday, May 31, 1912, the Dallas skies were clear and the temperature was moderate at 92 degrees Fahrenheit.[27] Dr. Nash discharged the last cerebrospinal meningitis patient from the City Hospital. The cerebrospinal meningitis epidemic of 1911 to 1912 in Dallas was over.

In a review of the cerebrospinal meningitis data he had collected, Dr. Nash announced that the hospital's staff had cared for 450 cerebrospinal meningitis patients since the hospital began caring exclusively for cerebrospinal meningitis patients on Monday, January 8, 1912. Dr. Nash earlier had received reports of another 100 cases of cerebrospinal meningitis in Dallas between October 1, 1911, and January 8, 1912. In addition to the 450 cerebrospinal meningitis patients treated at the City Hospital and the 100 additional cerebrospinal meningitis patients known to Dr. Nash between October 1, 1911, and January 8, 1912, were another 215 cerebrospinal meningitis patients in the city who had received their care at home. Summing the various numbers, Dr. Nash calculated a grand total of 765 known cases of cerebrospinal meningitis in Dallas from October 1911 to May 1912, inclusive. Of the 450 patients who received their care at the City Hospital, 125 died.[28]

The data cited by Dr. Nash yielded a prevalence rate for cerebrospinal meningitis in Dallas during the months of October 1911 through May 1912, inclusive, of *83.2 cerebrospinal meningitis cases per 10,000 Dallas residents*. The case fatality rate for the 450 cerebrospinal meningitis who received their care at the City Hospital was *27.8 percent*.

Also, on Friday, May 31, 1912, the Dallas County Register of Graduate Nurses hosted a moonlight picnic at Fair Park in Dallas to pay "a tribute of honor and love to the nurses, doctors, and hospital interns who sacrificed their health and lives in the recent prevalence of spinal meningitis in Dallas." Mayor Holland said at the picnic that he considered the spirit displayed by the nurses, doctors, and interns as much the courage of heroes as if "they had gone into battle on the field of war." The nurse Katherine Ott, who had contracted cerebrospinal meningitis while working at the City Hospital, said, "We were glad to do it. If it was helpful, it is a pleasure to us. We have gained more experience which will help us in ministering to afflicted humanity." The nurse Jessie Smith said that she had stood for two months in the operating room and finally had contracted the dreaded disease herself.[29]

On Tuesday, June 4, 1912, Dr. Sophian presented "Prophylactic Vaccination against Epidemic Meningitis" to his peers at the American Medical Association's Sixty-Third Annual Session (June 4–7, 1912) in Atlantic City, New Jersey,[30-32] Dr. Sophian said, "The utilization of active immunity as a means of preventing meningitis, has not, we believe, been previously used." He compared prophylactic meningitis vaccination to the "wonderful results obtained by extensive prophylactic typhoid vaccination." Dr. Sophian reviewed the experimental data obtained from studies of the ten medical-student volunteers in Dallas and stated that the experimental evidence demonstrated the efficacy of the injection of dead meningococcus received in three specific doses, separated of intervals of one week, in the prevention of cerebrospinal meningitis. The paper received little attention in the following months.[33] Although the lack of response frustrated Dr. Sophian, he did not give up.

Also, in early June 1912, Dr. Steiner and Dr. Hartman installed the diagnostic, limited biologics, and pure food department laboratories in the rooms in the west wing of the Texas State Capitol building. Funds remained tight, even though earlier, on May 17, 1912, the Texas State Senate sent to the Texas State House a bill with an appropriation of $20,000 for carrying through the work of the state laboratory.[34] On Saturday, June 8, 1912, the Texas state attorney general granted Dr. Steiner permission to use the state's profits obtained from the sale of antimeningitis serum to physicians during the winter of 1911–1912 to help fund the state laboratories. The Texas State Board of Health had purchased antimeningitis serum from the Research Laboratory in New York City and had resold it to Texas physicians at a price "slightly above cost."[35]

On Tuesday, June 11, 1912, Mayor Holland and Dr. Nash arranged for payment to eleven nurses who had contracted cerebrospinal meningitis while serving at the City Hospital for the time they were sick with the disease. The stricken nurses' names, the amount of time they were ill, and the amounts paid to them at $2.50 per day were as follows: M. E. Grier (ten days, $25); E. Fitzgerald (ten days, $25), E. Bierbaum (Brierbaum) (seven days, $17.50), Jessie Smith (twenty-six days, $65), A. C. Kimball (eleven days, $27.50), A. M. Sankey (twenty days, $50), Blanche Merrill (twenty-three days, $57.50), G. H. Topping (fifteen days, $37.50), Katherine Ott (sixteen days, $40), Margaret Howard (nineteen days, $47.50), and Rose Emma Nielsen (twenty-two days, $55).[36]

On Sunday, June 16, 1912, Dr. Hartman announced that he was manufacturing a typhoid vaccine in the new biologics laboratory in the Texas State Capitol building.[37] On Friday, June 21, 1912, Dr. Steiner and Dr. Hartman advertised in the *Texas State Journal of Medicine* the opening of the state-run diagnostic laboratory:

> The laboratory to be conducted in connection with or as a part of the state health department is in operation and ready, so far as it is incumbent upon a State laboratory as a public health agency to make or render assistance in making the following examinations: Swabs for diphtheria, spinal fluid, stools for parasites and ova, blood for Widal test,[38] malaria, smears for differential count, water examinations, bacteriological and chemical investigation of typhoid outbreaks, and microscopic examination of post mortem tissue.[39]

The announcement added,

> In addition to the above, an exceedingly important part of the work will be the examination and standardization, a bacteriological standardization, of the commercial disinfectants now being offered

for sale in the state. It will be but a matter of several weeks before the disinfectant value of these various preparations will have been determined and a list published in the bulletin of the Texas State Board of Health ... The laboratory will also be prepared to furnish antimeningitis serum, diphtheritic antitoxin, and typhoid vaccines at the cost of production.[39]

An unnamed pharmacist soon complained that the state's involvement in producing biologics would interfere with biologics sales from licensed entities through established pharmacy channels. Dr. Steiner and Dr. Hartman responded, "The diphtheria antitoxin and meningitis serum are expensive and beyond the reach of some people, but when the state makes same the cost will be considerably reduced and all profits eliminated."[39] On Sunday, July 21, 1912, Dr. Hartman announced the availability of a typhoid vaccine that he had prepared in the state laboratory. He sent small, hermetically sealed glass receptacles of the vaccine to Manor, Travis County, Texas, to control a typhoid epidemic there.[40]

On August 17, 1912, Dr. Sophian and Dr. Black published their seminal paper, titled "Prophylactic Vaccination against Epidemic Meningitis," in the *Journal of the American Medical Association.*[41] Five weeks later, on Tuesday, September 24, 1912, Dr. Sophian presented "Preventive Measures against Epidemic Meningitis"[42] at the Fifteenth Congress of the International Congress on Hygiene and Demography[43] in Washington. He described his and Dr. Black's discovery of protective substances in the sera of volunteers inoculated with the meningococcal vaccine, pointing out that these protective substances provided actual evidence of the acquisition of a high degree of immunity against the infective agent of cerebrospinal meningitis.[42] Dr. Sophian argued passionately for the use of the meningococcal vaccine to prevent a resurgence of cerebrospinal meningitis during the upcoming winter of 1912–1913[41] and was happy when newspapers throughout the United States covered the paper he had delivered at the International Congress.[44]

CHAPTER 7 NOTES

1   "Will Complete Experiments, Dr. Sophian Returns to Study Value of Vaccination against Meningitis," *Dallas Morning News*, April 20, 1912, 9.

2   The number of deaths from pneumonia and tuberculosis in Texas in April 1912 were 246 and 236, respectively. "Meningitis Leads in Cause of Deaths," *El Paso Herald-Post*, May 28, 1912, 2.

3   Dr. Nash's exact words were, "I am not prepared to say that I believe vaccination is a sure preventive, but I shall certainly give it a fair trial should another epidemic threaten, and I am sure that if the required number of doses of the vaccine are taken, there will be quite a little immunity established. Some of our nurses who contracted the disease, took the vaccine, but only one took the required dosage." Albert Ware Nash, "Epidemic Cerebrospinal Meningitis," *Medical Herald* 32, no. 1 (January 1913): 10.

4   Abraham Sophian, *Epidemic Cerebrospinal Meningitis* (St. Louis, MO: C. V. Mosby, 1913), 197.

5   Ibid., 192.

6   Dr. David John Davis (1875–1954) was born in Racine, Racine County, Wisconsin, as the youngest of the six children of David William Davis (1821–1894), a farmer, and Catherine Davis (1833–1894). His parents were natives of Wales. He completed high school at Racine Academy in 1894; earned his bachelor's degree from the University of Wisconsin in 1898; taught high school science for two years; enrolled in Rush Medical College, Chicago, in 1900; and earned his medical degree in 1903 and his doctorate in 1905 from the University of Chicago. He performed research for two years at the McCormick Memorial Institute for Infectious Diseases. He served an internship at Presbyterian Hospital and worked as a pathologist in various places in Chicago until 1910–1911, when he studied in Europe. When he returned to the United States, he became the hospital pathologist for St. Luke's Hospital, Chicago, and an assistant professor of pathology at Rush Medical College. In 1913, he became chairman and head of the departments of pathology and bacteriology at the College of Medicine, located in Chicago. He next became dean of the College of Medicine, a position he served from 1924 until he retired in 1943. He married Almira "Myra" Helen Jones (1875–1956) in 1908; they had two children. See "David J. Davis Papers, 1913–1955," University Library, University of Illinois

at Chicago, accessed January 24, 2018, http://findingaids.library.uic. edu/ead/lhsc/016-01-01-20-02b.html.

7   David J. Davis, "Studies in Meningococcus Infections," *Journal of Infectious Diseases* 4, no. 4 (November 15, 1907): 558–681.

8   The opsonic index is the ratio of the phagocytic activity of neutral or washed leukocytes (white blood cells) in the patient's serum for a given bacteria type, as compared with the leukocytes in a normal or a control serum. "Inasmuch as a neutral phagocyte will ingest the same number of bacteria, provided the two sera possess identical qualities, the normal or base line is arbitrarily taken as one. If, in the case of the patient's serum, it is found that 100 leukocytes contain 900 bacteria, while the same number of leukocytes treated with the control serum contain 1,000 bacteria, we have the proportion of 900:1000 as x:1, in which x, the opsonic index, equals 0.9. The technic of the opsonic index is a rather intricate laboratory procedure, which, to be reliable or trustworthy at all, involves much practice in mastering the details ... It demands that the opsonist shall be a thorough bacteriologist as well as an experienced laboratory worker." B. A. Thomas and R. H. Ivy, *Applied Immunology: The Practical Application of Sera and Bacterins Prophylactically, Diagnostically, and Therapeutically* (Philadelphia, PA: J. B. Lippincott Company, 1915), 229–30; and James Wesley Jobling, "Standardization of the Antimeningitis Serum," *Journal of Experimental Medicine* 11, no. 4 (July 17, 1909): 614–21.

9   Abraham Sophian, *Epidemic Cerebrospinal Meningitis* (St. Louis, MO: C. V. Mosby, 1913), 192–96.

10 Dr. Archibald Alexander McNeil (1874–1919) was a serologist and Dr. Sophian's colleague at the Research Laboratory in New York City. He was born in St. Joseph, Buchanan County, Missouri, as one of the eight sons of William D. McNeil (born in 1848) and Jane McPhee (1844–1930). His parents were natives of Canada. Archibald earned his medical diploma from Ensworth Medical College in St. Joseph, Buchanan County, Missouri, in 1898. He worked at the Research Laboratory, New York City Board of Health, from at least 1911 to 1918. He married Nellie (Ellen) Nash (1888–1964) in 1917. They had no children. He died in 1919 of influenza and cerebral meningitis at the age of forty-five years.

11 Abraham Sophian, *Epidemic Cerebrospinal Meningitis* (St. Louis, MO: C. V. Mosby Company, 1913), 192–94.

12 Ibid., 196–99.

13 J. Henderson Smith and Ralph St. John Brooks, "The Effects of Dosage in Typhoid Vaccination of Rabbits," *Journal of Hygiene (London)* 12, no. 1 (May 1912): 77–107.

14 Abraham Sophian, *Epidemic Cerebrospinal Meningitis* (St. Louis, MO: C. V. Mosby Company, 1913), 198–99.

15 On April 26, 1913, Dr. James Harvey Black published the one-year follow-up study on the immune status of the Dallas medical students inoculated with the meningococcal vaccine in April 1912. Dr. Black wrote, "With the desire to establish the value of prophylactic vaccination against epidemic cerebrospinal meningitis, experiments were undertaken by Dr. Abraham Sophian and myself during the month of April 1912 … Eleven months after the vaccinations were made, I repeated the former experiments to determine what, if any, immunity could be demonstrated after the lapse of this length of time. Eight of the original ten vaccinated students were accessible. The technic used was identical with that reported in the former communication. In addition to the blood of a normal individual acting as a negative control, the blood of a student who had recovered from a severe case of meningitis just prior to the time of these vaccinations was used as a positive control. It will be noted that some of those vaccinated gave higher fixation than he." Dr. Black continued, "While it is recognized that experimental vaccination of healthy individuals in the absence of an epidemic and the detection of immune bodies in their blood is an indirect way of proving its efficacy and that the method must finally be judged by its clinical application, we feel that we are justified in drawing the following conclusions from these studies." The first conclusion was "Prophylactic vaccination produces a high degree of immunity in most cases, this immunity being demonstrable at the end of one year. It seems a justifiable conclusion that most individuals prophylactically vaccinated may safely consider themselves immune for at least one year. Exceptions to this will, of course, be found." The second conclusion was "Some individuals may show an actual increase in immune bodies at the end of one year over those demonstrable soon after vaccination." The third conclusion was "Fixation occurred with the serum of the positive control who has recovered from meningitis but this fixation did not reach as high dilutions as did that of some of those vaccinated. This has previously been found also in some others recovered from the disease." The fourth conclusion was "Experimental evidence warrants us in concluding

that prophylactic vaccination is a measure of the greatest value in the control of epidemic meningitis." James Harvey Black, "Prophylactic Vaccination against Epidemic Meningitis," *Journal of the American Medical Association* 60, no. 17 (April 26, 1913): 1,289–90.

16 On December 12, 1914, Dr. James Harvey Black published the two-year follow-up study on the immune status of the Dallas medical students inoculated with the meningococcal vaccine in April 1912. Dr. Black wrote, "In April, 1912, Dr. Abraham Sophian, then of the Research Laboratory of the New York Board of Health, and I conducted a series of experiments to determine, as well as laboratory methods will permit, the value of prophylactic vaccination against epidemic meningitis. Injections of meningococcic vaccine were made on ten medic al students who volunteered for the work. Eleven months later I repeated these experiments ... With the effort to make this work as nearly complete as possible, I undertook in May, 1914, twelve and twenty-four months from the second and first examinations, respectively, a repetition of the complement-fixation studies ... All but one of the seven students at hand gave decided fixation in a dilution of 1:20, this, two years after the date of vaccination ... While it is recognized that experimental vaccination of healthy individuals in the absence of an epidemic and the detection of immune bodies in their blood is an indirect way of proving its efficacy and that the method must finally be judged by its clinical application, we feel that we are justified in drawing the following conclusions from these studies ... 1. Prophylactic vaccination produces a high degree of immunity in most cases, this immunity being demonstrable at the end of one year. It seems a justifiable conclusion that most individuals prophylactically vaccinated may safely consider themselves immune for at least one year. Exceptions to this will, of course, be found. 2. Some individuals may show an actual increase in immune bodies at the end of one year over those demonstrable soon after vaccination. 3. Fixation occurred with the serum of the positive control who has recovered from meningitis but this fixation did not reach as high dilutions as did that of some of those vaccinated. This has previously been found also in some others recovered from the disease. 4. Experimental evidence warrants us in concluding that prophylactic vaccination is a measure of the greatest value in the control of epidemic meningitis. James Harvey Black, "Prophylactic Vaccination against Epidemic Meningitis, A

Supplementary Note," *Journal of the American Medical Association* 63, no. 24 (December 12, 1914): 2,126.

17 "'I Do Not Want to Tear Down and Destroy, but to Build Up,'—O. B. Colquitt," *Houston Daily Post*, April 28, 1912, 27.

18 "Forty-Fourth Annual Meeting Waco, May 7, 8, 9, 1912," *Texas State Journal of Medicine* 7, no. 12 (April 1912): 319.

19 "'Some Studies in Epidemic Meningitis,' Dr. Abraham Sophian, New York City, Section on Medicine and Diseases of Children, May 9, 1912," *Texas State Journal of Medicine* 7, no. 12 (April 1912): 334; "Dr. Sophian Spoke before Medicos; State Association Elected Dr. Turner President and Adjourned until San Antonio Convention," *Houston Post*, May 10, 1912, 10; "Typhoid Fever and Meningitis," *Dallas Morning News*, June 16, 1912, 11.

20 Dr. William Spencer Carter (1869–1944) was born in Greenwich, Warren County, New Jersey, as the younger of the two sons of William Carter (1830–1879), a farmer, and Ann Carter. He earned his medical degree from the University of Pennsylvania (1890) and served an internship at Philadelphia General Hospital (1890) and a residency at Presbyterian Hospital, Philadelphia (1891). He worked as an assistant in physiology at the University of Pennsylvania (1889–1892); as an assistant demonstrator in pathology at the University of Pennsylvania (1892–1896); and as an assistant professor of comparative physiology and demonstrator in physiology (1896–1897). He then moved to Galveston to become professor of physiology and hygiene at the University of Texas Medical Branch. He established one of the earliest research and teaching laboratories in physiology in the South; taught hygiene and public health for several years; and encouraged his assistant, Oscar Plant, to offer the first course in pharmacology at the school. In 1903, Dr. Carter became the school's fourth dean. Fellow deans elected Dr. Carter as vice president in 1916 and as president of the University of Texas Medical Branch in 1917. In 1922, he joined the division of medical sciences of the Rockefeller Foundation. For the next twelve years, he led the development of medical schools in the Philippines, Australia, South Africa, Java, New Zealand, China, and India. In China, he was acting director of Peking Union Medical College (1925). He helped organize the School of Tropical Medicine in Calcutta in 1926. Dr. Carter retired in 1934 but came out of retirement to serve again as dean of the University of Texas Medical Branch (1935–1938). He married Lillian V. McCleary (1870–1964) in 1895; they had two

children. He died in Auburndale, Newton, Massachusetts, at the age of seventy-five years. See "The History of the UTMB School of Medicine," *UTMB Health*, accessed October 29, 2017, https://som.utmb.edu/About/history.asp; *General Alumni Catalogue of the University of Pennsylvania* (Philadelphia, PA: Alumni Association of the University of Pennsylvania, 1917), 753; and "William Spencer Carter, Dean of the Faculty of Medical Department; Professor of Physiology and Hygiene," *Cactus Yearbook 1907* (Galveston, TX: University of Texas Medical Branch, 1907), 344.

21 "The Effect of Injecting Ringer's Solution into the Spinal Canal in Varying Amounts and Under Varying Pressures, Dr. W. S. Carter, Galveston, Section on Medicine and Disease of Children, May 9, 1912," *Texas State Journal of Medicine* 7, no. 12 (April 1912): 335; and "Typhoid Fever and Meningitis," *Dallas Morning News*, June 16, 1912, 11.

22 "'Diphtheria,' Dr. Ralph Steiner, Austin, Section on Ophthalmology, Otology, Rhinology and Laryngology, Second Day, Wednesday, May 8, 1912," *Texas State Journal of Medicine* 7, no. 12 (April 1912): 334.

23 In April 1912, Dr. Steiner had started to collect data and information for a presentation on cerebrospinal meningitis that he intended to give at the Texas State Medical Association convention in Waco in May 1912. For example, on Thursday, April 11, 1912, he sent a letter to county and city health officers in Texas to request that they "supply him as soon as possible with all information bearing on the epidemic of cerebrospinal meningitis in Texas." Dr. Steiner specifically requested "frank statements of opinions regarding the immunity or susceptibility to meningitis of 'smokers' and 'alcoholics.'" For unknown reasons, he did not give the talk. See "Asks Meningitis Data from Cities; State Health Department Trying to Prevent Recurrence of Disease," *El Paso Herald*, April 11, 1912, 8; "Steiner Is after Meningitis Data; Report of Texas Epidemic Will Be Given to Medical Association Convention," *Fort Worth Star-Telegram*, April 11, 1912, 5; Information on Meningitis; Dr. Steiner Will Use Data before State Medical Association," *Galveston Daily News*, April 12, 1912, 6; "Steiner Seeks Information; All City and County Health Officers Asked to Report on Cases of Meningitis," *Dallas Morning News*, April 12, 1912, 14.

24 "Nervous Diseases, Illustrated by Moving Pictures, Dr. S. N. Key, Austin, Section on Mental and Nervous Diseases and Medical

Jurisprudence, Wednesday, May 8, 1912," *Texas State Journal of Medicine* 7, no. 12 (April 1912): 333.

25 "No title," *Houston Post*, May 2, 1912, 3.

26 "Mayor Has Prepared Annual Statement; Optimistic Resume of Affairs of City during Past Years Given; Suggestions Are Made," *Dallas Morning News*, May 20, 1912, 4.

27 "Temperature More Moderate," *Dallas Morning News*, May 31, 1912, 3.

28 "Says Meningitis Is Wholly Stamped Out; Last Patient Soon to Be Discharged from Hospital; Total of 450 Treated at Hospital, with Death Rate of 27 Per Cent; Grand Total, 765 Cases," *Dallas Morning News*, May 31, 1912, 16.

29 "Friends Remember Heroism of Nurses; Meningitis Fighters Tendered Picnic Last Night; Mayor Holland Spoke of Spirit Displayed during Dread Epidemic Last Winter," *Dallas Morning News*, June 1, 1912, 7.

30 The total number of registrants at the American Medical Association's Sixty-Third Annual Session, held at Atlantic City, New Jersey, June 4–7, 1912, was 3,598. Of these 3,598 attendees, 109 identified as pathologists and physiologists. Five registrants were from Kansas, seventy were from Missouri, 567 were from New York, and twenty-six were from Texas. "Association News, Proceedings of the Atlantic City Session," *Journal of the American Medical Association* 58, no. 25 (June 22, 1912): 1,981.

31 "Prophylactic Vaccination against Epidemic Meningitis," *Transactions of the Section on Pathology and Physiology of the American Medical Association at the Sixty-Third Annual Session, Held at Atlantic City, NJ, June 4 to 7, 1912* (1912): 48–64.

32 Dr. Sophian apparently was scheduled to present his paper "Blood Pressure Observations in Epidemic Meningitis: Use of Blood Pressure in Controlling the Administration of Serum" before his pathologist peers on Tuesday, June 4, 1912. He apparently substituted "Prophylactic Vaccination against Epidemic Meningitis" for "Blood Pressure Observations," or he presented both papers. See "Association News, Proceedings of the Atlantic City Session," *Journal of the American Medical Association* 58, no. 25 (June 22, 1912): 1,992.

33 The authors were unable in newspaper databases a single article mentioning Dr. Sophian's and Dr. Black's paper "Prophylactic

Vaccination against Epidemic Meningitis" following the Atlantic City session of the American Medical Association in June 1912.

34 "Hunt Will Call Extra Session," *El Paso Herald*, May 17, 1912, 7.

35 "Funds for State Laboratory," *Texas State Journal of Medicine* 8, no. 3 (July 1912): 96.

36 "Half Pay for Nurses Stricken at Hospital: Eleven Meningitis Victims Are Paid by City," *Dallas Morning News*, June 11, 1912, 16.

37 "Begins New Laboratory Work; Dr. Henry Hartman Now Cultivating Typhoid Germs for Anti-Vaccine Experiment Work," *Dallas Morning News*, June 16, 1912, 11.

38 The Widal test is a serological test to detect the present of typhoid fever due to *Salmonella typhi*. See L. A. Olopoenia and A. L. King, "Widal Agglutination Test—100 Years Later: Still Plagued by Controversy," *Postgraduate Medical Journal* 76, no. 892 (February 2000): 80–84.

39 "Work on State Laboratory; Health Officer Steiner and Dr. Hartman Issues [*sic*] Statement Explaining Manufacture of Serums," *Dallas Morning News*, June 21, 1912, 7; and "A Diagnostic Laboratory for the State Health Department," *Texas State Journal of Medicine* 8, no. 3 (July 1912): 1,912.

40 "State Laboratory Makes First Serum; Anti-Typhoid Product Is Sent to Manor for Use; The New Department, under Dr. Hartman's Work, Accomplishing Speedy and Satisfactory Results," *Dallas Morning News*, July 21, 1912, 1; and "First Serum Manufactured; New Vaccine Factory at Austin at Work; First Product Was Anti-Typhoid Serium [*sic*] Which Was Sent to Monor [*sic*] for Use in Threatened Typhoid Cases," *Houston Post*, July 21, 1912, 3.

41 Abraham Sophian and James Harvey Black, "Prophylactic Vaccination against Epidemic Meningitis," *Journal of the American Medical Association* 59, no. 7 (August 17, 1912): 527–32.

42 Dr. Sophian's twelve-page speech, "Preventive Measures against Epidemic Meningitis, by Dr. A. Sophian, Kansas City, Mo." was published in *Transactions of the Fifteenth International Congress on Hygiene and Demography* (Washington, DC: Government Printing Office, 1913), 54–66. See also "Sanitary Measures against Cerebrospinal Meningitis," *Journal of the American Medical Association* 59, no. 16 (October 19, 1912): 1,482.

43 The International Congress on Hygiene met for the first time in 1852 in response to the great pandemic of cholera in Europe. The purpose of the congress was to discuss scientific problems among eminent

scientists of different nationalities and countries. President William Howard Taft was the honorary president of the fifteenth congress, held in Washington, DC, September 23–28, 1912. "International Congress of Hygiene and Demography," *Nature* 43 (January 15, 1891): 241–42; "Fifteenth International Congress on Hygiene and Demography," *Journal of Hygiene* 11, no. 2 (July 1911): 301–6; and "International Congress of Hygiene to Meet in America," *Texas State Journal of Medicine* 7, no. 12 (April 1912): 337.

44 See, for example, "Meningitis Vaccine as Preventive Is Urged," *Santa Ana Register* (Santa Ana, CA), September 24, 1912, 3; "Scientists Clash on Typhoid Rules; Dr. Gaertner Insists That Bacteriological Tests Are Not Sufficient Guard; Need Sanitary Land Survey; Takes Issue with Prof. Jordan—Dr. Flexner Tells of Meningitis Cure," *New York Times*, September 25, 1912, 10; "Vaccination Favored as Guard against Dread Scourge of Childhood," *Washington Times*, September 24, 1912, 2; "Scourge of Rabies Could Be Blotted Out; Dr. Caroline Hedger Tells Congress of the Stock Yards Child; and Meningitis Vaccine as Preventative Strong Urged before the Members," *Eau Claire Leader* (Eau Claire, WI), September 25, 1912, 2.

CHAPTER 8

MENINGITIS VISITS THE TEXAS STATE CAPITOL BUILDING, FEBRUARY 1913

In the late summer of 1912, Dr. Hartman was hard at work manufacturing a meningococcal vaccine in the new Texas State Board of Health biologics laboratory inside the Texas State Capitol building.[1] He wanted to be prepared for the possible recurrence of cerebrospinal meningitis during the upcoming winter months (1912–1913). Dr. Hartman planned to test his meningococcal vaccine for efficacy and safety in volunteers using the methods proffered by Dr. Sophian and Dr. Black in their paper titled "Prophylactic Vaccination against Epidemic Meningitis."[3] However, when the time came to test his meningococcal vaccine on volunteers, Dr. Hartman could find no volunteers.[4] He was at an impasse and did not know what to do.

On Saturday, October 26, 1912, Dr. Steiner learned about a case of cerebrospinal meningitis—the first case of the new season. A local Texas druggist notified Dr. Steiner that he had received an order for antimeningitis serum for a child in Joshua, Johnson County, Texas.[5] The same day, Dr. Steiner learned of a second case of cerebrospinal meningitis in Temple, Bell County, Texas.[5] The man, a farmer, died of his disease. Dr. Steiner did not know whether the two cases were sporadic (non-epidemic) or signaled the dreaded return of the cerebrospinal meningitis epidemic in Texas. On Friday, November 8, 1912, he notified county and city health officers in Texas to be prepared, writing,

> From the history of the disease, there is a possibility of the reappearance of cerebrospinal meningitis in Texas during the colder months. The disease is a contagious and infectious one, due ... to the meningococcus, infection being conveyed by contact with the sick and by carriers. There are approximately ten otherwise healthy carriers to every case of cerebrospinal meningitis.[6]

Dr. Steiner instructed health officials to respond to a cerebrospinal meningitis case in their jurisdiction by isolating the infected individual, his or her direct contacts, and contacts who were healthy carriers of the meningococcus as demonstrated by assessment of their nasal and throat secretions. He also advised the centralization of all active cases in one place, if possible, and their quarantining in that place until bacteriological examination of cultures made from their nose and throat secretions became negative. Furthermore, he counselled that healthy carriers should remain in quarantine until their culture examinations, made every two to four days, proved negative for the presence of the meningococcus.[6]

Dr. Steiner added that Dr. Hartman was available to examine meningococcal cultures sent to him in Austin and that there would be no charge for the service. Dr. Hartman instructed county and city health officers to collect material from the noses and throats of contacts, examine the material under a microscope for the presence of Gram-negative diplococci, inoculate the material in Loeffler's blood serum tubes, incubate the cultures, examine the cultures for meningococcal colonies, and send the tubes containing meningococcal cultures to him in Austin.[6]

Finally, Dr. Steiner recommended the use of antiseptic nose sprays and throat applications and vaccination with the meningococcal vaccine. He offered vials of meningococcal vaccine manufactured in the Texas State Board of Health biologics laboratory and free directions on how to apply it to all who were interested. The cost of the meningococcal vaccine was twenty cents per dozen ampoules. He promised that the Texas State Health Board would "make every effort to keep on hand a full supply of antimeningitis serum" and would sell it to buyers at cost.[6] Dr. Steiner concluded, "I would urge upon you not only to carry out the above measures, but immediately to place your city or town in first-class sanitary condition."[6]

On Friday, November 15, 1912, Dr. Steiner offered to physicians across Texas free copies of "Prophylactic Measures against Epidemic Meningitis," the paper written by Dr. Sophian and Dr. Black. Dr. Steiner expressed his sincere "hope [that] the pamphlet [would] be generally read and the suggestions heeded."[7]

Twelve days passed. On Wednesday, November 27, 1912, the Texas State Board of Health met[8] in the Texas State Capitol building to discuss the return of cerebrospinal meningitis to Texas. Present at the meeting were Dr. Benjamin Franklin Calhoun[9] of Beaumont, Dr. Beall of Fort Worth, and Dr. Lister of Houston. Absent were Dr. Worsham of El Paso, Dr. McLaurin of Dallas, and Dr. Fly of Galveston. Dr. Steiner announced that he had procured an ample supply of antimeningitis serum from New York City[8] and that Dr. Hartman had manufactured a plentiful supply of meningococcal vaccine in the new biologics laboratory. Unfortunately, Dr. Hartman remained unable to test the vaccine for a lack of volunteers.

As the board discussed these issues, Dr. Steiner received word that a boy at the State Institute for Juvenile Training in Gatesville, a hundred miles north of Austin, had died of cerebrospinal meningitis.[10] The boy's death motivated Dr. Steiner and other unnamed persons of the Texas State Board of Health and the Texas State Capitol building to volunteer to test Dr. Hartman's meningococcal vaccine.[4]

On Tuesday, December 3, 1912, Dr. Steiner reported that he had received a shipment of antimeningitis serum and that Dr.

Hartman had received a live meningococcal culture with which to manufacture his meningococcal vaccine.[11] No other information about the meningococcal culture shipment is available. On Friday, December 6, 1912, Dr. Steiner announced the arrival of a second shipment of antimeningitis serum from New York City. He said that he was amassing quantities of the antimeningitis serum only as a precaution, because conditions were normal except for a few sporadic cases of cerebrospinal meningitis in Texas. He avowed that fifty years of experience had shown that cerebrospinal meningitis epidemics did not come in successive years. He did not say where he obtained this information.[12-13]

Also, on Friday, December 6, 1912, Dr. Steiner announced to the public that he, other members of the Texas State Board of Health, and some state officials in the capitol building had received Dr. Hartman's meningococcal vaccine without problems. The blood tests accompanying their vaccinations showed that the vaccine conferred "some degree of immunity."[4] The news that Dr. Steiner and others had survived their vaccinations encouraged some people in Austin to seek meningococcal vaccinations from Dr. Hartman.[4] Dr. Steiner projected a rosy future, saying that everything was in "splendid condition to meet the appearance of meningitis" that "was not expected."[12]

On Monday, December 9, 1912, Governor Colquitt climbed the stairs (the elevator was out of service) of the Texas State Capitol building, entered the third-floor biologics laboratory of the Texas State Board of Health, and received the first of three meningococcal vaccine inoculations from Dr. Morris H. Boerner,[14] the head of the Texas Hookworm Commission.[15] On Tuesday, December 17, 1912, Governor Colquitt received his second inoculation of the meningococcal vaccine.[16] It is unknown when or whether Governor Colquitt received the third dose to complete the vaccination series.

Four weeks passed. At noon on Tuesday, January 14, 1913, Chester Hunter Terrell,[17] the newly elected forty-third speaker of the Texas State House of Representatives, convened the Thirty-Third regular session[18] of the House in the House (Great) Hall, the largest room in the Texas State Capitol building. Dr. Steiner,

Dr. Hartman, and Mr. Babcock, situated in their suite of rooms on the third floor of the capitol building, adjacent to the House Hall, were unaccustomed to the myriad sounds coming from the 150 state representatives and their staff below. Recall that the House of Representatives had not convened in the hall during the year of 1912.[19]

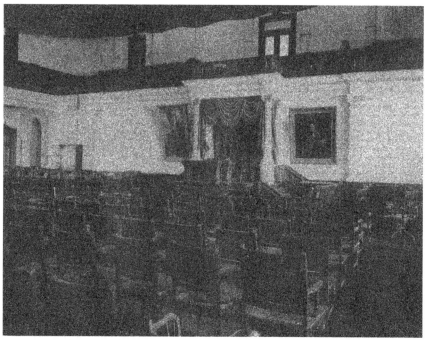

View, facing west, inside the Great Hall of the House of Representatives, Texas State Capitol building, Austin, Travis County, Texas, 1894. Rows of wooden chairs face the front and two painted portraits hang on the walls on the west side of the hall. Two sets of doors above the gallery near the top of the image lead into the warren of committee and other rooms on the west side of the capitol building. The image is held by the University of North Texas Libraries, Denton, Texas.

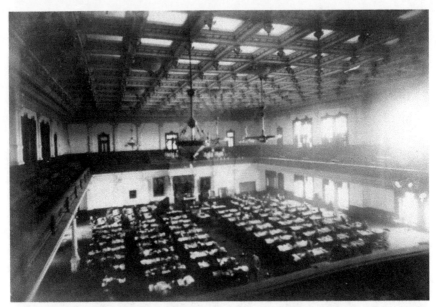

View (facing west) from the gallery (balcony) of the Great Hall of the House of Representatives, Texas State Capitol. The date of the image is unknown. The image is held by the University of North Texas Libraries, Denton, Texas.

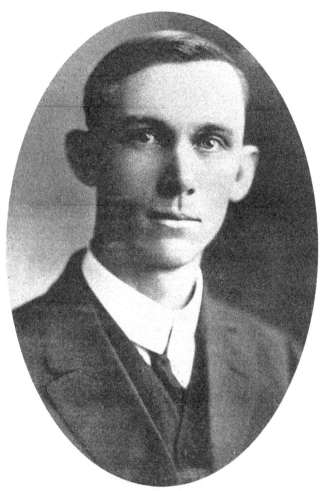

Chester Hunter Terrell (1882–1920), Thirty-Third House Speaker, Texas State Legislature House of Representatives, circa 1913. Detail from the Thirty-Second House Composite (CHA #1989.526). Courtesy of the Texas State Preservation Board, Austin, Texas, January 30, 2018.

Also, on January 14, 1913, Dr. Steiner learned that Archer W. Koons,[20] a cadet at the Texas Agricultural and Mechanical College[21] (Texas A&M College), had died of cerebrospinal meningitis. Texas A&M College was located in College Station, Brazos County, Texas, about a hundred miles west of Austin. Archer Koons had returned to college eight days before his death from his home in Nada, Colorado County, Texas, to attend a short winter course,[22] which began on Monday, January 6, 1913. He had been well on Saturday, January 11, 1913; had become ill on Sunday, January 12, 1913; and had died on Monday, January 13, 1913.

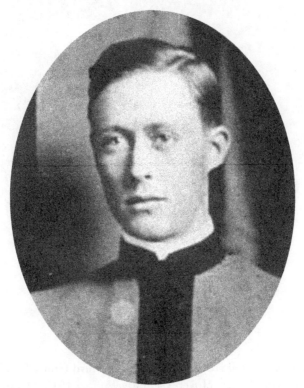

Archer W. Koons (1892–1913), circa 1913, "In Memory of Our Classmates," *Longhorn Texas A&M Yearbook*, 1914, p. 127.

Two days after the death of Cadet Koons, Fisher Younger Rawlins,[23] another cadet at Texas A&M College, died from cerebrospinal meningitis. He had returned to college from his home in Ardmore, Carter County, Oklahoma, to attend the college's short winter course, too. The two deaths prompted Dr. Steiner to send Dr. Hartman to College Station with a supply of meningococcal vaccine.[24]

On reaching the college, Dr. Hartman confirmed the two fatal cases of cerebrospinal meningitis. The two cadets had returned to the college eight and ten days before their deaths. Dr. Hartman announced that these two spans of time were within the incubating period for cerebrospinal meningitis, and therefore, in his opinion, the two victims had acquired their disease while visiting home.[25] In other words, the disease had developed within too short a time after the boys returned to the college for them to have acquired it at the college. Dr. Hartman's opinion was not shared by Dr. Sophian, who earlier had said that the incubation period of cerebrospinal meningitis was "a variable, unknown quantity."[26] Dr. Otto Ehlinger,[27] the Texas A&M College surgeon, had hospitalized the two cadets after they became ill, thereby minimizing the number of exposures, averred Dr. Hartman. Two hundred students fled the Texas A&M College campus following the two deaths, but seven hundred stayed. Dr. Ehlinger inoculated 316 students with the meningococcus vaccine.[28] Dr. Steiner said that students were safer at college than at home.[26]

Three weeks passed. Unexpectedly, on Friday, February 7, 1913, Dr. Wade Hampton Frost,[29–30] a US Public Health Service physician who previously had published a long primer[31] on cerebrospinal meningitis in January 1912, published a second meningitis-related paper titled "Anti-meningitis Vaccination."[32] In his second paper, Dr. Frost savaged "Prophylactic Vaccination Against Epidemic Meningitis," the seminal meningococcal vaccine paper published on August 17, 1912, by Dr. Sophian and Dr. Black. Dr. Frost accused Dr. Sophian and Dr. Black of failing to demonstrate convincingly the efficacy of the meningococcal vaccine. He also listed the untenable (in his opinion) risks and costs of meningococcal vaccination and strongly advised against the wholesale use of meningococcal vaccination except "in communities where the disease was epidemic, or where an epidemic seemed likely to occur, especially of physicians and nurses caring for patients with the disease."[32] In his earlier primer, Dr. Frost had written differently. To wit, he wrote, "The high mortality of cerebrospinal meningitis, its peculiarly distressing clinical course, and the frequency of most serious after-effects render it imperative that *every possible measure be taken to protect the public from its ravages*" [emphasis added].[30]

Four days later, on Tuesday, February 11, 1913, cerebrospinal meningitis invaded the Texas State Capitol building, infecting Representative Thomas McNeal.[33] Representative McNeal was a previously healthy sixty-two-year-old attorney, judge, farmer, husband, and father of five children from Lockhart, Caldwell County, about thirty-three miles south of Austin. He had taken an active part in the House of Representatives' proceedings for the previous five weeks.[34]

On that Tuesday, February 11, 1913, Representative McNeal experienced a chill. On the advice of his colleagues, he returned to his boardinghouse room at 208 East Ninth Street, Austin. On Wednesday morning, February 12, 1913, his son found him unconscious in bed and called Dr. Ernest Krueger,[35] a local physician, who diagnosed cerebrospinal meningitis and administered antimeningitis serum. Representative McNeal's wife and a daughter traveled from Lockhart to be at his bedside.

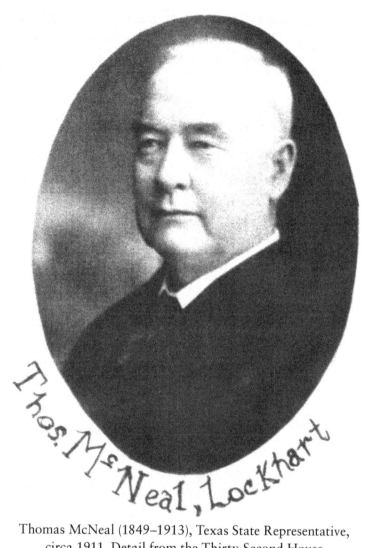

Thomas McNeal (1849–1913), Texas State Representative, circa 1911. Detail from the Thirty-Second House Composite (CHA #1989.526). Courtesy of the Texas State Preservation Board, Austin, Texas, January 30, 2018.

The next day, Wednesday, February 12, 1913, Representative Albert Leroy "Lee" Killingsworth was stricken with cerebrospinal meningitis in Austin. He was a previously healthy farmer, landowner, husband, and father of five children[36] from Marshall, Harrison County, Texas, about 340 miles northeast of Austin. He retired at about eight o'clock in the evening on Wednesday, February 12,

1913, after telling his roommate, Representative Clifford Lemuel Stone[37] of Rusk County, that he felt ill. Representative Stone urged him to call a doctor, but Representative Killingsworth refused, insisting that he had the grippe and that it would wear off. At two o'clock in the morning, Representative Killingsworth awakened Representative Stone and told him that he was in great pain but again refused to see a doctor. Representative Stone went to the Texas State Capitol building in the morning, answered roll call for Representative Killingsworth, explained to Speaker Terrell that Mr. Killingworth was ill, and obtained an excused absence for him.

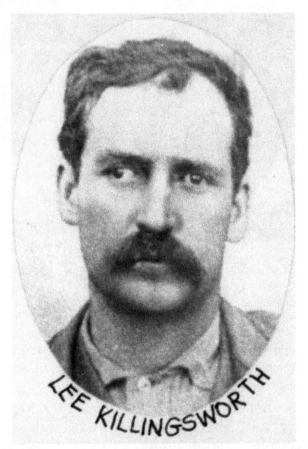

Albert Leroy "Lee" Killingsworth (1859–1913), Texas State Representative, circa 1913. Detail from the Thirty-Third House Composite (CHA #1989.527). Courtesy of the Texas State Preservation Board, Austin, Texas.

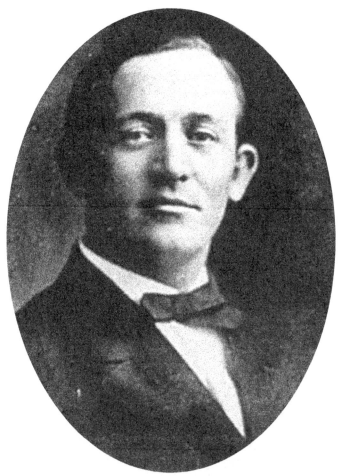

Clifford Lemuel Stone (1881–1940), Texas State Representative, circa 1913. Detail from the Thirty-Third House Composite (CHA #1989.527). Courtesy of the Texas State Preservation Board, Austin, Texas.

Representative Stone returned to the boardinghouse room later in the morning, found Lee Killingsworth in an alarming condition, and called Dr. Steiner, who arrived with another physician, probably Dr. Hartman. The two physicians examined Representative Killingsworth, diagnosed cerebrospinal meningitis, and prepared to administer a dose of intraspinal antimeningitis serum. However, Representative Killingsworth died before they could do so on the afternoon of Thursday, February 13, 1913.[38-39] Dr. Hartman performed an autopsy on Mr. Killingsworth, which confirmed the diagnosis of cerebrospinal meningitis. Dr. Steiner, shaken, ordered fumigation of the Texas State Capitol building.[40]

On Friday morning, February 14, 1913, Representative McNeal succumbed to cerebrospinal meningitis.[41-44] Speaker Terrell arranged for two groups of state representatives to accompany the bodies of Representatives McNeal and Killingsworth to their respective hometowns for burial. He also excused Representative George Herder Sr.[45] to return to his home in Weimar (Weimer), Colorado County, Texas, about eighty miles southeast of Austin, to tend to his ill wife. Speaker Terrell then adjourned the House until the next day, Saturday, February 15, 1913, at two o'clock.[43]

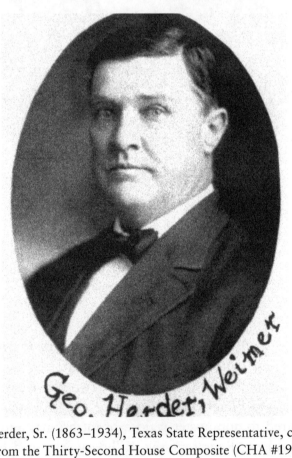

George Herder, Sr. (1863–1934), Texas State Representative, circa 1911. Detail from the Thirty-Second House Composite (CHA #1989.526). Courtesy of the Texas State Preservation Board, Austin, Texas.

The unexpected deaths from cerebrospinal meningitis of Representatives Killingsworth and McNeal alarmed Texas legislators, government officials, and employees who worked in the Texas State Capitol building. There was only one other case of cerebrospinal meningitis in Austin at the time of the deaths of Representatives Killingsworth and McNeal, according to Dr. Steiner. In addition, there had been only twenty-five cases of cerebrospinal meningitis in Austin thus far that winter and a paucity of cases across Texas in mid-February 1913. Dr. Steiner attributed the paucity of cerebrospinal meningitis cases across Texas to weather that was "unfavorable for the disease."[46]

Some people asked Dr. Steiner to explain why two people in the west wing of the Texas State Capitol building had developed cerebrospinal meningitis within days of each other. Dr. Steiner responded, "The germs were probably brought to the city and carried into the House by a member whose system is in perfect order and who is able to throw them off without injury to himself, with the result that the victims whose general conditions were not in such perfect condition, contracted them with fatal results."[47] Dr. Steiner said he could account for the two deaths in no other way.

Even as Dr. Steiner advised the legislators that there was "absolutely no danger from meningitis in the Legislature,"[48] he offered to vaccinate all representatives and their attachés at no cost to themselves. He instead charged the vaccinations to the state contingency fund.[49] About one hundred representatives, including Representative Joseph Clark Hunt[50] of Canyon City, Randall County, Texas, received an inoculation of Dr. Hartman's meningococcal vaccine on Friday, February 14, 1913.[49] After receiving the inoculation, Representative Hunt became ill and returned to his boardinghouse room. Dr. Steiner attributed Representative Hunt's illness to the judge's "nervous condition." Later, however, Dr. Steiner said the judge was "suffering a reaction from the meningitis vaccine administered to him."[51-52]

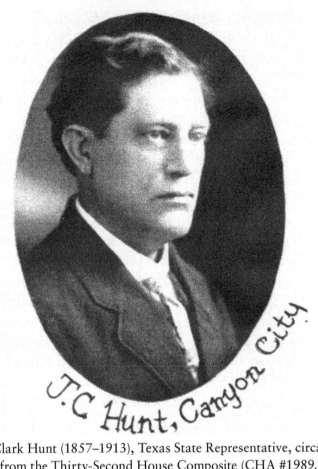

Joseph Clark Hunt (1857–1913), Texas State Representative, circa 1911.
Detail from the Thirty-Second House Composite (CHA #1989.526).
Courtesy of the Texas State Preservation Board, Austin, Texas.

On Saturday, February 15, 1913, Representative Hunt slid into
a coma to become the third Texas state representative to develop
cerebrospinal meningitis in four days. Representative William
Benjamin Goodner,[53] a physician from Dublin, Erath County,
Texas, suggested that Representatives Hunt, Killingsworth, and
McNeal might have contracted cerebrospinal meningitis as a result
of "the practice of the health department in developing the cultures
of the germs in the laboratory on the balcony floor of the House
chamber." He continued, "Committee rooms are located on this
[third] floor, and the halls and stairways there are in constant use
by members and employees."[54]

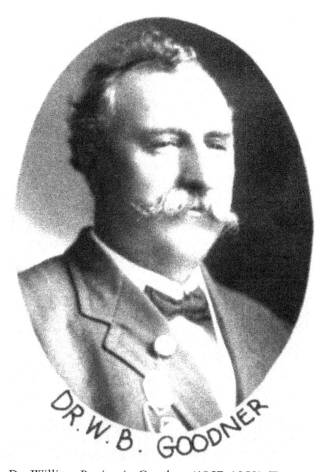

Dr. William Benjamin Goodner (1857–1950), Texas
State Representative, circa 1913. Detail from the Thirty-
Third House Composite (CHA #1989.527). Courtesy of
the Texas State Preservation Board, Austin, Texas.

Representative John Jeptha Stephens,[55] a newspaper publisher
and editor from Upshur County, Texas, further observed that
the stricken legislators had been seated in the Great Hall a short
distance in front of him, right behind him, and across the aisle
on the south side of the hall.[56] On learning of the illness of Judge
Hunt, Speaker Terrell excused all House members from attendance
until Monday, March 3, 1913. However, he changed the date
back to Monday, February 24, 1913, when Representative Hunt

emerged from his coma in his boardinghouse room in Austin on Sunday, February 16, 1913.[57]

On Monday, February 17, 1913, more bad news erupted in the Texas State Capitol building. Speaker Terrell learned that Representative George Herder was ill with cerebrospinal meningitis at home in Weimer.[58-59] Recall that Speaker Terrell had excused Representative Herder to return home on Friday, February 14, 1913, to care for his ill wife. On hearing of Representative Herder's diagnosis, Speaker Terrell abandoned his plan to reconvene the House on Monday, February 24, 1913.[60] In only six days (Tuesday, February 11, 1913, through Monday, February 17, 1913, inclusive), four state representatives working in the Great Hall of the Texas State Capitol building had contracted cerebrospinal meningitis and two of them had died.

On Wednesday, February 19, 1913, House Speaker Terrell learned of yet another Texas state representative—the fifth—who was ill with cerebrospinal meningitis. Representative David C. Kelley,[61] a farmer, husband, and father of six children, was diagnosed with cerebrospinal meningitis at his home in Kaufman, Kaufman County, Texas, about 220 miles northeast of Austin. Representative Kelley had left the Texas State Capitol on Wednesday, February 12, 1913, to care for his ailing wife in Kaufman. He had started to make the return trip to Austin from Kaufman on Sunday, February 16, 1913. When he reached Dallas, about thirty-three miles west of Kaufman, he learned that Speaker Terrell had adjourned the House subject to call. He turned around and headed back to Kaufman on Monday, February 17, 1913, and fell ill. His physician diagnosed cerebrospinal meningitis and administered antimeningitis serum on the night of Tuesday, February 18, 1913.[62]

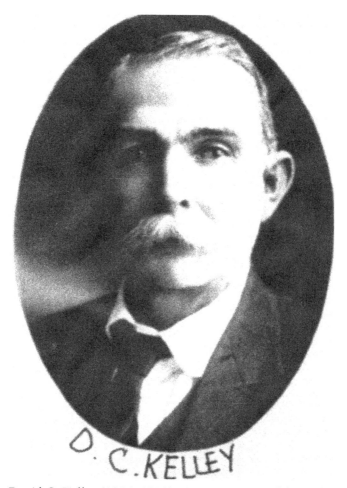

David C. Kelley (1856–1913), circa 1913. Detail from the
Thirty-Third House Composite (CHA #1989.527). Courtesy
of the Texas State Preservation Board, Austin, Texas.

Also, on Wednesday, February 19, 1913, Dr. Hartman suffered
a mental and physical breakdown, could not work, and remained
confined in his Austin home until further notice. Dr. Boerner
operated the laboratory in Dr. Hartman's absence. A newspaper
reported,

> [Dr. Hartman] has suffered a breakdown following
> arduous labor. Dr. Hartman has been devoting
> his best efforts to state work for several months,

culminating in increased duties incident to the present of cerebrospinal meningitis in the House of Representatives and locally. Not only was he making examinations and giving treatments, but he administered scores of inoculations of vaccine ... Dr. Morris Boerner, Texas State Director of the National Hookworm, has been working in conjunction with State Health Officer Steiner and Dr. Hartman and he, too, is almost incapacitated for work, so great has been the strain.[63]

On Saturday, February 22, 1913, at four o'clock in the afternoon, Representative David C. Kelley died.[64] Three representatives had died within less than two weeks. A great pall descended over the Texas State Capitol building as the legislators and Dr. Steiner tried to figure out what to do.[65-66]

CHAPTER 8 NOTES

1 "Prepares to Make Vaccine: Department to Manufacture Meningitis Vaccine to Combat Possible Recurrence of Epidemic," *Dallas Morning News*, August 28, 1928, 14.

2 Images of the preparation of the typhoid vaccine (which was similar to the preparation of the meningococcal vaccine) at the US Army Medical School in 1917 are available at "Typhoid Vaccine Preparation, US Army Medical School, 1917," Harris and Ewing Photographs Collection, Library of Congress Prints and Photographs Division, Washington, DC, accessed March 9, 2018, http://www.loc.gov/pictures/search/?q=typhoid%20vaccine.

3 Abraham Sophian and James Harvey Black, "Prophylactic Vaccination against Epidemic Meningitis," *Journal of the American Medical Association* 59, no. 7 (August 17, 1912): 527–32.

4 "Meningitis Vaccine Does Its Work Well; Paper Read at San Antonio by Dr. Henry Hartman; Deals with Results from Experiments Made in Austin at Session of Legislature," *Dallas Morning News*, May 11, 1913, 10.

5 "Meningitis at Joshua," *Cleburne Morning Review*, October 26, 1912, 8; and "Meningitis Death near Rogers," *Dallas Morning News*, October 26, 1912, 3.

6 "Prevent Advent of Meningitis; State Health Officer Takes Precautionary Steps; Addresses Letter to Every County Health Officer in State as to Means of Preventative," *Rice Belt Journal* (Welsh, LA), November 8, 1912, 3.

7 "Papers Ready for Distribution; Dr. Abraham Sophian Written Article on Meningitis Epidemic," *Dallas Morning News*, November 16, 1912, 6.

8 "State Health Board Meets: Physicians Discuss Recurrence in Texas of Meningitis Epidemic," *Dallas Morning News*, November 27, 1912, 2.

9 Dr. Benjamin Franklin Calhoun (1848–1922) was born in Laurens County, South Carolina, as one of the thirteen children of Patrick Ludlow Calhoun III (1814–1863), a farmer, and Martha Ella Teague (1816–1858). He attended public schools until fifteen years of age, joined the Confederate Army, and moved to Texas in 1866 to work on a farm in Brazoria County. In 1868, he began the study of medicine under his uncle by marriage, Dr. W. D. Jennings, and he earned his medical degree from Texas Medical College and Hospital

in Galveston in 1875. He first practiced medicine at Sandy Point, Brazoria County, and later moved to Beaumont, Jefferson County, Texas, in 1892. He served as mayor of Beaumont in 1886 and as Beaumont city health officer, 1888–1894. He married Lela Grist (1871–1943) in 1892; they had three children. He died at the age of seventy-three years. See "Dr. B. F. Calhoun," *Texas Magazine* 4, no. 1 (May 1911): 52.

10 "Training School Hybrid Institute; Reformatory Prisoners Still There, Contrary to Expectations of Advocates," *Dallas Morning News*, December 1, 1912, 1.

11 "Meningitis Serum Available," *Dallas Morning News*, December 3, 1912, 11.

12 "Health Conditions Normal; Another Consignment of Vaccine and Serum to Fight Meningitis Received at Austin," *Dallas Morning News*, December 6, 1912, 11.

13 Dr. Steiner cited the same cerebrospinal meningitis epidemic periodicity information in his annual report published in early December 1912. See "Texas Is a Living State, Data Proves; Health Officer Steiner Submits Annual Report to Governor; Births Double Deaths; Interesting Part of Statement Is That Dealing with Campaign against Hookworm," *Dallas Morning News*, December 8, 1912, 9.

14 Dr. Morris Hirschfeld Boerner (1885–1932) was born in Austin, Travis County, Texas, as one of the two sons of Louis Boerner (1854–1930) and Anna Morrison (1863–1941). He earned his bachelor's degree from the University of Texas at Austin and his medical degree from the University of Texas Medical Department at Galveston in 1909. On June 25, 1912, Dr. Steiner appointed him director of the Hookworm Commission in Texas (1912–1915). Dr. Boerner also succeeded Dr. Hartman as assistant state health officer (1913–1915). Dr. Boerner married Alma Rhodes (1901–1993) in 1923; they had no children. He died at the age of forty-seven years. W. J. Maxwell and John A. Lomax, *General Register of the Students and Former Students of the University of Texas, 1917* (Austin, TX: University of Texas Ex-Students' Association, 1917), 379; and "Seventeen Die on Weekend," *Marshall News Messenger*, June 28, 1932, 5.

15 "Governor Is Vaccinated against Meningitis Attack; Other State Officials and Department Officials Taking Treatment to Ward Off Disease," *Bryan Daily Eagle*, December 11, 1912, 7.

16 "Pardoned by the Governor; Fifty-One Christmas Pardons Were Granted; O. B. Colquitt Celebrated His Fifty-First Birthday by

Bringing Joy to That Number of Convicts," *Houston Daily Post*, December 17, 1912, 4.

17 Chester Hunter Terrell (1882–1920) of San Antonio, Bexar County, Texas, served in the Texas House of Representatives, 1909–1915, and as House speaker, 1913–1915. He was born in Terrell, Kaufman County, Texas, as one of the five children of Jonathan Olynthus Terrell (1855–1923), a lawyer and the Republican state senator from Kaufman County, 1885–1889, and Mattie S. Simpson (1857–1935). Jonathan O. Terrell also was the 1910 Republican nominee for governor, losing to Oscar Branch Colquitt. Chester H. Terrell moved from Terrell to Alamo City at the age of twelve years. He attended San Antonio Academy and the University of Texas at Austin, where he played baseball. He obtained his law degree from the university in 1904 and returned to San Antonio to join his father's law firm. Five years later, he won election to the Texas House of Representatives (1909) as a Democrat at the age of twenty-six years. During his second term, he chaired the House Committee on Jurisprudence, and in 1913, he became speaker when a split between the Prohibitionists over tactics allowed him, a so-called wet (against Prohibition), to win the gavel. At the age of thirty years, he was the second-youngest man ever to serve as speaker. In 1915, he considered running for governor, but his failing health caused him instead to leave the House of Representatives and return to San Antonio to rejoin his family's law firm. He married Gladys E. Bentley (1886–1981) in 1904; they had three children. He died of an incurable illness at the age of thirty-eight years. See "Chester H. Terrell," in *Presiding Officers of the Texas Legislature, 1846–2016* (Austin, TX: Texas Legislative Council, 2016), 176–77; "Chester Terrell Dies at His Home in San Antonio," *Galveston Daily News*, September 14, 1920, 2; and "On Deathbed, Pleads for US to Kill League; Former Speaker of House in Texas Sends His Last Word to Harding; A Lifelong Democrat; Internationalism of Wilson Drove Him into GOP for American Ideals; Reply Goes Too Late; Stanch [*sic*] Patriot Dead When Message from Marion Is Despatched [*sic*]," *New York Herald*, September 20, 1290, 1.

18 The thirty-third regular session of the Texas State Legislature House of Representatives met from January 14, 1913, to April 1, 1913. See *Legislative Reference Library of Texas*, accessed December 2, 2017, http://www.lrl.state.tx.us/sessions/sessionSnapshot.cfm?legSession=33-0.

19 Drawings of the second and third floors of the Texas State Capitol building, showing the relationship of the laboratory rooms to the House of Representatives Great Hall, are available at the "Texas State Capitol Project 1988," National Park Service, US Department of the Interior, US Government, 1988, HABS TEX, 227-AUST,13, 1988, Historic American Buildings Survey Program, Library of Congress Prints and Photographs Division, Washington, DC, accessed January 20, 2018, http://www.loc.gov/pictures/search/?q=texas%20state%20capitol%20drawing.

20 Archer W. Koons (1892–1913) was born in Tennessee as the second of the five children of Frederick Clifton Koons (1864–1949), a traveling salesman, and Mary Millicent Archer (1861–1943).

21 "Cadet Koons Died at A&M College; Was Stricken with Meningitis on Sunday Morning and Lived Only Forty-Eighth [*sic*] Hours," *Bryan Daily Eagle*, January 14, 1913, 3; "Two Deaths at the College; About 100 Students Leave Because Fatalities from Meningitis; No More Cases," *Waco Morning News*, January 16, 1913, 1; and "No New Cases of Meningitis: State Health Officer Believes Two Victims at A&M Contracted Disease Elsewhere," *Dallas Morning News*, January 18, 1913, 3.

22 "College Calendar," *Thirty-Sixth Annual Catalogue, Bulletin of the Agricultural and Mechanical College of Texas, April 1912* 9, no. 16 (1912): front pages.

23 Fisher Younger Rawlins (1892–1913) was born in Ardmore, Carter County, Oklahoma as the youngest of the seven children of Alexander Bledsoe Rawlins (1855–1937), a retail furniture merchant, and Ida Virginia "Virgie" Fisher (1857–1892). "Obituary of Fisher Younger Rawlins," *Lancaster Herald* (Lancaster, TX), January 17, 1913, 5; "Fisher Rawlins Dead," *Daily Ardmoreite* (Ardmore, OK), January 15, 1913, 5; "A&M Cadet Dies," *Dallas Morning News*, January 16, 1913, 15; and "Sophomore History," *Longhorn* Yearbook (College Station, TX: Texas A&M, 1913), 148.

24 "No Cause for Alarm," *Bryan Daily Eagle*, January 15, 1913, 3.

25 "Addresses Doctors at Night Meeting; Dr. Sophian Speaks at Session of Dallas County Medical Society; Situation Not Serious; Declares Presence of One Hundred Cases No Cause for Alarm—Suggests Immunitization [*sic*]," *Dallas Morning News*, January 7, 1912, 4.

26 "No New Cases of Meningitis; State Health Officer Believes Two Victims at A&M Contracted Disease Elsewhere," *Dallas Morning News*, January 18, 1913, 3.

27 Dr. Otto Ehlinger (1865 or 1871–1921) was born in Ehlinger, Fayette County, Texas, as one of the ten children of Charles Ehlinger (1826–1872) and Maria Wilhelmina Mueller or Miller (1832–1883). He graduated from Vanderbilt University in 1890 and earned his medical degree from Tulane University Medical Department in 1900. He worked as the college physician of Texas A&M University, 1911–1921. He married Sallie R. Goodwin (1874–1892) in 1892; they had one child. Dr. Ehlinger died of heart disease at the age of fifty-two years. See "Dr. Otto Ehlinger Dead; A&M College Physician Expires Suddenly Today," *Bryan Daily Eagle*, February 28, 1912, 1.

28 "Health Department," *Nineteenth Biennial Report of the Board of Directors of the Agricultural and Mechanical College of Texas for the Fiscal Years Ending August 31, 1913, and August 31, 1914* (Austin, TX: A. C. Baldwin and Sons, 1914), 10.

29 Dr. Wade Hampton Frost (1880–1938) was born in Marshall, Fauquier County, Virginia, as one of the eight children of Dr. Henry Rutledge Frost Jr. (1839–1917) and Sabra Jane Walker (1839–1917). His mother tutored him before he spent two years at unnamed boarding schools. Wade H. Frost earned his bachelor's and medical degrees from the University of Virginia in 1901 and 1903, respectively. He served in the US Public Health Service (1905–1929), studying water pollution, poliomyelitis, yellow fever, influenza, diphtheria, and tuberculosis. He resigned from the public health service to serve full-time as a professor of epidemiology and dean (1931–1934) at Johns Hopkins University School of Hygiene and Public Health. He married Susan Noland Haxall (1876–1965) in 1915; they had one child. He died at the age of fifty-eight years at Johns Hopkins University Hospital. See Thomas M. Daniel, *Wade Hampton Frost, Pioneer Epidemiologist 1880–1938: Up to the Mountain* (Rochester, NY: University of Rochester Press, 2004); and "Dr. W. H. Frost Dies at Johns Hopkins," *Columbia Record* (Columbia, SC), May 2, 1938, 11.

30 Dr. Frost had had direct experience with a cerebrospinal meningitis epidemic in Georgia earlier in his career. Thomas M. Daniel, *Wade Hampton Frost; Pioneer Epidemiologist, 1880–1938; Up to the Mountain* (Rochester, NY: University of Rochester, 2004), 69–70.

31 Wade Hampton Frost, "Epidemic Cerebrospinal Meningitis; A Review of Its Etiology, Transmission, and Specific Therapy, with Reference to Public Measures for Its Control," *Public Health Reports* 27 no. 4 (January 26, 1912): 97–112.

32 Wade Hampton Frost, "Anti-meningitis Vaccination," *Public Health Reports* 28, no. 6 (February 7, 1913): 252–54.

33 Thomas McNeal (1849–1913) was born in Washington County, Texas, as the only child of William Wallace McNeal (1821–1870), a merchant, and Elizabeth Walker Berry (1824–1898). He grew up in Lockhart, Caldwell County, Texas. In 1872, he attended the University of Mississippi. He returned to live in Lockhart, where he owned a large cotton-growing farm and practiced law for decades. He served in both the Thirty-Second and the Thirty-Third Texas State Legislatures. He married Mary Virginia Field (1851–1926) in 1878; they had five children. See "Thomas McNeal," *Legislative Reference Library of Texas*, accessed December 3, 2017, http://www.lrl.state.tx.us/legeLeaders/members/memberdisplay.cfm?memberID=2861; and *Historical and Current Catalogue of the Officers and Students of the University of Mississippi* (Oxford, MS: University of Mississippi, 1887), 53.

34 See "Legislator Stricken; M'Neal of Caldwell County Is Down with Meningitis; Took Active Part in the Deliberations up to Noon Tuesday—Many Members Leave," *Waco Morning News*, February 13, 1913, 1.

35 Dr. Ernest Krueger (1868–1946) was born in Germany as a son of Henry Krueger. He immigrated to the United States in 1882; became naturalized in 1892 in Cleveland, Ohio; worked in Kansas City, Missouri; married Annie Bornefeld (1873–1957) of Texas in 1894; and practiced general medicine in Austin from the early 1900s to his death in 1946. He and Annie had two children.

36 Albert Leroy "Lee" Killingsworth (1859–1913) was born in East Side Cahaba River, Bibb County, Alabama, as one of the twelve children of John Albert Killingsworth (1826–1906), a farmer, and Mary Margaret Rebecca Garner (1833–1881). The family moved to Harrison County, Texas, around 1869. Lee Killingsworth married Sarah Valula Reed (1867–1917) in Gregg County, Texas, and became a large landowner and farmer in the western section of Harrison County, on the line between Gregg and Harrison Counties. He took an interest in public matters to secure good service for his constituents. He was a county commissioner from his district before entering the race to represent the district composed of Harrison and Gregg Counties in the Texas State Legislature. He and Sarah had five children. See "Lee Killingsworth," *Legislative Reference Library of Texas*, accessed December 3, 2017, http://www.lrl.state.

tx.us/legeLeaders/members/memberdisplay.cfm?memberID=2856; and "Lee Killingsworth Died Suddenly; Flotorial Representative from This District Was Attacked by Meningitis at Austin," *Marshall Messenger*, February 14, 1913, 1.

37 Clifford Lemuel Stone (1881–1940) was born in Rusk County, Texas, as one of the eight children of William Dodson Stone (1855–1899) and Martha Jane Noble (1856–1941). He served as the Rusk County sheriff at the age of twenty-one years, the Texas state representative from Rusk County for two terms, and assistant attorney general during the Governor Daniel James Moody administration (1927–1931). He practiced law in Henderson, Rusk County, Texas. He married Nanette (Nannette) I. Wallace (1893–1990) in 1916; they had two children. He died of acute nephritis at the age of fifty-eight years. See "Clifford L. Stone, Prominent Texas Attorney, Is Dead," *Times* (Shreveport, LA), June 8, 1940, 2.

38 "Legislator Dies of Meningitis; Representative Lee Killingsworth Is Taken Off by the Disease; Is Ill But a Few Hours; Roommate Has Him Excused from Attendance and Returns to Find Him Dying," *Waco Morning News*, February 14, 1913, 1; and "Lee Killingsworth Died Suddenly; Flotorial Representative from This District Was Attacked by Meningitis at Austin," *Marshall Messenger,* February 14, 1913, 1.

39 "Meningitis Invades State Legislature; Representative Killingworth Dead, and Hon. T. J. McNeal Seriously Ill," *Bryan Daily Eagle*, February 14, 1913, 2.

40 "Legislator Dies of Meningitis; Representative Lee Killingsworth Is Taken Off by the Disease; Is Ill But a Few Hours; Roommate Has Him Excused from Attendance and Returns to Find Him Dying," *Waco Morning News*, February 14, 1913, 1; "No title," *Houston Post*, February 16, 1913, 52; "Call to Be Issued; Members of House Will Be Asked to Return by Monday," *Houston Post*, February 19, 1913, 9; Tom Finty Jr., "For Closed Season on 'Magnificent'; Term Not Appropriate as Applied to Texas Capitol; Cleaning Up Promised; In Meantime House May Hire Hall or Buy a Tent for Sessions," *Dallas Morning News*, February 19, 1913, 2.

41 "Hon. Thomas McNeal Dies; The Sudden Death of Two Members of the Body Has Telling Effect on Others," *Bryan Daily Eagle*, February 14, 1913.

42 "Dies of Meningitis; Representative T. S. M'Neal Second House Member to Succumb; Many Have Left Austin, and the Capitol

Is Being Fumigated—No Session Held," *Waco Morning News*, February 15, 1913, 3.

43 "House Member Dies Suddenly at Austin; Hon. Lee Killingsworth Succumbs to Attack of Meningitis; Funeral at Longview; House Adjourns as Mark of Respect and Names Committee to Accompany Body to His Home," *Dallas Morning News*, February 14, 1913, 3.

44 "Hon. Thomas M'Neal, House Member, Dies; Was Native Texan, 63 Years Old and Long Member of Caldwell County Bar; Funeral at Lockhart; Special Committee of Fellow-Representatives Named by Speaker as Escort for Body," *Dallas Morning News*, February 15, 1913, 9; and "Lawmakers Near Demoralization; Legislature May Adjourn for Sixty Days; Meningitis Spreads; Another Death from This Dread Malady and Illness," *Amarillo Daily News*, February 15, 1913, 2.

45 George Herder Sr. (1863–1934) was born at High Hill, near Schulenburg, Fayette County, Texas, as one of the eleven children of George Heinrich Herder (1818–1887), a farmer, and Wilhelmina "Minna" Wolters (1824–1878). George Heinrich Herder and Wilhelmina Wolters were natives of Germany. George Herder Sr. was a merchant who held many public offices, including alderman and mayor of Weimer, chief of the Weimer Fire Department, and Texas state representative. He married Mary Hefner (1864–1942) in 1885; they had three children. See "George Herder Sr., Passes Away, Funeral Saturday," *Weimar Mercury*, April 6, 1934, 20.

46 The Texas state vital statistics registrar received ninety-three reports of meningitis deaths for the month of February 1913. "Report of Vital Statistics; Registrar Gives Out the Figures for January," February 27, 1913, 8; "Pneumonia Leads in Deaths," *Dallas Morning News*, February 28, 1913, 5; and "Pneumonia's Death Toll Heavy in Texas," *El Paso Herald-Post*, March 1, 1913, 17.

47 H. E. Ellis, "Texas Solons Leave Austin, Legislators Excused on Account of Meningitis; House Members to Return March 3, and Senators February 24—Representative J. C. Hunt Is Critically Ill," *Houston Post*, February 16, 1913, 6.

48 "Meningitis Fatal in Legislature, Two Members Succumb to Disease in Twenty-Four Hours; Members Very Uneasy; Adjournment Talked of—Representatives McNeal and Killingsworth Are Victims," *Wichita Daily Times* (Wichita Falls, TX), February 14, 1913, 1.

49 "Legislator Dies of Meningitis; Representative Lee Killingsworth Is Taken Off by the Disease; Is Ill But a Few Hours; Roommate Has

Him Excused from Attendance and Returns to Find Him Dying," *Waco Morning News*, February 14, 1913, 1.

50 Joseph Clark Hunt (1857–1913) was born in Marshall County, Kentucky, as one of the eight children of Owen E. Hunt (1812–1868), a farmer, and Angeline Jane Turner (1820–1884). In 1880, Joseph C. Hunt moved to Paris, Lamar County, Texas, where he earned admission to the bar in 1893 at the age of thirty-six years. In 1894, he began serving the first of two terms as the elected county judge of Lamar County. In 1900, he moved to Randall County, where he practiced law in both state and federal courts. He was elected to the Texas State Legislature in 1910 and again in 1912. He was a candidate for House speaker of the Thirty-Third Legislature (he lost to Representative Terrell) and was always a prominent man on the floor of the House. He married Corinne Bomparte (1879–1936); they had two children. See "Representative Hunt Dies of Meningitis; Body Will Be Buried at His Old Home, Paris, Probably Monday," *Dallas Morning News*, March 23, 1913, 1; "Judge Hunt Active in Politics," *Dallas Morning News*, March 23, 1913, 1; and "Speaker Appoints Committee," *Dallas Morning News*, March 23, 1913, 2.

51 "Lawmakers near Demoralization; Legislature May Adjourn for Sixty Days; Meningitis Spreads; Another Death from This Dread Malady and Illness," *Amarillo Daily News*, February 15, 1913, 2.

52 "Funeral at Lockhart; Special Committee of Fellow-Representatives Named by Speaker as Escort for Body," *Dallas Morning News*, February 15, 1913, 9

53 Dr. William Benjamin Goodner (1857–1950) was born in Polk, Montgomery County, Arkansas, as one of the eleven children of James Monroe Goodner (1833–1893), a farmer, and Elizabeth Jane Logan (1835–1877). He grew up on his father's farm and received his formal education in Bellefonte, Arkansas. He worked as a tanner. At the age of sixteen years, he married his fourteen-year-old cousin, Lucy Ann Goodner (1859–1954). At the age of twenty-one years, he began to study medicine (1883). It is unknown where he earned his medical degree. He opened a medical practice at Mount Ida, Montgomery County, Arkansas, for two years and then moved to Black Springs, Montgomery County, Arkansas. He moved to Dublin, Erath County, Texas, with his family at an unknown time. He served as Dublin's mayor in 1907 before serving in the Texas State Legislature. He and Lucy had one child. He died of a cerebral hemorrhage at the age of ninety-two years. See "W. B. Goodner," in *Biographical and*

Historical Memoirs of Western Arkansas (Chicago, IL: Southern Publishing Company, 1891), 481; and "Ex-Dublin Mayor Dies," *Denton Record-Chronicle* (Denton, TX), February 28, 1950, 8.

54 "Scattered Are the Legislators; Third Case of Meningitis Has Frightened Them from Capital; No Session until March 3; Speaker Excuses All Members of the House and Lieutenant Governor Agrees to Plan—Hunt Is Ill," *Waco Morning News*, February 16, 1913, 6.

55 John Jeptha Stephens (1865–1947) was born in Heard County, Georgia, as one of the ten children of Isaac Newton Davis Stephens (1841–1924), a farmer, and Teresa Faver (1845–1928). He moved with his family from Georgia to Upshur County, Texas, when he was two years old. He graduated from Sam Houston Normal School in Huntsville, Walker County, Texas, in 1887; taught school in Upshur and neighboring counties for many years; and served as publisher and editor of the weekly *Upshur County Echo* in Gilmer, Upshur County, Texas, 1899–1925. He served two terms in the Texas House of Representatives, 1913–1916. After selling his newspaper, he served as justice of the peace in Precinct 1 for a number of years. He married Levici Della Wheeler (1871–1953) in 1891; they had two children. He died at the age of eighty-two years. See "J. J. Stephens Published Upshur County 'Echo,'" *Gilmer Mirror* (Gilmer, TX), August 15, 1968 [*sic*], 24; and "Gilmer Justice Ties 104 Couples; J. J. Stephens of Gilmer Performs Record Number of Marriage Ceremonies," *Longview News-Journal* (Longview, TX), January 2, 1942, 4.

56 "Providing for Memorial Services," and "Tributes to Deceased Members," *Journal of the House of Representatives of the Regular Session of the Thirty-Third Legislature of Texas, Convened at the City of Austin, January 14, 1913, and Adjourned without Day, April 1, 1913* (Austin, TX: Von Boeckmann-Jones, 1913), 1,469–85. (Representative Stephens's quote is on page 1,483.)

57 "Legislators Desert Austin; Spread of Meningitis the Cause of Sudden Leave Taking; Review of Work Done; Body Has Transacted Much Important Business during Time It Has Been in Session," *Amarillo Daily News*, February 16, 1913, 2; "House Adjourned to March 3 or Longer if Conditions Do Not Improve," *Bryan Daily Eagle*, February 15, 1913, 2; and "Legislators Anxious to Resume Work; Both Houses Are Expected to Get to Work Week from Today," *Dallas Morning News*, February 17, 1913, 1.

58 "Another Has Meningitis; Representative George Herder Reported Very Ill at His Home in Weimar," *Dallas Morning News*, February 18, 1913, 12.

59 The physician who notified Speaker Terrell about Representative Herder's meningitis was Dr. Charles "Dr. Charlie" Gilliam Cook (1875–1946), who was born in Sedan, Fayette County, Texas, as one of the two children of Dr. Thomas Chappelle Cook (1836–1906) and Judith Frances "Fannie" Gilliam (1839–1884). Charles Cook earned his medical degree from Tulane University Medical Department in 1895; took postgraduate work in New York; served in the Spanish-American War as an infantry lieutenant; and returned to Weimar, Texas, to open a medical practice. He married Berry Hall in 1902; they had no children. He died of a stroke at the age of seventy-one years. See "Final Rites for Dr. Chas. G. Cook, 71, Here Today," *Weimar Mercury* (Weimar, TX), November 8, 1946, 1.

60 "Another Solon Has Meningitis, Speaker Terrell Decides Not to Reassemble the Texas Legislature," *El Paso Herald-Post*, February 18, 1913, 6; and "Colquitt to Call National Guard; Governor Is Determined to Protect Texas Border," *Amarillo Daily News*, February 18, 1913, 2.

61 David C. Kelley (1856–1913) was born in Opelika, Lee County, Alabama, as the son of D. Kelley and Mary Campbell. In 1872, he moved to Dallas County, Texas. After living there for five or six years, he moved to Kaufman County, where he devoted his attention almost exclusively to farming for the rest of his life. He served as president of the County Farmers' Union and president of the Kaufman Clearing House, a mercantile concern. He was elected to the Texas State Legislature in November of 1912. He married Sarah Elizabeth Clark (1857–1942) in 1876; they had six children. See "Hon. D. C. Kelley Dies at Kaufman; Is Victim of Meningitis after Illness of Less Than Week; Funeral at 3 P.M. Today; Was Elected Member of Lower House of Texas Legislature Last November," *Dallas Morning News*, February 23, 1913.

62 "Fifth Legislator Reported Stricken Lives near Kaufman," *Fort Worth Star-Telegram*, February 19, 1913, 7.

63 "Heavy Strain on Physicians," *Dallas Morning News*, February 19, 1913, 13.

64 "Hon. D. C. Kelley Dies at Kaufman; Is Victim of Meningitis after Illness of Less Than Week; Funeral at 3 P.M. Today; Was Elected Member of Lower House of Texas Legislature Last November,"

Dallas Morning News, February 23, 1913; and "Kelley Funeral at Kaufman; Representatives Savage and Lewelling Deliver Addresses at Grave," *Dallas Morning News*, February 24, 1913, 16.

65 "Legislature Faces Jammed Calendars; Night Sessions May Be Held; Two Consolidation Bills to Come Up; Inspection Agreed Upon; Physicians to Examine All Members of House; Third Legislator Dies," *Fort Worth Star-Telegram*, February 23, 1913, 1.

66 "Quorum Is Expected in Each House Today; Health Officer Has Found No Trace of Meningitis in Members Examined," *Dallas Morning News*, February 24, 1913, 1.

CHAPTER 9

THE TEXAS MENINGITIS EPIDEMIC DISSIPATES, FEBRUARY-JULY 1913

On Saturday, February 22, 1913, the same day that Representative David C. Kelley died in Austin of cerebrospinal meningitis, the *Dallas Morning News* published a long editorial[1] detailing the cerebrospinal meningitis crisis in the Texas State Capitol building. The editors expressed their concern for the safety of the Texas legislators, especially because Speaker Terrell expected all representatives to report to the House Hall in the capitol building two days hence (Monday, February 24, 1913). The editors of the *Dallas Morning News* argued,

> We have no doubt it will be proposed to continue the sessions in the present Hall of Representatives; but this ought not be done save by unanimous consent, and the test should be by ballot in order that every member may unabashed express his real feeling and judgment. To go into the presence of contagious or infectious diseases for the purpose of alleviating human suffering requires bravery; but to needlessly go into and stay in an infected room is not an evidence of bravery, but, instead, of foolhardiness or cowardice—the lack of nerve to say "no" for

fear that cowardice may be charged. Such being the case, it would be wrong to force the resumption of sessions in the Hall of Representatives "by the will of the majority."[1]

The editors continued,

It is true that there has been some superficial cleansing of the Hall of Representatives, and indirect announcements made that State Health Officer Steiner considers the situation safe. But, with all due respect to that official, we recall the fact that doctors differ. We do not consider the House wing of the Capitol safe, and we say this with a fairly accurate knowledge of its condition and the remedies which have been applied ... Disinfection and the closing of hot and cold air registers in the floors amount to little. Such closing may exclude some of the foul air, but the problem of proper ventilation and heating will remain.[1]

The editors added,

Sessions in the Hall of Representatives ought to be completely abandoned until the place can be thoroughly overhauled. As a part of such overhauling, we beg to suggest the removal of the laboratories of the Health Department and the Pure Food Department from the Capitol. There may be no actual danger in the handling of germs and tainted foods in the building, but the psychic effect is bad, and there is positive danger in the chemicals and explosives employed.[1]

The editors concluded,

> Not only are the members of the Legislature, as well as laborers, entitled to the protection of their health, but it is essential to proper legislation that they be kept sound in body and easy in mind. These requirements we feel sure cannot be met in the House of Representatives. It may now be free from meningitis infection, but it is insanitary; this is sufficient to condemn it. If the Hall of Representatives were private property, human occupancy of it would be prohibited; the fact that it is state property ought not immunize it from sanitary regulations.[1]

Speaker Terrell was under great pressure to convene the House on Monday, February 24, 1913, because of the jammed House calendar.[2] On Monday, February 24, 1913, a sufficient number of legislators showed up in the Texas State Capitol building to achieve a quorum in both houses of the Texas State Legislature, thus paving the way to conduct pressing business for the first time in ten days.[2] However, immediately after the sessions began, members of both the House and the Senate introduced resolutions to adjourn the legislature until Thursday, May 1, 1913, because of the cerebrospinal meningitis situation.

In the House, representatives spoke fervently for and against the resolution to adjourn. Representative John Cunningham,[3] an elderly, wheelchair-bound physician from Fannin County, argued against adjournment, noting that the forty members who had shown up each day in the Texas State Capitol building during the ten-day suspension had not contracted the disease, the Great Hall had been fumigated time and again, and there was no more danger in Austin than in any other place in Texas.[1]

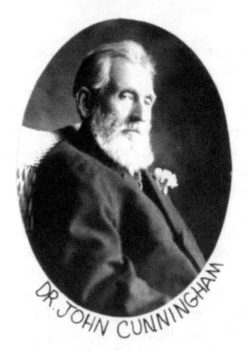

Dr. John F. Cunningham (1836–1924), circa 1913. Detail from
the Thirty-third House Composite (CHA #1989.527). Courtesy
of the Texas State Preservation Board, Austin, Texas.

Representative Almoth Dowden Rogers,[4] an insurance agent
with nine children, favored adjournment, announcing that

> he had obtained advice from the Texas state attorney
> general as to the legality of the proposed proceeding,
> commented upon the high mortality rate among the
> members from meningitis, referred to the fact that
> Representative Hunt's condition had become worse,
> argued that the members would feel remorseful
> if they insisted upon remaining and other deaths
> should occur, and declared that if adjournment were
> taken everybody would come back in better frame
> of mind to properly legislate.[2]

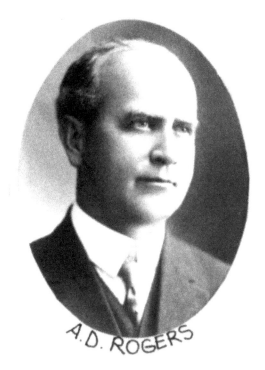

Almoth Dowden Rogers (1866–1931), circa 1913. Detail from
the Thirty-Third House Composite (CHA #1989.527). Courtesy
of the Texas State Preservation Board, Austin, Texas.

Representative Louis J. Wortham,[5] the editor of the *Fort
Worth Star-Telegram* in Tarrant County, supported Representative
Rogers, saying that he was "unwilling to enforce the attendance
of men in a place which they regarded as the focus of disease."[2]
Representative Wortham expressed his friendship and admiration
for State Health Officer Steiner but remarked, "The nature of
meningitis was such that doctors disagreed over many things
concerning it. Moreover, he denied that Dr. Steiner had advised
anybody that the conditions in the House of Representatives were
free from danger and declared that he would not have the nerve to
ask that official if they were." Representative Wortham cited a high
authority on sanitation who said that "the House wing ought not
be used again until the heating, ventilation, and plumbing systems
underwent remodeling."[2]

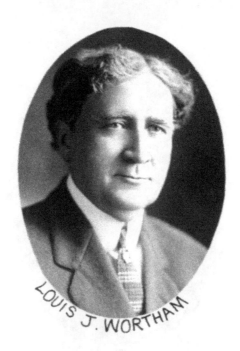

Louis J. Wortham (1858–1927), circa 1913. Detail from the
Thirty-Third House Composite (CHA #1989.527). Courtesy
of the Texas State Preservation Board, Austin, Texas.

Representative Rogers' resolution to adjourn was voted down in
the House on Monday, February 24, 1913. The legislators dutifully
returned to the Great Hall the next morning, only to find that
both the House and Senate chambers "were chilly because much
of the heat was choked off by the closing of the floor radiators to
trap the suspect vapors." Many of the legislators "worked in their
overcoats and got cold feet." There was plenty of ventilation, "as
the windows were kept down from the top."[2]

During Tuesday, February 25, 1913, the representatives
adopted a resolution to pay all the medical expenses incurred
by Representatives McNeal, Killingsworth, Kelley, Hunt, and
Herder and any other members who should become ill, and
the funeral expenses of Representatives McNeal, Kelley, and
Killingsworth.[6] The House then adopted a second resolution
providing for the appointment by Speaker Terrell of a committee

of five representatives to join a like committee of five senators to investigate the sanitary condition of the House and the Senate and report on the advisability of an adjournment.[6] Of note, none of the senators, who met in the east wing of the Texas State Capitol building, had contracted cerebrospinal meningitis.

The joint committee of the Texas State House of Representatives and the Texas State Senate turned to State Health Officer Steiner and six physicians of his choosing to provide information in a written report that addressed three points: (1) the situation confronting the Texas Legislature by the presence of cerebrospinal meningitis in Austin, (2) the effect of the sanitary conditions of the Capitol Building upon this situation, and (3) advice as to how legislators could best avoid contracting meningitis.[8] Dr. Steiner quickly recruited six Austin physician colleagues for his physician committee. Three of them—Dr. Robert McNutt Wickline,[9] Dr. Franklin Pierce McLaughlin,[10] and Dr. James Wharton McLaughlin Jr.[11]—rented medical offices in the same building (Scarborough Building at 101 West Sixth Street, Austin) as did Dr. Steiner. Dr. Wickline was also the Austin city health officer (beginning in 1911). The three other physicians were Dr. Steiner's colleagues Dr. Goodall Harrison Wooten,[12] Dr. Joseph Sil Wooten,[13] and Dr. Boerner.

The members of the Texas State Legislative Joint Committee interviewed the members of the physician committee about the meningitis situation that same afternoon of Tuesday, February 25, 1913. A *Houston Post* reporter witnessed and wrote about the discussion. The physicians stated many things, wrote the reporter, including,

> It would be safer for the members if the Legislature met in April or June [1913] rather than in February [1913], since meningitis is a cold weather disease. They thought there might be less danger to the legislators if the body now adjourned and they all went to their homes, though they pointed out that this procedure might result in the spread of the

> disease to the members' families and others [on] the trains and in the cities of Texas to which the members would return, and where the disease is more prevalent than in Austin.[14]

The reporter further noted that Dr. Steiner believed that the representatives who were susceptible had already contracted the disease and that he predicted no further cases if the legislature remained at work. The physicians admitted that they did not know many things about cerebrospinal meningitis. For example, they did not know "but that a person who is not susceptible this week might become so next week." They agreed that cerebrospinal meningitis was not related to bad sanitation, since more cases were found in the homes of the well-to-do than in the hovels of the poor. The disease also was not "in the air" but was communicated by personal contact of sick persons or "carriers" who had been near the sick. Relatively few persons were susceptible to the disease. Vaccination with the meningococcal vaccine was prudent because the vaccine conferred immunity.[14]

On the question of whether the legislature should adjourn, six of the seven physicians were evasive or noncommittal, believing that danger existed if the legislators remained in the Texas State Capitol building or if they went home. Only Dr. Wooten declared that if he were a legislator, he would remain in Austin, noting, "If there is anything at all in the quarantine theory it would certainly be the part of sense to keep the members of the House where they are," though "it would probably take a regiment of the National Guard to do this." The physicians agreed the disease was no more prevalent in Austin than across the state generally.[14] (In reality, Dr. Steiner's office later reported the following cerebrospinal meningitis data for the month of February 1913: four new cases in Dallas, one new case in Lamesa [Dawson County], one new case in Somervell County, and twelve new cases in Austin.[15])

The physician committee presented to the chairman of the joint committee a report that said,

Dear sir: We, the undersigned physicians, appointed by your joint committee under this resolution; Moved, that this joint committee requested the State Health Officer, Dr. Ralph Steiner, and the other physicians who have been before the committee this afternoon to give us their opinion upon the situation confronting the Legislature by the prevalence of meningitis in Austin, advising us fully as to the effect of sanitary conditions of the Capital, and advising us as to what is best to be done to avoid the danger to members of contracting meningitis, beg leave to report as follows. [16]

The report continued,

We are of the opinion that the meningitis situation at Austin is without cause for undue alarm. There have been 41 cases in Austin during the past two years, and at no time has the disease assumed epidemic proportions. There were 21 cases in January and February of 1913, with four deaths, two of which were among the legislators. Five members acquired the disease. The apparent *pro rata* increase occurring in the House is to be accounted for, in our opinion, by the fact that the members came from all parts of the State and represent the entire population of Texas, thereby increasing the probability of "carriers." [16]

The report added,

We are of the opinion that the sanitary condition of the House had no bearing on the production of this particular disease, but that it was due to a "carrier" or "carriers" among the legislators, employees, or visitors. We believe that the members of the

Legislature are in no more danger from assembling in the Capitol, than they would be in assembling in any other building in Austin or city in Texas. While we confessedly admit epidemic meningitis to be a cold weather disease and the members obviously in more danger now than during the summer months, we are of the opinion that if the members of the Legislature are properly vaccinated with antimeningitis vaccine, thereby diminishing individual susceptibility and limiting "carriers," there would be no necessity of adjourning on the ground of health conditions.

The seven physicians signed their names: Ralph Steiner, chairman; R. M. Wickline; E. P. [*sic*] McLaughlin (his correct initials are F. P.); J. M. [*sic*] McLaughlin (his correct initials are J. W.); G. H. Wooten; J. S. Wooten; and Morris Boerner.[82] On motion made by a representative, the report was adopted.[17]

Representative Harry Phillip Jordan Sr,[18] the son of the well-known Texas physician Dr. Powhatan Jordan,[19] disagreed with the viewpoints expressed by the seven physicians. Representative Jordan attributed the cause of the cerebrospinal meningitis epidemic in the west wing of the Texas State Capitol building to the Texas State Board of Health biologics laboratory located there.

Representative Jordan's opposing resolution said,

Whereas, It appears that besides the insanitary conditions of this [west] wing of the Capitol, it is believed that the epidemic probably arose from local conditions, and it is believed that the proximity of the Board of Health's experimental station and Pure Food Commission's chemical laboratories situated adjacent to and opening into the Hall of Representatives, from which no doubt these fatal disease germs make their exodus in countless herds, and incubated, nurtured and developed by the fearful insanitary condition of the heating plant, the atmosphere is rendered absolutely poisonous to mankind, and to further remain in the Hall and committee rooms under such circumstances and conditions would be a reckless disregard of life and health.[20]

The resolution continued,

> Therefore, be it resolved, that hereafter no fire be built in this heating plant; that the radiators be securely covered, but before doing so thoroughly cleansed and disinfected; that the Board of Health remove its laboratories or experimental station from the Capitol building and to thoroughly disinfect and cleanse the room or rooms vacated by them after removal; that all the windows of this Hall, corridors and committee rooms be opened and be kept partially open at all times; that when the weather is too cold and inclement to transact business in this manner that the House stand recessed until the weather shall permit a resumption of duties; and that we conclude this session at the earliest possible date.

The resolution was read a second time.[20]

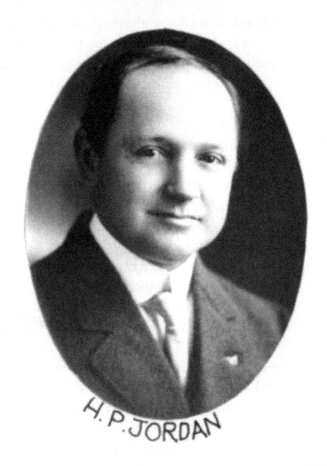

Harry Phillip Jordan, Sr. (1875–1965), circa 1913. Detail from the Thirty-Third House Composite (CHA #1989.527). Courtesy of the Texas State Preservation Board, Austin, Texas.

The question was asked, "Shall the resolution be adopted?" On the motion of Speaker Terrell, the resolution was tabled.[20] Thus, on February 25, 1913, the House members voted to continue to work in the capitol building despite the cerebrospinal meningitis outbreak.

A month passed without further cases of cerebrospinal meningitis emerging among those working in the Texas State Capitol building. On Saturday, March 22, 1913, after fighting for his life for five weeks, Representative Hunt, still living in his

Austin boardinghouse room, surrendered to his disease.[21] He joined Representatives McNeal, Killingsworth, and Kelley as victims of cerebrospinal meningitis. On Sunday, March 23, 1913, the Texas House of Representatives held a session of sorrow in memory of Representatives McNeal, Killingsworth, Kelley, and Hunt. Speaker Terrell and twelve state representatives paid tribute in moving orations.[22]

The state of Texas had only sixteen new meningitis cases for the month of March 1913; Travis County reported only one case for that month.[23] In addition, Representative Herder, the fifth Texas state representative sick with cerebrospinal meningitis, was steadily improving at his home in Weimar, Texas. Three physicians had been attending him for two months. On Sunday, March 30, 1913, Dr. Franklin Pierce McLaughlin presented a medical bill on behalf of the three Weimar physicians for the amount of $3,434.44 (about $100 per patient visit). The House members gasped and postponed action until Dr. Steiner and Dr. McLaughlin could intervene to lower the charge.[24]

On Tuesday, April 1, 1913, the regular session of the Thirty-Third Texas State Legislature concluded, with the expectation of meeting again that year for further sessions.[25] Four days later (Saturday, April 5, 1913), Dr. Hartman was well enough to return to work as state bacteriologist. He accepted Dr. Steiner's conferral of a promotion to assistant state health officer.[26] Dr. Hartman had been absent from work for six and a half weeks (February 19, 1913, to April 5, 1913).

The Texas meningitis epidemic of 1911 to 1913 ended with the onset of hot weather in 1913. On Wednesday, May 7, 1913, Dr. Hartman described his meningococcal vaccine experience before his peers at the Texas State Medical Society in San Antonio.[27] In February 1913, he vaccinated around 3,500 individuals—about 3,000 in Austin (including 1,000 university students); 400 in Manor; and 100 physicians, nurses, and family members tending to someone with the disease. He noted, "Following the rapid invasion of the ranks of the Legislature there were no further cases of meningitis among the members of that body after a large majority of their number had received the second injection." In no case did he observe a serious reaction after injecting an individual with the meningococcal vaccine, adding, "What was observed in the way of a reaction was very similar to that occurring in the use of typhoid vaccine."[27]

Dr. Hartman performed blood tests on volunteers, including Dr. Steiner and others, during his clinical trial of the meningococcal vaccine. He found that these individuals developed "a rather high degree of immunity in nearly every case 12 days after the last injection of the treatment and that three months later a slightly smaller per cent still showed evidence of a high degree of immunity."[27] Although these test results were promising, Dr. Hartman acknowledged the need for further clinical and laboratory evidence of the efficacy of the vaccine before it could be classed, like the smallpox vaccination, as "highly salutary to the human race." In the meantime, he avowed that the efficacy of the meningococcal vaccine had been "established to such an extent and its harmlessness so clearly shown that it would not be wrong for us, as members of the medical profession, to contradict the great amount of misinformation that has been spread among the people and has aroused considerable opposition to vaccination." He concluded,

> We are mindful of the fact that the great majority of the body politic is willing to be guided by scientific medical opinion in matters medical, and that we owe it to the people to wait until it would be difficult to more strongly and conclusively prove any fact of medicine before recommending its use too highly. We feel that in the use of antimeningitis vaccine we are allowed to favor the argument "let those who will protect themselves."[27]

On July 26, 1913, Representative Herder, who had survived his meningitis in Weimar, Texas, refused to permit the state to pay his meningitis medical bill, which the state legislature had trimmed from $3,434.44 to $640. When the state treasury department sent a warrant for the amount, Mr. Herder sent it back.[28]

On Monday, September 8, 1913, Dr. Hartman resigned his position as assistant state health officer and state bacteriologist to chair the pathology department at his alma mater, the University of Texas Medical Branch at Galveston.[29] In January 1914, Dr. Steiner resigned as the state health officer and returned to his otolaryngology practice in the Scarborough Building in Austin. In his final annual report, he reviewed his accomplishments: the enactment of the Texas Sanitary Code; an increase in reports of births and deaths in the state of Texas; the erection of a sanatorium for the care and treatment of consumptives; and the "distribution of diphtheria antitoxin, antimeningitis serum and vaccine at less than one-third of their normal cost, a plan resulting in the saving of thousands of dollars to the poor and near-poor of the State." He considered his greatest achievement as the establishment and operation of a bacteriological laboratory.[30]

CHAPTER 9 NOTES

1   "Welfare of Legislators Due Consideration," *Dallas Morning News*, February 22, 1913, 14.

2   Tom Finty Jr., "House with Quorum Refuses to Adjourn; Resolution to Suspend Activity until May 1 Is Voted Down; Mexican Question Up; Senate Adopts Long Resolution, but Other Matters Prevent Definite Action in House," *Dallas Morning News*, February 25, 1913, 3.

3   Dr. John F. Cunningham (1836–1924) was born in Trigg County, Kentucky, as one of the ten children of John Cunningham (1796–1854), a farmer, and Mary Gresham (1803–1875). He attended Bethel College in Russellville, Logan County, Kentucky, and attended medical college in St. Louis, Missouri, before completing his medical education at the Galveston Medical College in 1873. After the American Civil War, he moved to Texas as "a tramp without money or friends, and settled in Fannin County, near Ravenna," where he practiced medicine and became the owner and manager of several large farms and a partner in a mercantile house. He served in the Texas State House 1873–1874, 1901–1905, and 1913–1917. He married Ann Olivia Patterson (1841–1860) in 1859; they had one child. He married Fannie Agnew (1845–1930) in 1869; they had five children. See "Dr. John Cunningham," *Biographic Souvenir of the State of Texas* (Chicago, IL: F. A. Battey and Company, 1889), 224.

4   Almoth Dowden Rogers (1866–1931) was born in Pontotoc, Pontotoc County, Mississippi, as one of the three children of Reverend John D. Rogers (1825–1866) and his second wife, Jennie C. Allen (1837–1872). He worked as a clerk in Kentucky; a traveling salesman; and an insurance agent in San Antonio, Texas, in 1894. He settled in Decatur, Wise County, Texas, where he had interests in life insurance, real estate, and cattle and livestock businesses. In 1898, he won election as the Wise County treasurer. From 1910 to 1915, he served as the Wise County representative to the Texas State House. He ran unsuccessfully as the Democratic candidate for the US Congress from the Fourteenth District. He married Lila Stone (1870–1962) in 1889; they had nine children. In 1924, he died of a stroke at the age of sixty-five years. "Former Legislator, A. D. Rogers, Is Dead," *Dallas Morning News*, December 16, 1931, 2; and "Almoth Dowden Rogers (1866–1931)," *The Strangest Names in American Political*

History, accessed January 22, 2018, http://politicalstrangenames. blogspot.com/2015/11/almoth-dowden-rogers-1866-1931.html.

5   Louis J. Wortham (1858–1927) was born in Sulphur Springs, Hopkins County, Texas, as one of the six children of William Amos Wortham (1830–1910), the editor and publisher of the *Sulphur Springs Gazette*, and Elizabeth Adeline Ashcroft (1834–1905). Representative Wortham was editor of the *Fort Worth Star-Telegram* for many years, retiring in 1923. He represented Tarrant County in the Texas House of Representatives for four years. He wrote the five-volume *History of Texas from Wilderness to Commonwealth*, published in 1924. He married Faye Fruzanna "Fru" Becton (1858–1922) in 1880; they had two children. "Wortham, Louis J.," *Handbook of Texas Online*, accessed December 4, 2017, https://tshaonline. org/handbook/online/articles/fwo29; and "Louis J. Wortham Died in Greenville, Buried Fort Worth; Veteran Texas Editor, Writer, Statesman, and Historian Passes," *Corsicana Daily Sun*, September 12, 1927, 4.

6   "Verified Pleadings Bill Is Engrossed; Same Action Taken on Deficiency and Election Bills in House; Will Pay Doctor Bills; Expenses of Illness of Members Ordered Paid out of Contingent Fund," *Dallas Morning News*, February 25, 1913, 13.

7   "Texas Solons May Take Recess Again; Discussing Adjournment until April, Owing to Scare regarding Presence of Meningitis," *El Paso Herald-Post*, February 25, 1913, 5.

8   "Physicians Assert No Danger Exists; Consider Austin as Safe for Legislators as Any Other Place in State; Cold Weather Disease; Suggestion Made by Speaker That if Adjournment Is Taken at All It Be until Summer," *Dallas Morning News*, February 26, 1913, 14.

9   Dr. Robert McNutt Wickline (1864–1925) was born in Guadalupe County, Texas, as one of the eight children of Joseph Pernell Wickline (1825–1878), a carpenter, and Jennette Elizabeth McNutt (1829–1901). He married Sarah Virginia "Sallie/Jennie" Fry in San Marcos, Hays County, Texas, in 1890, and earned his medical degree from Memphis Hospital Medical College (in existence from 1876 to 1911) in 1891 at the age of twenty-seven years. He and Jennie had two children in Johnson City, Blanco County, Texas. Around 1900, the family moved to Austin, Travis County, where Dr. Wickline practiced medicine for the rest of his professional career. In 1908, he accepted an appointment as a trustee of the State Blind Institute Board and as the Austin city health officer in 1911. He died at the age of sixty

years. See "Texas," *Journal of the American Medical Association* 56, no. 1 (February 11, 1911): 521; and William Benjamin Hamilton, *Social Survey of Austin* (Austin, TX: University of Texas, 1913), 64–70.

10 Dr. Franklin Pierce McLaughlin (1855–1935) was born in Springfield, Clark County, Ohio, as one of the six children of Cyrus Duncan McLaughlin (1814–1897) and Sarah J. Wharton (1816–1892). His much older brother was Dr. James Wharton McLaughlin Sr. (1840–1909). Dr. Franklin Pierce McLaughlin's medical training is unknown. In 1887, he worked at the Austin City Hospital. He later became affiliated with the Texas School for Defectives and Sanitarium for Mental Nervous Diseases, along with Dr. Ralph Steiner and Drs. Goodall Harrison Wooten and Joseph Sil Wooten. Dr. Franklin Pierce McLaughlin shared a medical office with his older brother, Dr. James Wharton McLaughlin Sr, and with his nephew, Dr. James Wharton McLaughlin Jr., at 700 Congress Street, Austin. Dr. Franklin Pierce McLaughlin lived with his niece, Miss Sarah Evelyn McLaughlin, the daughter of Dr. James Wharton McLaughlin Sr. and the younger sister of Dr. James Wharton McLaughlin Jr. Dr. Franklin Pierce McLaughlin died at the age of eighty years. He was buried with his niece, Sarah Evelyn McLaughlin, who died later the same year (1935). See "The M'Millan Case," *Austin Weekly Statesman*, February 10, 1887, 2; and *Austin, Texas, City Directory 1906* (Austin, TX: J. B. Stephenson, 1907), 322.

11 Dr. James Wharton McLaughlin Jr. (1877–1942) was born in Austin, Travis County, Texas, as one of the seven children of Dr. James W. McLaughlin Sr. (1840–1909) and Tabitha Byrd Moore (1847–1922). He earned his bachelor's degree at the University of Texas in 1898 and his medical degree from Tulane University Medical Department in 1903. He practiced medicine in Austin with his renowned father, Dr. James Wharton McLaughlin Sr, and his uncle, Dr. Franklin Pierce McLaughlin. Dr. James Wharton McLaughlin Sr, a national medical expert in immunity and infection, said a physician is "morally, if not legally" obligated to employ a microscope in the diagnosis of disease; he died in 1909. Dr. James Wharton McLaughlin Jr. married Florence Alberta Askew (1879–1942) in 1907; they had no children. W. J. Maxwell and John A. Loman, *General Register of the Students and Former Students of the University of Texas, 1917* (Austin, TX: University of Texas Ex-Students' Association, 1917), 370; and "What Texan Thought," *Houston Post*, February 10, 1906, 6.

12 Dr. Goodall Harrison Wooten (1869–1942) was born in Paris, Lamar County, Texas, as one of the seven children of Dr. Thomas Dudley Wooten (1829–1906) and Henrietta Goodall (1829–1906). He earned his bachelor's and master's degrees at the University of Texas in 1891 and 1892. He earned his medical degree from the College of Physicians and Surgeons of New York City and returned to Austin to practice medicine with his father. He became affiliated with the Texas School for Defectives and Sanitarium for Mental Nervous Diseases with Drs. Ralph Steiner and Franklin Pierce McLaughlin. He was an entrepreneur, philanthropist, and president of the Austin Chamber of Commerce, 1936–1937. In 1934, he presented to the Boy Scouts of the Central Texas area a camp located on Bull Creek and named it in honor of his son, Tom D. Wooten. He also helped found the Texas Memorial Museum on the University of Texas campus and left his extensive gun collection to the museum. He married Ella Newsome (1878–1972) in 1897; they had three children. See "Dr. G. H. Wooten Dies in Austin," *Dallas Morning News*, January 31, 1942, 4; and "Wooten, Goodall Harrison," *Handbook of Texas Online*, accessed December 5, 2017, https://tshaonline.org/handbook/online/articles/fwo22.

13 Dr. Joseph Sil Wooten (1872–1949) was born in Paris, Lamar County, Texas, as one of the seven children of Dr. Thomas Dudley Wooten (1829–1906) and Henrietta Goodall (1829–1906). He earned his bachelor's degree at the University of Texas in 1892 and his medical degree from the College of Physicians and Surgeons of New York City in 1895. He moved back to Austin to join the medical practice of his brother, Dr. Goodall Harrison Wooten, and their father, Dr. Thomas Dudley Wooten, in Austin. He married Blossom Lydia Greenwood (1875–1946) in 1897; they had two children. See "Joe Sil Wooten," in W. J. Maxwell and John A. Lomax, *General Register of the Students and Former Students of the University of Texas, 1917* (Austin, TX: University of Texas Ex-Students' Association, 1917), 24; and "Wooten, Joe Sil," *Handbook of Texas Online*, accessed December 5, 2017, https://tshaonline.org/handbook/online/articles/fwo23.

14 Lloyd P. Lochridge, "The Doctors Are Evasive; Advise Members of Legislature Remain in Austin; and Would Depend upon Vaccination, but Admit They Do Not Know Much about Meningitis," *Houston Post*, February 26, 1913, 8.

15 "Cerebrospinal Meningitis State Reports," *Public Health Reports* 28, no. 15 (April 11, 1913): 691.

16 The *Dallas Morning News* published a separate report. See "Physicians Assert No Danger Exists; Consider Austin as Safe for Legislators as Any Other Place in State; Cold Weather Disease; Suggestion Made by Speaker That if Adjournment Is Taken at All It Be Until Summer," *Dallas Morning News*, February 26, 1913, 14.

17 "Relative to Adjournment of Legislature," *Journal of the House of Representatives of the Regular Session of the Thirty-Third Legislature of Texas, Convened at the City of Austin, January 14, 1913, and Adjourned without Day, April 1, 1913* (Austin, TX: Von Boeckmann-Jones, 1913), 691–92.

18 Harry Phillip Jordan Sr. (1875–1965) was born in the British Honduras, Central America, as the youngest of the three children of Dr. Powhatan Jordan (1828–1904) and his second wife, Mary Ada Hoskins (1841–1890). Harry Jordan grew up in Beaumont, Jefferson County, Texas; attended Texas public schools; earned his bachelor's degree from the Agricultural and Mechanical College in College Station, Texas; and earned his law degree from the University of Texas at Austin. In 1898, immediately after securing his supreme court license, he moved to Waco; opened a law practice; and received an appointment as assistant county attorney, an office he held for four years. In 1912, he was elected representative from Jefferson County. He was reelected in 1914 for a second term. He practiced law in Waco thereafter. He married Vara Higginson (1880–1976) in 1908; they had three children. He died of a coronary occlusion at the age of ninety years. "Harry P. Jordan Gets into Race for State Senate: Resident of Waco Since 1898; Former Colonel of National Guard; Is Kiwanis Secretary," *Waco News-Tribune*, February 25, 1924, 60; "Jordan, Harry Phillip Sr.," *Waco News-Tribune*, June 8, 1965, 14; and "Jordan, Harry Philip," in *Who's Who on the Pacific Coast*, Franklin Harper, ed. (Los Angeles, CA: Harper Publishing Company, 1913), 309.

19 Dr. Powhatan Jordan (1828–1904) was born in Norfolk, Virginia, as the son of Merit Jordan (1792–1872), a citizen of the Isle of Wight County, Virginia, and Paulina Voynard (born in 1801) of Petersburg, Fauquier, Virginia. Powhatan Jordan earned his bachelor's degree from the Virginia Military Academy (founded in 1839) and studied medicine in 1847–1848 with Drs. R. W. Sylvester and John P. Young in Norfolk County, Virginia. He attended a course of lectures at the

University of Pennsylvania Medical Department (session of 1848–1849) and two courses at Columbia College Medical Department (the precursor of George Washington University Medical School) in Washington, DC (1849–1850), graduating from the latter institution on April 6, 1850. He practiced medicine in Washington City until 1856, when he became an acting assistant surgeon of the United States. He moved to Fort Inge, Uvalde County, Texas, and served as surgeon to the State Rangers with Captain John Salmon Ford (1815–1897). During this service, Dr. Jordan fought the Comanche during three engagements. He resigned in 1857 and moved to San Antonio to become surgeon to the state troops during Cortina's War on the Rio Grande. In 1861, he joined the Confederate States Army and served the last two years as the head of the hospitals. He married Jessie Alberta Edwards of Alabama in 1864. They went to Mexico in 1866, where he declined a position in the Imperial Army. They returned to Texas in 1867; went through the yellow fever epidemic of Indianola, Calhoun County (1867 and 1868); and moved to Guatemala, Central America, where he joined the Guatemala Army (1869–1870). When a revolution broke out in Guatemala, he moved to the British Honduras, where, from 1871 to 1876, he served as surgeon to the Northern District. In 1876, he returned to Texas and settled in Beaumont, Jefferson County, where he practiced medicine and lived for the rest of his life. See "Dr. Powhatan Jordan," in Lewis E. Daniell, *Types of Successful Men of Texas* (Austin, TX: Eugene von Boeckmann, 1890), 484–85.

20 "Relative to Adjournment of Legislature," *Journal of the House of Representatives of the Regular Session of the Thirty-Third Legislature of Texas, Convened at the City of Austin, January 14, 1913, and Adjourned without Day, April 1, 1913* (Austin, TX: Von Boeckmann-Jones, 1913), 692–93.

21 "Representative Hunt Dies of Meningitis; Body Will Be Buried at His Old Home, Paris, Probably Monday," *Dallas Morning News*, March 23, 1913, 1; and "Death Claimed Judge J. C. Hunt; Representative from Randall County Fourth Member of Legislature to Die of Meningitis," *Houston Post*, March 23, 1913, 4.

22 "Memorial Services for Four Legislators; Lower House Hears Tributes to Memory of Meningitis Victims in Session of Sorrow," *Fort Worth Star-Telegram*, March 24, 1913, 7; and "Providing for Memorial Services" and "Tributes to Deceased Members," *Journal of the House of Representatives of the Regular Session*

of the Thirty-Third Legislature of Texas, Convened at the City of Austin, January 14, 1913, and Adjourned without Day, April 1, 1913 (Austin, TX: Von Boeckmann-Jones, 1913), 1,469–85.

23 "State Reports for Cerebrospinal Meningitis, March 1913," *Public Health Reports* 28, no. 19 (May 9, 1913): 894.

24 "Direct Legislation Killed Second Time; Increased Pay Wanted; House Pauses Resolution to Give Legislators Straight Salary of $1,200 for First Year," *Dallas Morning News*, March 30, 1913, 10; and "The Milkin' Was Good," *Bryan Daily Eagle*, April 3, 1913, 3.

25 The Thirty-Third Texas State Legislature would meet for further sessions July 21, 1913–August 19, 1913; August 24, 1914–September 22, 1914; and September 23, 1914–October 22, 1914. See "Overview, 33rd Regular Session, January 14, 1913–April 1, 1913," Legislative Reference Library of Texas, accessed December 7, 2017, http://www. lrl.state.tx.us/sessions/sessionSnapshot.cfm?legSession=33-0 and http://www.lrl.state.tx.us/sessions/sessionYears.cfm.

26 "Austin Departmental News," *Dallas Morning News*, April 6, 1913, 6.

27 "Meningitis Vaccine Does Its Work Well; Paper Read at San Antonio by Dr. Henry Hartman; Deals with Results from Experiments Made in Austin at Session of Legislature," *Dallas Morning News*, May 11, 1913, 10; and "Vaccination to Halt Meningitis; Report on Results during Past Winter by State Bacteriologist; People at First Are Afraid; Several Thousand Are Finally Persuaded and Efficacy of Method Is Proved," *Waco Morning News*, May 8, 1913, 14.

28 "Legislator Won't Let State Pay His Meningitis Bill," *Fort Worth Star-Telegram*, July 27, 1913, 5.

29 Dr. Hartman chaired the pathology department, 1913–1926, and served as the dean of the University of Texas Medical Branch at Galveston, 1926–1928. "Graham Is Appointed State Bacteriologist," *El Paso Herald*, September 8, 1913, 4; and "The History of the UTMB School of Medicine," *UTMB Health History*, accessed December 7, 2017, https://som.utmb.edu/About/history.asp.

30 "State Health Officer Steiner Makes Report; Retiring Official Commends Efforts of Board; Plague Prevention, Erecting of Tubercular Sanatorium and Sanitary Code among Accomplishments," *Dallas Morning News*, December 11, 1914, 3.

CONCLUSION

A MONSTROUS TEXAS MENINGITIS EPIDEMIC

The Texas cerebrospinal meningitis epidemic of 1911 to 1913 struck people wantonly, caused untold agony for its victims, and stressed and disordered city life. The collection and analysis of epidemiological data was in its infancy, resulting in cerebrospinal meningitis data caches of unreliable accuracy and completeness except in isolated instances. One of those instances was the data collected for Dallas, whose health officer and head of the City Hospital, Dr. Nash, counted 765 known cases of cerebrospinal meningitis between October 1, 1911, and Friday, May 31, 1912.

Based on the case count of 765, the prevalence rate of cerebrospinal meningitis in Dallas between October 1, 1911, and Friday, May 31, 1912, calculates to *83.2 cerebrospinal meningitis cases per 10,000 Dallas residents*. This rate was much greater than the prevalence rate for cerebrospinal meningitis in New York City during its 1905 epidemic, i.e., *12.5 cerebrospinal meningitis cases per 10,000 New York City residents*.[1] Recall that the 1905 cerebrospinal meningitis epidemic in New York City so alarmed the city's health department officials that they convened a cerebrospinal meningitis commission to study the contagiousness of the disease for the first time. Based on the findings of that commission, the disease became reportable and medical researchers initiated studies to find a cure for the first time. The cure, of course, was antimeningitis serum, the first treatment ever devised for cerebrospinal meningitis.

In the days before the advent of antimeningitis serum, victims of cerebrospinal meningitis either survived their disease on their own or not at all. The advent of antimeningitis serum saved lives but created a new set of issues. For example, patients receiving antimeningitis serum required prolonged, intensive care by medical and nursing staff whose close contact with their patients placed them at risk for contracting the disease. Nowhere was this reality better illustrated than at the City Hospital in Dallas, where almost a dozen nurses eventually developed the disease in 1912.

The initial solutions to this problem were barrier precautions (heavy clothing and masks) and subcutaneous antimeningitis serum. The latter was a short-term solution that lasted only days to weeks and carried its own risk of horse serum sickness upon repeated doses. Physicians and nurses required repeated doses because the duration of the cerebrospinal meningitis epidemic was many months. The solution to the limitations of subcutaneous antimeningitis serum was a meningococcal vaccine, which three physicians—Dr. Sophian, Dr. Thayer, and Dr. Black—originated and tested in Dallas in 1912.

Medical social behavior was in full color in Dallas during the cerebrospinal meningitis epidemic. The courageous private physician community in Dallas, who cared for most of the victims before the designation of the City Hospital for the exclusive care of cerebrospinal meningitis patients in early January 1912, organized to persuade the municipal physician health leaders to seek outside help from a New York City meningitis expert. The private and municipal physician groups rapidly found common ground to fight the epidemic together while receiving the unflinching support of the municipal government and the business community.

Government social behavior also was in full color in Austin in February 1913, when federal and state health officials and state legislators faced the terrible cerebrospinal meningitis predicament inside of the Texas State Capitol building, where five previously healthy legislators developed cerebrospinal meningitis and four died from it. The governor and state health officials, dedicated to bettering the lives of poor Texans by installing and operating a state biologics laboratory inside the Texas State Capitol building, were stunned and overwhelmed by the enormity of what they had undertaken and possibly had wrought.

The people of Dallas, Austin, Waco, and other Texas cities and towns doggedly worked through the dreadful cerebrospinal meningitis epidemic of 1911 to 1913 with grit and grace. The hardship and grief that people suffered during the crisis may have been the reason they so quickly relegated the experience to the dustbin of history while not realizing the state's significance as the origin of the meningococcal vaccine to prevent cerebrospinal meningitis in the United States.

CONCLUSION NOTE

1   No cerebrospinal meningitis case counts were available in New York City in 1905. We used the death count of 1,511, which was available for that year in New York City; the New York City population of 2,390,382 for that year; and a mortality rate of 50 percent. From these three data points, we estimated a prevalence rate of *12.5 cerebrospinal meningitis cases per 10,000 New York City residents* for 1905.

BIBLIOGRAPHY

Newspapers

Abilene Daily Chronicle (Abilene, TX)

Abilene Reporter-News (Abilene, TX)

Abilene Semi Weekly Farm Reporter (Abilene, TX)

Amarillo Daily News (Amarillo, TX)

Amarillo Globe-Times (Amarillo, TX)

Arkansas Gazette (Little Rock, AR)

Austin American-Statesman (Austin, TX)

Austin Daily Statesman (Austin, TX)

Austin Weekly Statesman (Austin, TX)

Bonham Daily Favorite (Bonham, TX)

Boston Traveler (Boston, MA)

Brooklyn Daily Eagle (New York, NY)

Bryan Daily Eagle (Bryan, TX)

Chillicothe Morning Constitution (Chillicothe, MO)

Cleburne Morning Review (Cleburne, TX)

Columbia Record (Columbia, SC)

Corpus Christi Caller-Times (Corpus Christi, TX)

Corpus Christi Times (Corpus Christi, TX)

Corsicana Daily Sun (Corsicana, TX)

Corsicana Semi-Weekly Light (Corsicana, TX)

Courier Gazette (McKinney, TX)

Courier-News (Bridgewater, NJ)

Daily Ardmoreite (Ardmore, OK)

Daily Courier-Gazette (McKinney, TX)

Dallas Morning News (Dallas, TX)

Democrat and Chronicle (Rochester, NY)

Democrat Gazette (McKinney, TX)

Denton Record-Chronicle (Denton, TX)

Eau Claire Leader (Eau Claire, WI)

El Paso Herald (El Paso, TX)

El Paso Herald-Post (El Paso, TX)

Evening News (Ada, OK)

Evening Star (Washington, DC)

Fort Wayne Sentinel (Fort Wayne, IN)

Fort Worth Star-Telegram (Fort Worth, TX)

Galveston Daily News (Galveston, TX)

Gazette Globe (Kansas City, KS)

Houston Daily Post (Houston, TX)

Houston Post (Houston, TX)

Jewish Herald (Houston, TX)

Kansas City Star (Kansas City, MO)

Kansas City Times (Kansas City, MO)

Lancaster Herald (Lancaster, TX)

Longview News-Journal (Longview, TX)

Los Angeles Times (Los Angeles, CA)

Macon Telegraph (Macon, GA)

Marshall Messenger (Marshall, TX)

Marshall News (Marshall, TX)

Marshall News Messenger (Marshall, TX)

McKinney Weekly Democrat-Gazette (McKinney, TX)

New Orleans Item-Tribune (New Orleans, LA)

News and Observer (Raleigh, NC)

New York Times (New York, NY)

New York Tribune (New York, NY)

Omaha World-Herald (Omaha, NE)

Pensacola Journal (Pensacola, FL)

Philadelphia Inquirer (Philadelphia, PA)

Rice Belt Journal (Welsh, LA)

Salt Lake Telegram (Salt Lake, UT)

San Antonio Express (San Antonio, TX)

San Antonio Express-News (San Antonio, TX)

San Francisco Call (San Francisco, CA)
Santa Ana Register (Santa Ana, CA)
Springfield Republican (Springfield, MA)
St. Louis Post-Dispatch (St. Louis, MO)
St. Louis Star and Times (St. Louis, MO)
Tammany Times (New York, NY)
Taylor Daily Press (Taylor, TX)
Times-Picayune (New Orleans, LA)
The Times (Shreveport, LA)
Waco Morning News (Waco, TX)
Waco News-Tribune (Waco, TX)
Washington Times (Washington, DC)
Waxahachie Daily Light (Waxahachie, TX)
Weimar Mercury (Weimar, TX)
Wheeling Daily Intelligencer (Wheeling, WV)
Whitewright Sun (Whitewright, TX)
Wichita Daily Eagle (Wichita Falls, TX)
Wichita Daily Times (Wichita Falls, TX)

Websites

Ancestry at https://www.ancestry.com/.
Baylor Scott and White Health at http://news.bswhealth.com/pages/history.
Biographical Directory of the United States Congress at http://bioguide.congress.gov/biosearch/biosearch.asp.
Collin County, Texas History at https://www.collincountyhistory.com/doctors.html.
Find a Grave at https://www.findagrave.com.
Flashback: Dallas at https://flashbackdallas.com/contact/.
Grayson County TX GenWeb at http://txgenwebcounties.org/grayson/.
Handbook of Texas Online at https://tshaonline.org/handbook.
Legislative Reference Library of Texas at http://www.lrl.state.tx.us/.

Library of Congress Prints and Photographs Division at https://www.loc.gov/pictures/.

Rockefeller University at http://digitalcommons.rockefeller.edu/hospital-of-institute/15/ngs.

Texas Almanac: City Population History of Selected Cities, 1850–2000 at https://texasalmanac.com/sites/default/files/images/CityPopHist%20web.pdf.

Texas Archival Resources Online, Dallas Public Library, at http://www.lib.utexas.edu/taro/dalpub/08212/dpub-08212.html.

University of Texas Southwestern Medical Center Library at http://library.utsouthwestern.edu/speccol/archives/FindingAid_Parkland_Coll.pdf.

Wikipedia at https://en.wikipedia.org.

Urban Dictionary at https://www.urbandictionary.com.

US National Library of Medicine, National Institutes of Health, https://www.ncbi.nlm.nih.gov/.

YouTube at https://www.youtube.com/.

Waymarking at http://www.waymarking.com/.

Whonamedit at http://www.whonamedit.com.

Wikipedia at https://www.wikipedia.org/.

Web Articles, Blogs, Videos, and Images

Alexandra [*sic*]. "The End of St. Paul Medical Center." University of North Texas Libraries. Discovering the Southwest Metroplex. https://blogs.library.unt.edu/southwest-metroplex/2015/12/16/the-end-of-st-paul-medical-center/.

"Almoth Dowden Rogers (1866–1931)." *The Strangest Names in American Political History*. http://politicalstrangenames.blogspot.com/2015/11/almoth-dowden-rogers-1866-1931.html.

American College of Surgeons. "The Minimum Standard." https://www.facs.org/about-acs/archives/pasthighlights/minimumhighlight.

"Anton Weichselbaum." http://www.whonamedit.com/doctor.cfm/2874.html.

"Anton Weichselbaum." *Wikipedia.* https://en.wikipedia.org/wiki/ Anton_Weichselbaum.

"Baylor Scott and White Health—Our History—YouTube." https:// www.youtube.com/watch?v=ebo7lrW97no.

Bernstein, Robert. "Texas Department of Health." *Handbook of Texas Online.* https://tshaonline.org/handbook/online/articles/ mdt40.

"Bluitt Sanitarium." Dallas Landmark Structures and Sites. Dallas Landmark. National Register of Historic Places. http:// dallascityhall.com/departments/sustainabledevelopment/ historicpreservation/Pages/Bluitt-Sanitarium.aspx.

Bosse, Paula. "The Marsalis House: One of Oak Cliff's 'Most Conspicuous Architectural Landmarks.'" Flashback: Dallas. https://flashbackdallas.com/2014/05/30/marsalis-house/.

Bosse, Paula. "St. Paul's Sanitarium." Flashback: Dallas. https:// flashbackdallas.com/2015/08/23/st-pauls-sanitarium-1910/.

Bridges, Jennifer. "Bluitt, Benjamin Rufus." *Handbook of Texas Online.* https://tshaonline.org/handbook/online/articles/fbl69.

"Burleson, Albert Sidney." *Biographical Directory of the United States Congress.* http://bioguide.congress.gov/scripts/ biodisplay.pl?index=B001110.

Connor, Seymour V. "Burleson, Albert Sidney." *Handbook of Texas Online.* https://tshaonline.org/handbook/online/articles/ fbu38.

"David J. Davis Papers, 1913–1955." University Library, University of Illinois at Chicago. http://findingaids.library.uic.edu/ead/ lhsc/016-01-01-20-02b.html.

"Demographics of Texas," *Wikipedia,* accessed August 18, 2018, https://en.wikipedia.org/wiki/Demographics_of_Texas.

"Fort Worth Medical College." http://www.waymarking.com/ waymarks/WM5V45_Fort_Worth_Medical_College_ Fort_Worth_Texas.

"Historical Note." Southern Methodist University Medical and Pharmacy School Records: A Guide to the Collection. *Texas Archival Resources Online.* http://www.lib.utexas.edu/taro/ smu/00088/smu-00088.html.

"History of the UTMB School of Medicine." *UTMB Health.* https://som.utmb.edu/About/history.

Huckaby, George P. Huckaby. "Oscar Branch Colquitt," *Handbook of Texas Online,* accessed August 18, 2018, https://tshaonline. org/handbook/online/articles/fco32.

Jakobi, Patricia L. "Brumby, William McDuffie." *Handbook of Texas Online.* https://tshaonline.org/handbook/online/articles/ fbrcx.

Kleiner, Diana J. "Sanger Brothers." *Handbook of Texas Online.* https://tshaonline.org/handbook/online/articles/ijsqj.

Manguso, John. "Fort Sam Houston." *Handbook of Texas Online.* https://tshaonline.org/handbook/online/articles/qbf43.

"Metropolitan." Grayson County TX GenWeb. http:// txgenwebcounties.org/grayson/Ethnic/AfricanAmerican/ TheMetropolitan_newspaper/Metropolitan.html.

Minor, David. "Carrick, Manton Marble." *Handbook of Texas Online.* https://tshaonline.org/handbook/online/articles/fca62.

Morens, David M., and Anthony S. Fauci. "The Forgotten Forefather: Joseph James Kinyoun and the Founding of the National Institutes of Health." *mBio* 3, no. 4 (July–August 2012): e00139-12, https://www.ncbi.nlm.nih.gov/pmc/articles/ PMC3388889/.

"Neisseria meningitidis." In NCBI Taxonomy, *EOL Encyclopedia of Life.* http://eol.org/pages/996566/names/synonyms.

Ornish, Natalie. "Sanger, Alexander." *Handbook of Texas Online.* https://tshaonline.org/handbook/online/articles/fsa54.

"Our History." Baylor Scott and White Health. http://news. bswhealth.com/pages/history.

"Overview, 33rd Regular Session, January 14, 1913–April 1, 1913." Legislative Reference Library of Texas. http://www.lrl.state. tx.us/sessions/sessionSnapshot.cfm?legSession=33-0 and http:// www.lrl.state.tx.us/sessions/sessionYears.cfm.

Perez, Joan Jenkins. "Charles McDaniel Rosser," *Handbook of Texas Online.* https://tshaonline.org/handbook/online/articles/ fro88.

Pinkney, Kathryn. "John Oliver McReynolds." *Handbook of Texas Online.* https://tshaonline.org/handbook/online/articles/fmccj.

Senate Journal. Thirty-Third Legislature. Regular Session, Friday, January 17, 1913, 70. http://www.lrl.state.tx.us/collections/journals/journals.cfm.

"SMU's Forgotten Medical School." *SMU Magazine.* http://blog.smu.edu/smumagazine/2011/12/smus-forgotten-medical-school/.

Snyder, Billie Jane Chandler. "Trimble, William Marshall." *Handbook of Texas Online.* https://tshaonline.org/handbook/online/articles/ftr31.

"Texas Legislative Sessions and Years." Legislative Reference Library of Texas. http://www.lrl.state.tx.us/sessions/sessionYears.cfm.

"Texas State Capitol Project 1988." National Park Service. United States Department of the Interior. 1988. HABS TEX, 227-AUST,13, 1988. Historic American Buildings Survey Program. Library of Congress Prints and Photographs Division. Washington, DC. http://www.loc.gov/pictures/search/?q=texas%20state%20capitol%20drawing.

"Typhoid Vaccine Preparation, US Army Medical School, 1917." Harris and Ewing Photographs Collection. Library of Congress Prints and Photographs Division. Washington, DC. http://www.loc.gov/pictures/search/?q=typhoid%20vaccine.

"Valleix, François Louis Isidore." *Comité des travaux historiques et scientifiques.* http://cths.fr/an/savant.php?id=106004.

"Wooten, Joe Sil." *Handbook of Texas Online.* https://tshaonline.org/handbook/online/articles/fwo23.

"Wortham, Louis J." *Handbook of Texas Online.* https://tshaonline.org/handbook/online/articles/fwo29.

Books

Abbott, Alexander Crever. *The Hygiene of Transmissible Diseases.* Philadelphia, PA: W. B. Saunders, 1899.

Aitken, William, and Meredith Clymer. *The Science and Practice of Medicine.* Philadelphia, PA: Lindsay and Blakiston, 1868.

Alumni of the Medical Schools, New York University Alumni Catalogue, 1833–1907. New York: General Alumni Society, 1908.

Alumni Roster of the University of Pennsylvania. Philadelphia, PA: University of Pennsylvania General Alumni Society, 1902.

Anderson, Adrian H. "Albert Sidney Burleson: A Southern Politician in the Progressive Era." PhD diss., Texas Tech University, 1967.

Announcement of the Medical School of Harvard University, 1909–1910. Cambridge, MA: Harvard University, 1909.

Annual Announcement, Baylor University School of Medicine and School of Pharmacy, Dallas, Texas, 1910–1911. Dallas, TX: Medical Department of Baylor University, 1910.

Annual Announcement and Catalogue of the College of Physicians and Surgeons, Baltimore, Maryland, 1890–1891. Philadelphia, PA: College of Physicians and Surgeons, 1891.

Annual Report of the Bureau of Vital Statistics for the Year 1917. Bureau of Vital Statistics. Texas State Board of Health. Austin, TX: Von Boeckmann-Jones Company, 1918.

Annual Report of the Surgeon General of the Public Health Service of the United States for the Fiscal Year 1912. Washington, DC: Government Printing Office, 1913.

Appletons' Cyclopedia of American Biography, 1600–1889. New York: D. Appleton and Company, 1888.

Austin, Texas, City Directory 1906. Austin, TX: J. B. Stephenson, 1907.

Baker, Marilyn Miller. *The History of Pathology in Texas.* Austin, TX: Texas Society of Pathologists, 1996.

Barnhart, Ryan, and Ryan Estes. *Mckinney.* Charleston, SC: Arcadia Publishing, 2010.

Beam, Harold Beam. "A History of Collin County, Texas." Master's thesis, University of Texas, 1951.

Besson, A. *Practical Bacteriology, Microbiology, and Serum Therapy: A Textbook for Laboratory Use.* London: Longmans, Green, and Company, 1913.

Biggs, Hermann M. *Brief History of the Campaign against Tuberculosis in New York City: Catalogue of the Tuberculosis*

Exhibit of the Department of Health, City of New York, 1908. New York: Department of Health, 1908.

Biographical and Historical Memoirs of Western Arkansas. Chicago, IL: Southern Publishing Company, 1891.

Biographic Souvenir of the State of Texas. Chicago, IL: F. A. Battey and Company, 1889.

Blochman, Lawrence G. *Doctor Squibb: The Life and Times of a Rugged Idealist.* New York: Simon and Schuster, 1958.

Bosanquet, William Cecil, and John William Henry Eyre. *Serum, Vaccines, and Toxines in Treatment and Diagnosis.* New York: Funk and Wagnalls Company, 1910.

Boyd, John W. *Parkland Hospital.* Charleston, SC: Arcadia, 2015.

Brock, Thomas D. *Robert Koch: A Life in Medicine and Bacteriology.* Berlin: Springer-Verlag, 1988.

Brown, E. Richard. *Rockefeller Medicine Men: Medicine and Capitalism in America.* Berkeley, CA: University of California Press, 1979.

Budd, Harrell J., Jr. "Geology of the McKinney Area, Collin County, Texas." Master's thesis, Southern Methodist University, 1950.

Cactus Yearbook 1907. Galveston, TX: University of Texas Medical Branch, 1907.

Capace, Nancy. *Encyclopedia of Texas.* St. Clair Shores, MI: Somerset Publishers, 1999.

Cassedy, James H. *The New Age of Health Laboratories, 1885–1915: An Exhibit, May–October 1987 Marking the Centennial of the Founding of the Pasteur Institute of Paris and the National Institutes of Health.* Bethesda, MD: National Library of Medicine, 1987.

Centers for Disease Control and Prevention. *Principles of Epidemiology in Public Health Practice, Third Edition: An Introduction to Applied Epidemiology and Biostatistics.* Atlanta, GA: US Department of Health and Human Services, 2006.

Chapman, John S. *The University of Texas Southwestern Medical School: Medical Education in Dallas, 1900–1975.* Dallas, TX: Southern Methodist University Press, 1976.

Childers, Sam. *Historic Dallas Hotels*. Charleston, SC: Arcadia Publishers, 2010.

Clymer, Meredith. *Epidemic Cerebro-Spinal Meningitis*. Philadelphia, PA: Lindsay and Blakiston, 1872.

Cooper, Page. *The Bellevue Story*. New York: Thomas Y. Crowell Company, 1948.

Corner, George Washington. *A History of the Rockefeller Institute, 1901–1953: Origins and Growth*. New York: Rockefeller Institute Press, 1964.

Daniel, Thomas M. *Wade Hampton Frost, Pioneer Epidemiologist 1880–1938: Up to the Mountain*. Rochester, NY: University of Rochester Press, 2004.

Daniell, Lewis E. *Personnel of the Texas State Government with Sketches of Representative Men of Texas*. San Antonio, TX: Maverick Printing House, 1892.

Daniell, Lewis E. *Types of Successful Men of Texas*. Austin, TX: Eugene von Boeckmann, 1890.

Davis, Ellis A., and Edwin H. Grobe. *The Encyclopedia of Texas*. Dallas, TX: University of North Texas, 1922.

Davis, Ellis A., and Edwin H. Grobe. *New Encyclopedia of Texas*. Dallas, TX: Texas Development Bureau, 1926.

Dixon, Samuel Houston. *The Men Who Made Texas Free*. Houston, TX: Texas Historical Publishing Company, c. 1924.

Duncan, Donald. *The University of Texas Medical Branch at Galveston: A Seventy-Five Year History*. Austin, TX: University of Texas Press, 1967.

Dunnill, Michael S. *The Plato of Praed Street: The Life and Times of Almroth Wright*. London: Royal Society of Medicine Press, 2001.

Ellis, Roy. *A Civic History of Kansas City, Missouri*. Springfield, MO: Press of Elkins-Swyers Company, 1930.

Fitzgerald, Hugh Nugent. *Governors I Have Known*. Austin, TX: Austin American-State, 1927.

Flexner, James Thomas. *An American Saga: The Story of Helen Thomas and Simon Flexner*. New York: Fordham University Press, 1993.

Fowler, Giles. *Deaths on Pleasant Street*. Kirksville, MO: Truman State University Press, 2009.

Fulmore, Zachary Fulmore. *The History and Geography of Texas as Told in County Names*. Austin, TX: Texas Historical Association, 1915.

Galambos, Louis. *Networks of Innovation: Vaccine Development at Merck, Sharp and Dohme, and Mulford, 1895–1995*. New York: Cambridge University Press, 1997.

General Alumni Catalogue of the University of Pennsylvania. Philadelphia, PA: Alumni Association of the University of Pennsylvania, 1917.

General Laws of the State of Texas Passed by the Thirty-First Legislature at Its Regular Session Convened January 12, 1909, and Adjourned March 13, 1909, at Its First Called Session, Convened March 13, 1909, and Adjourned April 11, 1919, and at Its Second Called Session, Convened April 12, 1909, and Adjourned May 11, 1909. Austin, TX: Von Boeckmann-Jones Company, 1909.

Griffith, Glenn, Sandy Bryce, James Omernik, and Anne Rogers. *Ecoregions of Texas*. Austin, TX: Commission on Environmental Quality, 2007.

Hafner, Arthur Wayne. *Directory of Deceased American Physicians, 1804–1929: A Genealogical Guide to Over 149,000 Medical Practitioners Providing Brief Biographical Sketches Drawn from the American Medical Association's Deceased Physician Masterfile*. Chicago, IL: American Medical Association, 1993.

Hahnemann, Samuel. *The Homoeopathic Medical Doctrine*. Dublin, Ireland: W. F. Wakeman, 1833.

Hamilton, William Benjamin. *Social Survey of Austin*. Austin, TX: University of Texas, 1913.

Hardy, Dremont H., and Ingham S. Roberts. *Historical Review of Southeast Texas*. Chicago, IL: Lewis Publishing Company, 1910.

Harper, Franklin. *Who's Who on the Pacific Coast*. Los Angeles, CA: Harper Publishing Company, 1913.

Health and Hospital Survey, Kansas City, Missouri. Kansas City, MO: Chamber of Commerce of Kansas City, 1931.

Historical Catalogue of the University of Mississippi (1849–1909). Nashville, TN: Marshall and Bruce Company, 1910.

Historical and Current Catalogue of the Officers and Students of the University of Mississippi. Oxford, MS: University, 1887.

History of the Long Island College Hospital and Its Graduates. Brooklyn, NY: Association of the Alumni, 1899.

Journal of the House of Representatives of the Regular Session of the Thirty-Third Legislature of Texas, Convened at the City of Austin, January 14, 1913, and Adjourned without Day, April 1, 1913. Austin, TX: Von Boeckmann-Jones, 1913.

Kelley, Dayton. *With Scalpel and Scope: A History of Scott and White*. Waco, TX: Library Binding Company, 1970.

Koch, Robert, *Die Ätiologie der Tuberkulose*. Berlin, Germany: Verlag von August Hirschwald, 1884.

Lindsley, Phillip, and Luther B. Hill. *A History of Greater Dallas and Vicinity*. Chicago, IL: Lewis Publishing Company, 1909.

Longhorn Yearbook. College Station, TX: Texas A&M, 1913.

Loughery, E. H. *Texas State Government: A Volume of Biographical Sketches and Passing Comment*. Austin, TX: McLeod and Jackson, 1897.

Major, Ralph Hermon, ed. *Classic Descriptions of Disease*. Springfield, IL: Charles C. Thomas, 1959.

Manguso, John. *Fort Sam Houston*. Charleston, SC: Arcadia Publishing, 2012.

Maxwell, W. J. *General Alumni Catalogue of Jefferson Medical College Alumni, 1890–1899*. Philadelphia, PA: Jefferson Medical College, 1917.

Maxwell, W. J. *General Alumni Catalogue of New York University*. New York: New York University, 1916.

Maxwell, W. J., and John A. Lomax. *General Register of the Students and Former Students of the University of Texas, 1917*. Austin, TX: University of Texas Ex-Students' Association, 1917.

McClintock, John, and James Strong. *McClintock and Strong Biblical Cyclopedia*. New York: Harper and Brothers, 1880.

McGarry, William A. *The Story of the House of Squibb*. New York: Doubleday, Doran, and Company, 1931.

Memorial and Biographical History of Ellis County, Texas. Chicago, IL: Lewis Publishing Company, 1892.

Miller, K. E. *A Survey of the Public Health Problems and Needs in the State of Texas*. Washington, DC: US Public Health Service, 1937.

Mooney, Booth. *More Than Armies: The Story of Edward H. Cary, MD*. Dallas, TX: Mathis, Van Nort Company, 1948.

Moursund, Walter Henrik. *A History of Baylor University, College of Medicine, 1900–1953*. Houston, TX: Gulf Printing Company, 1956.

Nineteenth Biennial Report of the Board of Directors of the Agricultural and Mechanical College of Texas for the Fiscal Years Ending August 31, 1913, and August 31, 1914. Austin, TX: A. C. Baldwin and Sons, 1914.

North, Elisha. *A Treatise on a Malignant Epidemic Commonly Called Spotted Fever*. New York: T. and J. Swords, 1811.

Oliver, Wade W. *The Man Who Lived for Tomorrow*. New York: E. P. Dutton, 1941.

Page, Walter Hines, and Arthur Wilson Page. *The World's Work: A History of Our Time, November 1911 to April 1912*. Garden City, NY: Doubleday, Page, and Company, 1912.

Polk's Medical Register and Directory of North America. Detroit, MI: R. L. Polk and Company, 1904.

Porta, Miquel, *A Dictionary of Epidemiology*. Oxford, England: Oxford University Press, 2014.

Porter, Gerald M. "A History of State Organization for Public Health Administration in Texas, 1718–1927." Master's thesis, University of Chicago, 1942.

Presiding Officers of the Texas Legislature, 1846–2016. Austin, TX: Texas Legislative Council, 2016.

Public Health Papers and Report 37, Presented at the Thirty-Ninth Annual Meeting of the American Public Health Association,

Havana, Cuba. Concord, NH: Rumford Printing Company, 1913.

Quebbeman, Frances E. *Medicine in Territorial Arizona.* Phoenix, AX: Arizona Historical Foundation, 1966.

Rhodes, Desha P. *A History of Flint Medical College, 1889–1911.* New York: iUniverse, 2007.

Scribner, Harvey. *Memoirs of Lucas County and the City of Toledo.* Madison, WI: Western Historical Society, 1910.

Segura, Judith Garrett. *Belo: From Newspapers to New Media.* Austin, TX: University of Texas Press, 2008.

Sherman, George Henry. *Vaccine Therapy in General Practice.* Detroit, MI: printed by the author, 1911.

Smith, Howard E. *History of Public Health in Texas.* Austin, TX: Texas State Department of Public Health, 1974.

Sophian, Abraham. *Epidemic Cerebrospinal Meningitis.* St. Louis, MO: C. V. Mosby, 1913.

Sou'wester Yearbook 1907. Georgetown, Texas: Athletic Association of Southwestern University, 1907.

Stambaugh, J. Lee, and Lillian J. Stambaugh. *A History of Collin County, Texas.* Austin, TX: Texas State Historical Association, 1958.

Stimson, Arthur Marston. *A Brief History of Bacteriological Investigations of the United States Public Health Service.* Washington, DC: US Government Printing Office, 1938.

Taylor, Dencil R. "The Political Speaking of Oscar Branch Colquitt, 1906–1913." PhD diss., Louisiana State University, 1979.

Thayer, Alfred Edward. *Compend of Pathology: General and Special; A Student's Manual in One Volume.* Philadelphia, PA: P. Blakiston's Son and Company, 1906.

Thayer, Alfred Edward. *Compend of Special Pathology.* Philadelphia, PA: P. Blakiston's Son and Company, 1902.

Thirty-Sixth Annual Catalogue, Bulletin of the Agricultural and Mechanical College of Texas, April 1912. Austin, TX: Austin Printing Company, 1912.

Thomas, B. A., and R. H. Ivy. *Applied Immunology: The Practical Application of Sera and Bacterins Prophylactically,*

Diagnostically, and Therapeutically. Philadelphia, PA: J. B. Lippincott Company, 1915.

Transactions of the Section on Pathology and Physiology of the American Medical Association at the Sixty-Third Annual Session, Held at Atlantic City, NJ, June 4 to 7, 1912. Chicago, IL: American Medical Association, 1912.

Turpin, Rees, George King, and Charles L. Shannon. *Charter and Revised Ordinances of Kansas City, 1909*. Kansas City, MO: Frank T. Riley Publishing Company, 1909.

University of Michigan General Catalogue of Officers and Students, 1837–1901. Ann Arbor, MI: University of Michigan, 1902.

Valleix, François-Louis-Isidore. *Guide Médecin Praticien or Résumé Général de Pathologie Interne et de Thérapeutique Appliqués*. Paris: J. B. Billière, 1847.

Vargo, Julia L. *McKinney, Texas—The First 150 Years*. Virginia Beach, VA: Donning Company Publishers, 1997.

Von Pirquet, Clemens F., and Béla Schick. *Serum Sickness*. Philadelphia, PA: Williams and Wilkins, 1951.

Wall, Cecil. *On Acute Cerebro-Spinal Meningitis Caused by the Diplococcus Intracellularis of Weichselbaum; A Clinical Study*. London: Royal Medical and Chirurgical Society, 1993.

Weichselbaum, Anton. *The Elements of Pathological Histology*. London: Longmans, Green, and Company, 1895.

Winslow, Charles-Edward Armory. *The Life of Hermann M. Biggs, Physician and Statesman of the Public Health*. Philadelphia, PA: Lea and Febiger, 1929.

Worley's 1912 Directory of Dallas, Texas. Dallas, TX: John F. Worley Directory Company, 1912.

Wright, Almroth Edward. *Vaccine Therapy: Its Administration, Value, and Limitations*. London: Longmans, Green, and Company, 1910.

Government Resources

"California, Occupational Licenses, Registers, and Directories (1919)." California State Archives. Sacramento, California. Board of Medical Examiners Registers of Licensed Physicians. 1901–39.

Jung, Kay. *Historical Census Statistics on Population Totals by Race, 1790 to 1990, and by Hispanic Origin, 1970 to 1990, for Large Cities and Other Urban Places in the United States.* US Census Bureau. Washington, DC. 2005.

US Department of Agriculture. *The Agriculture, Soils, Geology, and Topography of the Blacklands Experimental Watershed, Waco, Texas.* Washington, DC: Government Printing Office, 1942.

US States Census, 1910. *Agriculture, 1909 and 1910, Reports by States, with Statistics for Counties.* Washington, DC: United States Government Printing Office, 1913, 7:626–27, 682.

Professional Journals and Magazines

American Journal of Clinical Pathology
American Journal of Dermatology
American Journal of the Medical Sciences
Berliner Klinische Wochesnschrift
British Journal of Clinical Pharmacology
British Medical Journal
Canada Medical Record
Clinical Microbiology Reviews
Electric Traction
Fortschritte der Medizin
Johns Hopkins University Circular
Journal of Bacteriology
Journal of Experimental Medicine
Journal of Hygiene (London)
Journal of Infectious Diseases
Journal of Medical Biography
Journal of Pathology and Bacteriology

Journal of the American Chemical Society
Journal of the American Medical Association
Journal of the Oklahoma State Medical Association
Maryland Medical Journal: Medicine and Surgery
mBio
Medico-Chirurgical Transactions (London)
Medical Herald
Medical Record
Military Medicine
Morbidity and Mortality Weekly Report
Mount Sinai Hospital Reports (New York City)
Nature
New York Medical Journal
Postgraduate Medical Journal
Proceedings of Baylor University Medical Center
Public Health Reports
Red River Valley Historical Review
Review of Infectious Diseases
SMU Magazine
Southern Illinois Journal of Medicine and Surgery
Southwestern Historical Quarterly
Texas Magazine
Texas State Journal of Medicine
Texas State Journal of Medicine Transactions
Transactions of the American Clinical and Climatological Association
Verhandl Kong Innere Medizinisch Wiesbaden

Journal Articles

"About People." *Electric Traction* 14 (November 1918): 754.

"Aid to Texas Authorities in the Installation of a Laboratory." *Annual Report of the Surgeon General of the Public Health Service of the United States for the Fiscal Year 1912* (1913): 40.

Albrecht, Heinrich, and Anton Ghon. "About the Etiology and Pathological Anatomy of Meningitis Cerebrospinalis

Epidemica." *Vienna Klinische Wochenschrift* 14 (1901): 984–96.

Anderson, Adrian H. "President Wilson's Politician: Albert Sidney Burleson of Texas." *Southwestern Historical Quarterly* 77 (January 1974): 339–54.

"An Interesting Announcement Is Made in This Issue by the H. K. Mulford Company Concerning Meningo-Bacterin (Meningococcus Vaccine)." *American Journal of Dermatology* 16, no. 4 (April 1912): 222.

"Annual Conference of Health Officers." *Texas State Journal of Medicine* 7, no. 8 (December 1911): 228.

"Association News, Proceedings of the Atlantic City Session." *Journal of the American Medical Association* 58, no. 25 (June 22, 1912): 1,981.

"Banti's Disease or Syndrome." *Journal of the American Medical Association* 115, no. 17 (October 26, 1940): 1456–57.

Billings, John S. "Cerebrospinal Meningitis in New York City during 1904 and 1905." *Journal of the American Medical Association* 46, no. 22 (June 2, 1906): 1,670–76.

"Biological Products: Establishments Licensed for the Propagation and Sale of Viruses, Serums, Toxins, and Analogous Products." *Public Health Reports* 27, no. 2 (January 12, 1912): 40–41.

"Biological Products: Establishments Licensed for the Propagation and Sale of Viruses, Serums, Toxins, and Analogous Products." *Public Health Reports* 28, no. 2 (January 10, 1913): 61–62.

Black, J. H. "Prophylactic Vaccination against Epidemic Meningitis." *Journal of the American Medical Association* 60, no. 17 (April 26, 1913): 1,289–90.

Black, J. H. "Prophylactic Vaccination against Epidemic Meningitis, A Supplementary Note." *Journal of the American Medical Association* 68, no. 24 (December 12, 1914): 2,126.

Blailock, William R. "Meningitis in Texas and Indian Territory during First Three Months of 1899." *Transactions of the Texas State Medical Association, Thirty-First Annual Session Held at San Antonio, Texas* (1899): 121–38.

Bolduan, Charles F. "Cerebrospinal Meningitis from the Standpoint of Public Health." *Medical Times* 36, no. 7 (July 1908): 193–95.

Bolduan, Charles F. "Over a Century of Health Administration in New York City." *Department of Health of the City of New York Monograph Series* 13 (March 1916): 23–24.

Bulloch, W. "Waldemar Mordecai Wolff Haffkine." *Journal of Pathology and Bacteriology* 34, no. 2 (1931): 125–29.

"Bureau of Public Health and Marine Hospital Service." *Texas State Journal of Medicine* 7, no. 1 (May 1911): 31–32.

Cartwright, K. "Microbiology and Laboratory Diagnosis." *Methods of Molecular Medicine* 67 (2001): 1–8.

"Cerebrospinal Meningitis." *Public Health Reports* 29, no. 5 (January 30, 1914): 308.

"Cerebrospinal Meningitis." *Public Health Reports* 29, no. 11 (March 6, 1914): 574.

"Cerebrospinal Meningitis." *Public Health Reports* 29, no. 15 (April 10, 1914): 889.

"Cerebrospinal Meningitis." *Public Health Reports* 29, no. 31 (July 31, 1914): 2,025.

"Cerebrospinal Meningitis." *Public Health Reports* 29, no. 34 (August 21, 1914): 2,207.

"Cerebrospinal Meningitis State Reports, Texas." *Public Health Reports* 28, no. 15 (April 11, 1913): 691.

"Cerebrospinal Meningitis in Texas." *Public Health Reports* 27, no. 4 (January 26, 1912): 128.

Chase, Ira Carleton. "Flexner's Antimeningitis Serum." *Texas State Journal of Medicine* 5, no. 3 (July 1909): 105.

"Chester H. Terrell." In *Presiding Officers of the Texas Legislature, 1846–2016.* Austin, TX: Texas Legislative Council, 2016, 176–77.

Cirillo, V. J. "Arthur Conan Doyle: Physician during the Typhoid Epidemic in the Anglo-Boer War (1899–1902)." *Journal of Medical Biography* 22, no. 1 (2014): 2–8.

Colebrock, Leonard. "Sir Almroth Wright and Anti-Typhoid Inoculation." *British Medical Journal* 2, no. 4471 (September 14, 1946): 398.

"College Calendar." *Thirty-Sixth Annual Catalogue, Bulletin of the Agricultural and Mechanical College of Texas, April 1912* 9, no. 16 (1912): front pages.

"Communication: Serum Sickness." *Texas State Journal of Medicine* 7, no. 12 (April 1912): 336.

Comer, Lewis A. "The Technique of Lumbar Puncture." *New York Medical Journal* 71 (May 12, 1900): 723–25.

Councell, Clara E. "War and Infectious Disease." *Public Health Reports* 56, no. 12 (March 21, 1941): 547–73.

Coureuil, Mathieu, Olivier Join-Lambert, Hervé Lécuyer, Sandrine Bourdoulous, Stefano Marullo, and Xavier Nassif.t al. "Pathogenesis of Meningococcemia." *Cold Spring Harbor Perspectives in Medicine* 3, no. 6 (June 2013).

Creathe, Luther B. "Gelsemium." *Texas State Journal of Medicine Transactions* 17 (1885): 140–41.

"Dallas Medical Lunch Club." *Texas State Journal of Medicine* 7, no. 3 (July 1911): 99.

Danielson, L., and E. Mann. "The First American Account of Cerebrospinal Meningitis." *Review of Infectious Diseases* 5, no. 5 (September–October 1983): 969–72.

Davis, David J. "Studies in Meningococcus Infections." *Journal of Infectious Diseases* 4, no. 4 (November 15, 1907): 576–77.

"Deaths." *Journal of the American Medical Association* 70, no. 21 (May 25, 1918): 1,555.

"Deaths." *Journal of the American Medical Association* 76, no. 18 (April 30, 1921): 1,262.

"Deaths." *Texas State Journal of Medicine* 12, no. 6 (October 1916): 278.

"Diagnostic Laboratory for the Health Department." *Texas State Journal of Medicine* 8, no. 3 (July 1912): 97.

"'Diphtheria,' Dr. Ralph Steiner, Austin, Section on Ophthalmology, Otology, Rhinology, and Laryngology, Second Day, Wednesday, May 8, 1912." *Texas State Journal of Medicine* 7, no. 12 (April 1912): 334.

Dowling, Harry Filmore. "Field, Ward, and Laboratory: Where the Infectious Disease Physician Worked." *Journal of Infectious Diseases* 153, no. 3 (March 1986): 390–96.

"Dr. B. F. Calhoun." *Texas Magazine* 4, no. 1 (May 1911): 52.

"Dr. Thomas Darlington." *Tammany Times* 12, no. 12 (January 23, 1904): 4.

DuBois, Phebe L. "Differential Diagnosis and Treatment of Epidemic Cerebrospinal Meningitis." *Journal of the American Medical Association* 60, no. 11 (March 15, 1913): 822.

Dunn, Charles Hunter. "The Serum Treatment of Epidemic Cerebrospinal Meningitis." *Journal of the American Medical Association* 51, no. 1 (July 4, 1908): 15–21.

"Effect of Injecting Ringer's Solution into the Spinal Canal in Varying Amounts and Under Varying Pressures, Dr. W. S. Carter, Galveston, Section on Medicine and Disease of Children, May 9, 1912." *Texas State Journal of Medicine* 7, no. 12 (April 1912): 335.

"Epidemic and the Board of Health." *Texas State Journal of Medicine* 7, no. 10 (February 1912): 267–68.

"Epidemic Cerebrospinal Meningitis; Current Prevalence." *Public Health Reports* 32, no. 18 (May 4, 1917): 639–40.

"Epidemic Cerebrospinal Meningitis; Recorded Prevalence by States, 1916." *Public Health Reports* 32, no. 24 (June 15, 1917): 939.

"Epidemic Meningitis: Editorial." *Medical Herald* 32, no. 2 (February 1913): 75–77.

Ernst, Edzard. "A Systematic Review of Systematic Reviews of Homeopathy." *British Journal of Clinical Pharmacology* 54, no. 6 (December 2002): 577.

Erwin, John Caleb. "Report of Ten Cases of Epidemic Meningitis, Treated with Flexner Antimeningitis Serum." *Texas State Journal of Medicine* 5, no. 3 (July 1909): 124–25.

"Establishments Licensed for the Propagation and Sale of Viruses, Serums, Toxins, and Analogous Products." *Public Health Reports* 27, part 1, no. 28 (January 12, 1912): 40.

"Faithful Work." *Journal of the American Medical Association* 58, no. 9 (March 2, 1912): 641.

"Fifteenth International Congress on Hygiene and Demography." *Journal of Hygiene* 11, no. 2 (July 1911): 301–6.

Fisher, H. C. "Malaria—Its Treatment." *Southern Illinois Journal of Medicine and Surgery* 1, no. 7 (February 1901): 247–50.

Flexner, Simon. "Concerning a Serum Therapy for Experimental Infection with *Diplococcus intracellularis*." *Journal of Experimental Medicine* 9, no. 2 (March 14, 1907): 168–85.

Flexner, Simon. "Experimental Cerebrospinal Meningitis and Its Serum Treatment." *Journal of the American Medical Association* 47, no. 8 (August 25, 1906): 560–66.

Flexner, Simon. "Experimental Cerebro-Spinal Meningitis in Monkeys." *Journal of Experimental Medicine* 9, no. 2 (March 14, 1907): 142–67.

Flexner, Simon. "The Present Status of the Serum Therapy of Epidemic Cerebrospinal Meningitis." *Journal of the American Medical Association* 53, no. 18 (October 30, 1909): 1,443–45.

Flexner, Simon, and James Wesley Jobling. "An Analysis of Four Hundred Cases of Epidemic Meningitis Treated with the Antimeningitis Serum." *Journal of Experimental Medicine* 10, no. 5 (September 5, 1908): 690–733.

Flexner, Simon, and James Wesley Jobling. "Serum Treatment of Epidemic Cerebrospinal Meningitis." *Journal of Experimental Medicine* 10, no. 1 (January 1, 1908): 141–203.

Fordtran, John S. "Medicine in Dallas 100 Years Ago." *Proceedings of Baylor University Medical Center* 13, no.1 (January 2000): 34–44.

"Forty-Fourth Annual Meeting Waco, May 7, 8, 9, 1912." *Texas State Journal of Medicine* 7, no. 12 (April 1912): 319.

Freedman, Ben. "The First State Board of Health Laboratories in the United States." *Public Health Reports* 69, no. 9 (September 1954): 867–75.

Frost, Wade Hampton. "Anti-meningitis Vaccination." *Public Health Reports* 28, no. 6 (February 7, 1913): 252–54.

Frost, Wade Hampton. "Epidemic Cerebrospinal Meningitis; A Review of Its Etiology, Transmission, and Specific Therapy, with Reference to Public Measures for its Control." *Public Health Reports* 27 no. 4 (January 26, 1912): 97–121.

Fuller, William. "Treatment of Meningitis." *Canada Medical Record* 5 (June 1977): 237–39.

Geddings, H. D. "Research Work in the Hygienic Laboratory of the Public Health and Marine-Hospital Service." *Journal of the American Medical Association* 62, no. 26 (June 25, 1904): 1,686–87.

Graves, Marvin L. "Some Remarks on Cerebrospinal Meningitis." *Texas State Journal of Medicine* 3, no. 10 (February 1908): 261–63.

Green, Jerome Davis. "The Texas Meningitis Epidemic." *Journal of the American Medical Association* 58, no. 9 (March 2, 1912): 649.

Groschel, D. N., and R. B. Hornick. "Who Introduced Typhoid Vaccination: Almroth Wright or Richard Pfeiffer?" *Review of Infectious Diseases* 3, no. 6 (November–December 1981): 1,251–54.

Hand, Alfred, Jr. "A Critical Summary of the Literature on the Diagnostic and Therapeutic Value of Lumbar Puncture." *American Journal of the Medical Sciences* 120 (October 1900): 463–69.

Hawgood, Barbara J. "Waldemar Mordecai Haffkine, CIE (1860–1930): Prophylactic Vaccination against Cholera and Bubonic Plague in British India." *Journal of Medical Biography* 15, no. 1 (2007): 9–19.

"Health Department." *Nineteenth Biennial Report of the Board of Directors of the Agricultural and Mechanical College of Texas for the Fiscal Years Ending August 31, 1913, and August 31, 1914* (1914): 10.

Heiman, Henry. "The Technics of Lumbar Puncture in Children: With Particular Reference to the Pressure of the Cerebrospinal Fluid." *Mount Sinai Hospital Reports* 5 (1905–1906): 114–23.

Hillebrand, W. F., and W. T. Schaller. "The Mercury Minerals from Terlingua, Texas: Kleinite, Terlinguaite, Eglestonite, Montroydite, Calomel, Mercury." *Journal of the American Chemical Society* 29, no. 8 (1907): 1,180–94.

"In Memoriam, James Harvey Black, 1884–1958." *American Journal of Clinical Pathology* 32, no. 2 (August 1959): 172–73.

"International Congress of Hygiene and Demography." *Nature* 43 (January 15, 1891): 241–42.

"International Congress of Hygiene to Meet in America." *Texas State Journal of Medicine* 7, no. 12 (April 1912): 337.

Jacoby, George W. "Lumbar Puncture of the Subarachnoid Space." *New York Medical Journal* 62 (December 28, 1895): 813–18.

Jobling, James Wesley. "Standardization of the Antimeningitis Serum." *Journal of Experimental Medicine* 11, no. 4 (July 17, 1909): 614–21.

Jochmann, Gustav. "Versuche zur Serodiagnostic und Serotherapie der epidemischen Genickstarre." *Deutsch Medizinische Wochenschrift* 32 (1906): 788–93.

Jones, I. J. "The Epidemic of Cerebrospinal Meningitis in Texas during the Years 1898–1899." *Transactions of the Texas State Medical Association, Thirty-Third Annual Session Held at Galveston, Texas* (1899): 183–85.

Kere, J. W. "Federal Public Health Administration: Its Development and Present Status in the United States." *Public Health Reports* 28, no. 3 (January 17, 1913): 113.

Kolle, Wilhelm, and August Wasserman. "Versuch zur Gewinnung und Wertbestimmung eines Meningococcenserums." *Deutsch Medizinische Wochenschrift* 32 (1906): 609–12.

Kopetzky, Samuel Joseph. "Lumbar Puncture: A General Review of Its Value and Applicability." *American Journal of the Medical Sciences* 131 (April 1906): 648–74.

"Laboratory of Clinical Pathology." *Medical Herald* 32, no. 11 (November 1913): 431.

"List of Members." *Texas State Journal of Medicine* 8, no. 2 (June 2, 1912): 67.

Low, R. Bruce. "Epidemic Cerebrospinal Meningitis." *Transactions of the Epidemiological Society of London, New Series* 18 (January 20, 1899): 53–85.

Lynch, Thomas. "Cerebrospinal Meningitis—Treatment." *Medical Herald* 31, no. 6 (June 1912): 296–98.

Madani, Kaivon. "Dr. Hans Christian Jaochim Gram: Inventor of the Gram Stain." *Primary Care Update for OB/GYNS* 10, no. 5 (September–October 2003): 235–37.

Marcet, Alexander. "History of a Singular Nervous or Paralytic Affection Attended with Anomalous Morbid Sensations, Communicated by Dr. Marcet, Read Dec. 28, 1810." *Medico-Chirurgical Transactions* 2 (1811), 215–33.

Marsden, R. W. "Inoculation with Typhoid Vaccine as a Preventive of Typhoid Fever." *British Medical Journal* 1, no. 2052 (April 28, 1900): 1,017–18.

"Medical Colleges of the United States, Dallas." *Journal of the American Medical Association* 59, no. 8 (August 24, 1912): 632.

"Medical News, Alabama." *Journal of the American Medical Association* 68, no. 26 (June 29, 1912): 2,037.

"Medical News, Texas." *Journal of the American Medical Association* 57, no. 11 (September 9, 1911): 909.

"Meningitis Situation." *Texas State Journal of Medicine* 7, no. 10 (February 1912): 265.

Merrell, Woodson C., and Edward Shalts. "Homeopathy." *Medical Clinics of North America* 86, no. 1 (2001): 47–62.

Moore, John T. "The Laboratory of Clinical Pathology and Its Relation to the Practice of Medicine and Surgery." *Texas State Journal of Medicine* 2, no. 2 (June 1906): 61–62.

Morel, Harry. "Inoculation and Typhoid Fever." *Public Health Journal* 6, no. 5 (May 1915): 244–46.

Müllener, Eduard-Rudolf. "Six Geneva Physicians on Meningitis." *Journal of the History of Medicine and Allied Sciences* 20, no. 1 (January 1965): 1–26.

"M. Valleix." *Boston Medical and Surgical Journal* 53, no. 17 (November 22, 1855): 352–53.

Nash, Albert David. "Epidemic Cerebrospinal Meningitis." *Medical Herald* 32, no. 1 (January 1913): 10.

"Nervous Diseases, Illustrated by Moving Pictures, Dr. S. N. Key, Austin, Section on Mental and Nervous Diseases and Medical Jurisprudence, Wednesday, May 8, 1912." *Texas State Journal of Medicine* 7, no. 12 (April 1912): 333.

"New Books: 'Epidemic Cerebro Spinal Meningitis' by Abraham Sophian, MD, Kansas City, Mo., Formerly with the New York Research Laboratory, 272 Pages, 23 Illustrations, Cloth 272 Pages, Price $3. C. V. Mosby Co., St. Louis, Mo., 1913." *Journal of the Oklahoma State Medical Association* 5, no. 11 (April 1913): 550.

"Northern District, Society News." *Texas State Journal of Medicine* 7, no. 11 (March 1912): 313–14.

"Notable Contributions to Medical Research by Public Health Service Scientists." National Library of Medicine Reference Division (1960): 56–57.

"Notifiable Diseases: Prevalence during 1917 in Cities of over 100,000." *Public Health Reports* 33, no. 51 (December 20, 1918): 2,260.

"Notifiable Diseases: Prevalence during 1917 in Cities of over 100,000." *Public Health Reports* 34, no. 31 (August 1, 1918): 1,693.

"Obituary, Dr. Meredith Clymer." *British Medical Journal* 1, no. 2159 (May 17, 1902): 1,243.

"Obituary, Sir William Aitken, MD." *British Medical Journal*, vol. 2 for 1892 (July 2, 1892): 54–55.

Olopoenia, L. A., and A. L. King. "Widal Agglutination Test— 100 Years Later: Still Plagued by Controversy." *Postgraduate Medical Journal* 76, no. 892 (February 2000): 80–84.

Park, William Hallock, and Alfred Beebe. "Diphtheria and Allied Pseudo-Membranous Inflammations, A Clinical and Bacteriological Study." *Medical Record* 42 (July 30 and August 6, 1892): 113–25, 141–47.

Park, William Hallock, and Charles Bolduan, "The Communicability of Cerebro-Spinal Meningitis," *Public Health Reports* 31, Pt 1 (1905): 359–63.

"Personal." *Journal of the American Medical Association* 58, no. 7 (February 17, 1912): 492.

Quincke, Heinrich Ireneaus. "Die Lumbalpunktion des Hydrocephalus." *Verhandl Kong Innere Medizinisch Wiesbaden* 10 (1891): 321–31.

Quincke, Heinrich Ireneaus. "Uber Lumbalpunktion." *Berliner Klinische Wochesnschrift* 32 (1895): 861–62, 929–33.

Rackemann, Francis M. "Dr. Thomas Darlington." *Transactions of the American Clinical and Climatological Association* 58 (1946): lvii–lix.

"Relative to Adjournment of Legislature." *Journal of the House of Representatives of the Regular Session of the Thirty-Third Legislature of Texas, Convened at the City of Austin, January 14, 1913, and Adjourned without Day, April 1, 1913* (1913): 692–93.

Rice, George J., G. Weldon Tilley, and Peter A. Dysert. "A History of Pathology and Laboratory Medicine at Baylor University Medical Center." *Proceedings of Baylor University Medical Center* 17, no. 1 (January 2004): 42–55.

"Sanitary Measures against Cerebrospinal Meningitis." *Journal of the American Medical Association* 59, no. 16 (October 19, 1912): 1,482.

Schmelzer, Janet. "Thomas M. Campbell, Progressive Governor of Texas." *Red River Valley Historical Review* 3, no. 4 (Fall 1978): 52–63.

Sheets, Channing D., Kathleen Harriman, Jennifer Zipprich, Janice K. Louie, William S. Probert, Michael Horowitz Janice C. Prudhomme, Deborah Gold, and Leonard Mayer. "Fatal Meningococcal Disease in a Laboratory Worker, California, 2012." *Morbidity and Mortality Weekly Report* 63, no. 35 (September 5, 2014): 770–72.

Smith, J. Henderson, and Ralph St. John Brooks. "The Effects of Dosage in Typhoid Vaccination of Rabbits." *Journal of Hygiene (London)* 12, no. 1 (May 1912): 77–107.

"'Some Studies in Epidemic Meningitis,' Dr. Abraham Sophian, New York City, Section on Medicine and Diseases of Children, May 9, 1912." *Texas State Journal of Medicine* 7, no. 12 (April 1912): 334.

Sophian, Abraham. "A New Method of Controlling the Administration of Serum in Epidemic Meningitis: Preliminary Note." *Journal of the American Medical Association* 58, no. 12 (March 23, 1912): 843–45.

Sophian, Abraham. "Preventive Measures against Epidemic Meningitis." *Transactions of the Fifteenth International Congress on Hygiene and Demography* (1913): 54–66.

Sophian, Abraham, and J. Black. "Prophylactic Vaccination against Epidemic Meningitis." *Transactions of the Section on Pathology and Physiology of the American Medical Association at the Sixty-Third Annual Session, Held at Atlantic City, NJ, June 4 to 7, 1912* (1912): 48–64.

"State Bacteriologist Appointed." *Texas State Medical Journal* 7, no. 8 (December 1911): 227.

"Texas." *Journal of the American Medical Association* 56, no. 1 (February 11, 1911): 521.

"Texas." *Journal of the American Medical Association* 58, no. 3 (January 20, 1912): 206.

"Texas: The Meningitis Situation." *Journal of the American Medical Association* 58, no. 4 (January 27, 1912): 287.

Texas Senate Journal. Thirty-Third Legislature. Regular Session, Friday, January 17, 1913, 70.

Thayer, Alfred Edward. "The Dallas Epidemic of Meningitis; Preliminary Note on the Laboratory Work." *Texas State Journal of Medicine* 7, no. 11 (March 1912): 305–7.

"Travis County Medical Society." *Texas State Journal of Medicine* 7, no. 12 (February 9, 1912): 340.

"Vaccine Therapy." *Texas State Journal of Medicine* 8, no. 11 (March 1913): 311.

Van Deuren, Marcel, Petter Brandzaeg and Jos W. M. van der Meer, "Update on Meningococcal Disease with Emphasis on Pathogenesis and Clinical Management," *Clinical Microbiology Reviews* 13, no 1 (January 2000): 144–166.

Vieusseux, Gaspar. "*Mémoire sur La Maladie Qui a Règne à Genève, au Printemps de 1805.*" *Journal de Médecine, Chirurgie, Pharmacie, Etc.*, xii (1806): 163–82.

Von Ezdorf, Rudolph H. "Cerebrospinal Meningitis in Texas." *Public Health Reports* 27, no. 8 (February 23, 1912): 270–76.

Wall, Cecil. "On Acute Cerebro-Spinal Meningitis Caused by the Diplococcus Intracellularis of Weichselbaum: A Clinical Study." *Medico-Chirurgical Transactions* 86 (1903): 77–79.

Watson, David A., Daniel M. Musher, and Jan Verhoef. "A Brief History of the Pneumococcus in Biomedical Research: A Panoply of Scientific Discovery." *Clinical Infectious Diseases* 17, no. 5 (November 1993): 913–24.

Weichselbaum, Anton. "Über die Ätiologie der Akuten Meningitis Cerebrospinalis," *Fortschritte der Medizin* 5 (1887): 573–83.

Zinsser, Hans. "William Hallock Park 1863–1939." *Journal of Bacteriology* 38, no. 1 (July 1939): v-3–3.

INDEX

intraspinal injection of, xxiv–
xxvi, 11, 18n17
lumbar puncture procedure
administration of, 4,
7, 8, 9, 10, 15–16n8,
74, 78, 79, 83, 129,
192–193n39
manufacture of in Texas, 130–
131, 174–175, 199–200,
204, 217, 261
Mary Lou McCallum's
treatment with, 9–10
procurement of, 217
publication of outcome data
on, 11
scarcity of, 99, 130
subcutaneous administration
of, xxiv, 86, 90, 100,
142, 177, 270
as supplied free of charge by
Dr. Flexner, xxvi, 6, 7,
30–31, 47
use of antiseptics during
administration of, 151
use of as preventive measure,
142, 143, 153–154n7
use of in McKinney, Texas
outbreak, 11
"Anti-meningitis Vaccination"
(Frost), 223
antiseptic nose sprays and throat
applications, 143, 151, 216
Archer, Mary Millicent, 238n20
Aronson, Emile A. (E. A.), 51,
66–67n45
Aronson, Herman, 66–67n45
Arthur, Henry, 13–14n5
Ashcroft, Elizabeth Adeline, 263n5
Askew, Florence Alberta, 264n11
Associated Press, 89, 97

Austin, Texas, cerebrospinal
meningitis cases in, 88–89,
103, 128, 141–142, 229,
254, 255
autogenous vaccine, 178, 187–
188n19, 187n18

B

Babcock, Henry Dwight, 157n25
Babcock, John Robert, 136,
157n25, 219
Babcock, Robert Percy, 30, 40n33,
47, 104–105
Baird, Raleigh William, 49, 51,
64–65n41
Baird, William Leroy, 64–65n41
Baker, Andrew Jackson, 158n26
Baker, Rhodes Semmes, 136,
158n26
Baldwin, Sarah "Sadie" Letitia,
163n39
Banti, Guido, 162n36
Banti's disease, 162n36
Barbee, Nancy, 20–21n26
Barnes, Jesse, 113n33, 135
Barnes, Mrs., 102
Baylor University College of
Medicine, 68–69n50, 73,
186–187n17
Baylor University Hospital, 167n53
Beach, Hannah, xxviii–xxixn5
Beall, Elias James, 20n21
Beall, Khleher Heberden, 6, 20n21,
38n19, 88, 217
Becton, Edwin P., 65–66n43
Becton, Faye Fruzanna "Fru,"
263n5
Bedford, Sarah "Sally" Rebecca,
65n42
Beggs, Elnora Frances, 56n5

Brown, Nancy, 157n25
Brumby, George McDuffie, 33–34n2
Brumby, William McDuffie, 23, 24, 25, 26, 33–34n2
Bruner, Fannie Irene, 33n1
Bryan, F. A., 115–116n39
Bryan, Ruth, 60n23
Burkhalter, Ann Eliza, 36–37n15
Burleson, Albert Sidney, 175, 184n6
Burleson, Edward, Jr., 184n6
Busch, Adolphus, 107–108n6

C

Calhoun, Benjamin Franklin, 38n19, 217, 235–236n9
Calhoun, Ludlow, III, 235–236n9
Calloway, Miss, 113n33
calomel, 5, 16–17n12
Campbell, Mary, 245n61
Campbell, Thomas Duncan, 33n1
Campbell, Thomas Mitchell, 23, 24, 25, 33n1
Campbell, Victoria, 106n2
Card, C. F., 113n32
Carpenter, Sallie Willis, 193n41
Carrick, Manton Marble, 71, 84, 86, 107n4, 127, 132, 139
Carrick, White L., 107n4
Carter, Ann, 209–210n20
Carter, William, 209–210n20
Carter, William Spencer, 200, 209–210n20
Cary, Edward Henry, 49, 51, 63–64n40, 71, 83, 132
Cary, Joseph Milton, 63–64n40
case count
in Dallas between October 1, 1911 and May 31, 1912, 269

database of in Austin, 24
defined, xxiii
in Greater New York City in 1906, xxiii
use of to determine case fatality rate, xxv
case fatality rate
antimeningitis serum as reducing, 73
in Dallas, Fort Worth, and Waco between October 1911 and January 24, 1912, 128
in Dallas, Fort Worth, Houston, Austin, and Waco between October 1911 and January 20, 1912, 103
in Dallas during months of October 1911 through May 1912, 201
in Dallas in November 1911, 46–47
in Dallas in October/November and December 1911, 47
defined, xxv
discrepancy in regarding Dallas in October/November 1911, 48
in McKinney, Texas, 11
in Texas between October 1, 1911 and January 22, 1912, 131
cerebrospinal fluid, meningococci and inflammatory cells in, 8
cerebrospinal fluid space (a.k.a. subarachnoid space or thecal sac), 6, 18n17
cerebrospinal meningitis
1872 epidemic, xviii
1904 epidemic, xix

in Dallas, Fort Worth,
Houston, Austin, and
Waco between October
1911 and January 20,
1912, 103
in Dallas, Fort Worth,
Houston, Austin, and
Waco between October
1911 and January 24,
1912, 128
in Dallas between October
1, 1911 and May 31,
1912, 269
in Dallas during months of
October 1911 through
May 1912, 201
in Dallas in November
1911, 46
in Dallas in October/November
1911, 47
defined, xxiii
in New York City in 1905
epidemic, 269, 272n1
in Texas between October 1,
1911 and January 22,
1912, 131
"Preventive Measures against
Epidemic Meningitis"
(Sophian), 204, 212n42
prophylactic vaccination, 198,
207–208n15, 208–209n16
"Prophylactic Vaccination against
Epidemic Meningitis"
(Sophian and Black), 202,
204, 211–212n33, 211n32,
215, 217, 223
Prudden, T. Mitchell, xlii–xliiin49
Public Health Reports, 178

Q

quarantine, xxiii, 52, 77, 81, 85,
89, 90, 104, 126, 127, 129,
142, 151–152, 169–170n65,
216, 254
Quarantine Act of 1870 (Texas),
34n3
Quincke, Heinrich Ireneaus,
15–16n8
Quincke needle (spinal needle),
15–16n8

R

rabies virus research, 179, 189n24
Ralston, Lila Kirby, 33–34n2
rash of meningococcemia,
xxvii–xxviiin4
Rawlins, Alexander Bledsoe,
238n23
Rawlins, Fisher Younger, 222–223,
238n23
Reed, Sarah Valula, 240–241n36
Rembert, Edna M. "Pansy,"
158n26
Research Laboratory (New York
City Board of Health),
xxii, xxiii, xxiv, 31, xxxix–
xxxx36, 85, 87, 130, 169–
170n65, 174, 202
resolution (adopted by Dallas
Chamber of Commerce),
136–137, **137**
Reuss, J. H., 57n7
Rhodes, Alma, 236n14
Roach, Andrew Jackson, 119n51
Roach, Erskine Horton, 94–96,
119n51
Robbins, V. E., 113n32, 135
Roberts, Mrs., 113n33

V

vaccination, xxviin2, 86, 87–88,
148, 177, 178, 196, 198–199,
202, 205n3, 207–208n15,
208–209n16, 216, 218, 223–
224, 229, 254, 260. *See also*
immunization; inoculation
vaccines
autogenous vaccine, 178, 187–
188n19, 187n18
meningococcal vaccine. *See*
meningococcal vaccine
smallpox vaccine, 180, 183–
184n4, 196, 199
typhoid vaccine. *See* typhoid
vaccine
Valleix, François-Louis-Isidore,
xvi, xxix–xxxn8
Van Arsdale, Annie, 113n33
Van Cott, Joshua, xxxviin32
Vieusseux, Gaspard, xv, xxvii–
xxviiin4, xxviin2
vital statistics
reporting of in Texas, 23, 24,
25, 97–98, 242n45
in Texas Sanitary Code of
1911, 39n25
violations of Texas Sanitary
Code regarding, 28
von Ezdorf, Richard, 119–120n61
von Ezdorf, Rudolph Hermann, 99,
102, 103, 119–120n61, 126,
127, 131, 178
Von Pirquet, Clemens Freiherr,
118n46
Voynard, Paulina, 266–267n19

W

Waco, Texas

cerebrospinal meningitis cases
in, 48, 62n32, 97, 103,
127, 128, 129, 188n22
thank-you gift to Dr. Sophian,
170n66
Waco Morning News, 169n64
Walcott, Bess, 158–159n28
Walker, Sabra Jane, 239n29
Wallace, Nanette (Nannette) I.,
241n37
Wames, W. M., 115–116n39
Ware, Lillian Alice, 154–155n14
Wasserman, August von, xxiii–xxiv
Weichselbaum, Anton, xix,
xxxiiin18, xxxivn21
Weigert, Carl, xxxivn19
Welch, J. T., 115–116n39
Welch, William Henry, xxviiin33
Wharton, Sarah J., 264n10
Wheeler, Levici Della, 244n55
White, Raleigh Richardson, Jr.,
192n36
Whitney, Mary Eleanor,
121–122n67
Wickline, Joseph Pernell,
263–264n9
Wickline, Robert McNutt, 253,
256, 263–264n9
Widal test, 203, 211–212n33
Williams, Anna, xxxix–xxxx36
Williams, Margaret, 21n27
Wilson, Evelyn, 14–15n6
Wilson, Kate, 115n38
Wilson, Lucille, 114–115n37
Wilson, William E., 121–122n67
Wolters, Wilhelmina "Minna,"
242n45
Wood, Francis W., 67n46
Woodson, Lorena "Lunie" Ellen,
158–159n28

Wooten, Goodall Harrison, 253,
    254, 256, 264n10, 265n12
Wooten, Joseph Sil, 253, 256,
    264n10, 265n12
Wooten, Thomas Dudley, 265n12
Worsham, Benjamin Milton,
    38n19, 88, 114n36, 217
Worsham, James Albert, 114n36
Wortham, Louis J., 251, 252,
    263n5
Wortham, William Amos, 263n5
Worthington, Sarah "Sallie,"
    61–62n31
Worthy, Mary Belle, 12–13n3
Wright, Almroth Edward,
    110–111n17
Wright method, 197
Wyatt, Julia N., 59–60n19

Y

Young, John P., 266–267n19

Z

Zandt, Frances Cooke van, 20n21
Zeiss counting chamber, 176
Ziehl, Franz, xxxiiin17

MARGARET R. O'LEARY, MD

Dr. Margaret Rose O'Leary was born in Indianapolis, Marion County, Indiana, in 1952 as the second eldest of the five children of Dr. Gerald Philip Wiedman (1924–1995), an internist and cardiologist, and Margaret "Peg" Rose McGrath (1926–2008). Dr. O'Leary graduated from the Anna Head School (Oakland, Alameda County, California) in 1970; earned bachelor's degrees from both Smith College (Northampton, Hampshire County, Massachusetts; religion major; 1974) and the University of California, Berkeley (Berkeley, Alameda County, California; zoology major; 1976); and received her medical degree from the George Washington University School of Medicine (Washington, DC, 1980). She completed her emergency medicine residency at the Georgetown University Medical Center/George Washington University Medical Center/Maryland Institute of Emergency Medical Services program (1980–1984) and became one of the earliest residency-trained and board-certified emergency physicians in the US. She served as an assistant professor of emergency medicine and emergency department attending physician at both the George Washington University Medical Center (1984–1986) and the University of Chicago Hospitals (1987–1988) and as an attending emergency physician at Saint Therese Medical Center in Waukegan, Lake County, Illinois (1988–1989). She thereafter was a senior consulting writer at the Joint Commission on Accreditation of Healthcare Organizations (Oakbrook Terrace, DuPage County, Illinois, 1988–1995), where she wrote the *Primer on Indicator Development and Application*, *The Measurement Mandate*, *Clinical Data Interpretation*, the *Lexikon: Dictionary of Health Care Terms, Organizations, and Acronyms*, and two other books. In 1995, she returned to clinical emergency medicine as an attending physician at Northwest Community Hospital in Arlington Heights, Cook County, Illinois (1995–1998). In 1999, she earned her master of business administration degree at Benedictine University in Lisle, DuPage County, Illinois, and joined its academic faculty as an associate professor of management and the director of its MBA Programs (1999–2002). In the aftermath of the attack on the US on September 11, 2001, she accepted a large, unsolicited grant from the Grace Bersted Foundation, which she applied to the establishment of the Suburban Emergency Management Project (SEMP) in DuPage County, Illinois (2001–2010). The SEMP conducted community-based emergency preparedness activities for two years and produced three books (*The First 72 Hours, The Dictionary of Homeland Security,* and *Measuring Disaster Preparedness*), eight years each of the monthly online *Securitas Magazine* and the weekly online *SEMP Biots*. Dr. O'Leary served on the boards of the American Academy of Emergency Medicine and the Girl Scouts of DuPage County (Illinois). In 2007, Dr. O'Leary moved with her husband to the Kansas City area, where she enjoys gardening, playing her cello, and writing.

DENNIS S. O'LEARY, MD

Dr. Dennis Sophian O'Leary was born in Kansas City, Jackson County, Missouri, in 1938 as the eldest of the two sons of Theodore Morgan O'Leary (1910–2001), a writer, editor, sports correspondent, and literary critic, and Emily Sophian (1913–1994), the daughter of Dr. Abraham Sophian, a character in this book. Dr. O'Leary graduated from Shawnee Mission High School (Shawnee Mission, Johnson County, Kansas) in 1956; earned his bachelor's degree from Harvard College (1960); and received his medical degree from Cornell University Medical College in Manhattan (1964). He then completed an internal medicine residency at the University of Minnesota Medical Center (1964–1966) and at the University of Rochester Medical Center (1966–1968). Thereafter, he served in the US Army Medical Corps as the director of the blood coagulation laboratory at the Walter Reed Army Institute of Research (1968–1971) in Washington, DC, attaining the rank of major. He then joined the internal medicine faculty of the George Washington University Medical Center in Washington, DC, in 1971, rising in rank from assistant professor to full professor in 1979. In 1974, he was appointed acting medical director of the George Washington University Hospital, a position that he held until 1986. He was appointed dean for clinical affairs at the George Washington University Hospital in 1978, a position that he also held until 1986. In 1981, he achieved fame as the spokesman for the George Washington University Hospital following the attempted assassination of US President Ronald Reagan, reporting to the news media daily on the president's and Press Secretary James Brady's recovery from their wounds in the George Washington University Hospital. He subsequently served as the president of the Medical Society of the District of Columbia (1983). In 1986, he became president of the Joint Commission on Accreditation of Hospitals (now The Joint Commission) in Chicago, a position he held for twenty-one years, at which time he retired as president emeritus. In 1992, he was elected to the Institute of Medicine (now the National Academy of Medicine). He has served on many boards, including the National Advisory Council of the Agency for Healthcare Research and Quality (2001–2005), the Defense Health Board of the US Department of Defense (2009–2013), the National Patient Safety Foundation and the Lucian Leape Institute (2008–2013), the Truman Medical Center Board of Directors

(Kansas City, MO) (2008–2013), and the Institute for Healthcare Improvement (2008–2012). In 2007, Dr. O'Leary moved with his wife to his childhood home near Kansas City to run his family's farms and estate. He closely follows all sports, reads novels, and devours crossword puzzles.

CPSIA information can be obtained
at www.ICGtesting.com
Printed in the USA
BVHW031015020419
544363BV00001B/63/P

9 781532 054334